Quantification of
Neurologic Deficit

Quantification of Neurologic Deficit

Edited by

Theodore L. Munsat, M.D.

Professor of Neurology
New England Medical Center
Tufts University Medical School
Boston, Massachusetts

With 50 Contributing Authors

Butterworths
Boston London Singapore Sydney Toronto Wellington

Library of Congress Cataloging-in-Publication Data

Quantification of neurologic deficit / edited by Theodore L. Munsat.
  p. cm.
  Papers presented at a workshop entitled, Quantification in Clinical Neurology, held at Talloires, France, Sept. 29–Oct. 2, 1986.
  Bibliography: p.
  Includes index.
  ISBN 0-409-90152-0
  1. Nervous system—Diseases—Diagnosis—Congresses.
  2. Neurologic examination—Congresses. I. Munsat, Theodore L.
RC348.Q35   1989
616.8'0475—dc19   88-22604
                                          CIP

British Library Cataloguing in Publication Data

Quantification of neurologic deficit.
  1. Medicine. Neurology. Quantitative methods.
  I. Munsat, Theodore L.
616.8'01'8

ISBN 0-409-90152-0

Butterworth Publishers
80 Montvale Avenue
Stoneham, MA 02180

10 9 8 7 6 5 4 3 2 1

Printed in the United States of America

Contents

Contributing Authors

Patricia L. Andres, M.S., P.T.
Lecturer in Neurology
Tufts University School of Medicine
Research Physical Therapist
Neuromuscular Research Unit
New England Medical Center
Boston, Massachusetts

Kathryn A. Bamford, M.S.
Research Associate
Department of Psychiatry
University of Rochester
Rochester, New York

Jill Behr, R.N., M.S.
Instructor
Department of Neurology
University of Rochester
Rochester, New York

**Dorothy V.M. Bishop, M.A.,
M.Phil., D.Phil**
MRC Senior Research Fellow
Department of Psychology
University of Manchester
Manchester, England

Michael H. Brooke, M.D.
Director, Division of Neurology
University of Alberta
Edmonton, Alberta, Canada

Benjamin Rix Brooks, M.D.
Professor of Neurology and Medical
  Microbiology
University of Wisconsin—Madison
  Medical School;
Director, ALS Clinical Research
  Center
Chief, Neurology Service
William S. Middleton Memorial
  Veterans Administration Hospital
Madison, Wisconsin

Eric D. Caine, M.D.
Associate Professor of Psychiatry and
  Neurology
University of Rochester
Rochester, New York

Deborah L. Claman, Ph.D.
Office of Scientific Affairs, NIAAA
Alcohol, Drug Abuse and Mental
  Health Administration
Rockville, Maryland;
formerly, Postdoctoral Fellow
Department of Brain and Cognitive
  Science
Massachusetts Institute of Technology
Boston, Massachusetts

Jo Ann Clough, R.P.T.
Clinical Supervisor
Rehabilitation Medicine Service
William S. Middleton Memorial
  Veterans Administrative Hospital
Madison, Wisconsin

Jill Conrad, R.P.T.
Physical Therapist
Rehabilitation Medicine Service
William S. Middleton Memorial

Veterans Administrative Hospital
Madison, Wisconsin

Suzanne Corkin, Ph.D.
Professor of Behavioral Neuroscience
Massachusetts Institute of Technology
Cambridge, Massachusetts

Gena Desclos
Research Technician
Department of Neurology
Massachusetts General Hospital
Boston, Massachusetts

Peter James Dyck, M.D.
Professor of and Consultant in
    Neurology
Director of the Peripheral Neuropathy
    Center
Mayo Clinic
Rochester, Minnesota

Lynelle M. Erickson, M.S.
Research Psychologist
ALS Clinical Research Center
University of Madison—Madison
    Medical School
Madison, Wisconsin

Stanley Fahn, M.D.
H. Houston Merritt Professor of
    Neurology
Columbia University College of
    Physicians and Surgeons;
Attending Neurologist
Presbyterian Hospital
New York, New York

A.M. Ferrandez, Ph.D.
Research Assistant in Psychology
Department of Cognition and
    Movement
University of Marseilles
Marseilles, France

Clare J. Fowler, M.Sc., M.R.C.P.
Consultant Clinical Neurophysiologist

The Middlesex Hospital
London, United Kingdom

David Goldblatt, M.D.
Professor of Neurology
University of Rochester
Rochester, New York

John H. Growdon, M.D.
Associate Professor of Neurology
Massachusetts General Hospital
Harvard Medical School
Boston, Massachusetts

Judith Kennedy, M.S.
Associate
Department of Neurology
University of Rochester
Rochester, New York

Daniel K. Kido, M.D.
Associate Professor of Radiology
University of Rochester
Rochester, New York

Jon L. Kosanke
Programmer/Analyst
Information Services
Mayo Clinic
Rochester, Minnesota

George V. Kondraske, Ph.D.
Associate Professor of Electrical
    Engineering
University of Texas at Arlington;
Director
Human Performance Institute
Arlington, Texas

Roger Kurlan, M.D.
Associate Professor of Neurology
University of Rochester
Rochester, New York

**Anthony E.T. Lang, M.D.,
    F.R.C.P.(C.)**
Associate Professor of Neurology

University of Toronto Medical
  School
Director, Movement Disorders Clinic
Member, Division of Neurology
Toronto Western Hospital
Toronto, Ontario, Canada

Nicholas G. LaRocca, Ph.D.
Assistant Professor of Neurology
  (Psychology)
Albert Einstein College of Medicine
Bronx, New York

**Pamela M. Le Quesne, D.M.,
  F.R.C.P.**
Member
Medical Research Council
  Toxicology Unit
Honorary Member of Department of
  Neurological Studies
University College and
Middlesex School of Medicine;
Honorary Consultant in Neurology
Middlesex Hospital
London, United Kingdom

Ulf Lindblom, M.D.
Professor and Chairman
Neurology
Karolinska Institute;
Head, Neurology Department
Karolinska Hospital
Stockholm, Sweden

Charlyne Miller, R.N., M.S.
Instructor
University of Rochester
Rochester, New York

J. Philip Miller, Ph.D.
Associate Professor of Biostatistics
Washington University School of
  Medicine
St. Louis, Missouri

Peter C. O'Brien, Ph.D.
Professor of and Consultant in
  Biostatistics
Mayo Clinic
Rochester, Minnesota

Charles Odoroff, Ph.D.
(died December 29, 1987)
Professor of Biostatistics
University of Rochester
Rochester, New York

Jean Pailhous, Ph.D.
Director of Research in Psychology
Department of Cognition and
  Movement
University of Marseilles
Marseilles, France

N. Parkhouse, F.R.C.S.
Lecturer
Department of Surgical Studies
The Middlesex Hospital Medical
  School
London, United Kingdom

Sandra Plumb, B.S.
Senior Analyst Programmer
Division of Biostatistics
University of Rochester
Rochester, New York

Sigrid Poser, M.D.
Professor of Neurology
University Hospital
Gottingen, West Germany

Chris Anne Raymond, Ph.D.
Associate Editor
Journal of the American Medical
  Association
Chicago, Illinois

T. John Rosen
Research Scientist
Massachusetts Institute of Technology
Cambridge, Massachusetts

Allen J. Rubin, M.D.
Assistant Professor of Psychiatry and
  Neurology
Division of Neurology
Cooper Hospital/University Medical
  Center
Camden, New Jersey

Mohammed Sanjak, Ph.D.
Exercise Physiologist
ALS Clinical Research Center
University of Wisconsin—Madison
  Medical School
Madison, Wisconsin

Labe C. Scheinberg, M.D.
Professor of Neurology, Psychiatry,
  and Rehabilitation Medicine
Albert Einstein College of Medicine;
Attending Neurologist
Weiler Hospital of the Albert Einstein
  College of Medicine
Bronx, New York

Martha Schram, R.P.T.
Cardiac Rehabilitation Supervisor
Rehabilitation Medicine Service
William S. Middleton Memorial
  Veterans Administration Hospital

Georges Serratrice, M.D.
Professor of Neurology
Aix-Marseilles University;
Head of Neuromuscular Department
La Timone Hospital
Marscilles, France

Ira Shoulson, M.D.
Professor of Neurology, Pharmacol-
  ogy, and Medicine
University of Rochester;
Neurologist and Physician
Strong Memorial Hospital
Rochester, New York

Linda M. Skerry, P.T.A.
Research Physical Therapist Assistant
Neuromuscular Research Unit
New England Medical Center
Boston, Massachusetts

Robert L. Sufit, M.D.
Assistant Professor of Neurology
University of Wisconsin—Madison
  Medical School
Madison, Wisconsin;
Co-Director
MDA Neuromuscular Clinic
Assistant Chief, Rehabilitation
  Medicine Service
William S. Middleton Memorial
  Veterans Administration Hospital

Karl Syndulko, Ph.D.
Neuropsychologist
Veterans Administration Medical
  Center—Wadsworth;
Assistant Professor
Department of Neurology
University of California at Los
  Angeles
Los Angeles, California

Richard Tegnér, M.D., Ph.D.
Assistant Professor of Neurology and
  Registrar
Karolinska Hospital
Stockholm, Sweden

**Wallace W. Tourtellotte, M.D.,
Ph.D.**
Chief of Neurology
Veterans Administration Medical
  Center—Wadsworth;
Professor and Vice Chairman
Department of Neurology
University of California at Los
  Angeles
Los Angeles, California

Thomas A. Zeffiro, M.D., Ph.D.
Assistant Professor of Neurology
Director, Abnormal Movements Clinic
Department of Neurology
University of Wisconsin Hospital
Madison, Wisconsin;
formerly, Resident, Neurology
  Service
Massachusetts General Hospital
Boston, Massachusetts

Preface

A four-day workshop titled "Quantitation in Clinical Neurology" was held at the Tufts University European Center at Talloires, France, from September 29 to October 2, 1986. This workshop grew out of a perceived need to assess our current knowledge in the field and to make recommendations for the future. Support was generously provided by the Fondation Merrieux of Lyon, France, and by Tufts University. Participants were invited on the basis of a demonstrated interest and proficiency in the area of quantification of neurologic deficit. An attempt was made to invite clinical neuroscientists with experience in several diverse neurologic systems and various diseases, although not all areas could be covered in the time available. For example, the issues of quantification of function in head injury or coma and in stroke were not addressed. The boundaries of the term *quantification* were defined by clinical usefulness. Thus, procedures requiring expensive instrumentation, such as electroencephalography, electromyography, and neuro-imaging, were largely excluded from the scope of the discussions.

More accurate quantitation of clinical neurologic deficit is of considerable demonstrated and potential importance. Although the time-honored neurologic examination continues to be an effective method of lesion localization and clinical diagnosis, neurologists—particularly those interested in therapeutics—concur that the examination is seriously deficient in its ability to track deficit longitudinally and to determine accurately the effectiveness of therapeutic intervention. Its reproducibility from examiner to examiner is limited.

The subjective nature of the classic neurologic examination frequently leads to an inaccurate portrayal of the patient's functional disability and limits the examination's value in clinical trials, which require quantitative and reproducible measurement. Clinicians have therefore begun to search for a way to supplement the neurologic examination with more objective techniques that could also be used by non-neurologists, such as physical therapists.

During the workshop, several common themes were echoed in the various presentations and discussions. Although individual participants understandably came to the workshop convinced that their own quantitative approach was meaningful, it became apparent that the views of most of the presenters had been shaped in great part by discussions with like-minded colleagues working in the same neurologic system or disease. Thus, many of the most useful and insightful criticisms came from participants with quite different perspectives and experience.

Considerable discussion focused on whether quantitation beyond the classic neurologic examination would be acceptable or valuable to the average practicing neurologist. The consensus seemed to be that quantitation, as discussed in this workshop, would most likely remain the domain of the clinical researcher—at least for the near future. Most participants agreed that the workshop presentations and discussions would be most useful if published as a state-of-the-art document that could serve as a guide for the future, but that such a publication would most likely not change the practice patterns of most clinical neurologists, desirable as that goal may be.

Nonetheless, there was agreement that several trends in clinical medicine will continue to direct the practicing neurologist toward the use of more quantitative techniques in the day-to-day management of clinical problems. Of particular importance in this regard is the increasing pressure from health insurers, as well as from the lay public, to document the efficacy or lack of efficacy of therapeutic interventions. This trend, which has already affected the rehabilitation field, will most likely be an important driving force in establishing quantitation as an adjunct to the classic neurologic examination.

Several workshop discussions addressed the issue of whether a neurofunction laboratory, equipped to provide broad or even limited quantitative assessment, is desirable. The consensus was that although such a laboratory may currently be effective in limited situations in certain institutions, its broader application will require more time. Several participants were concerned about the use of a global approach to such testing. They thought that a neurofunction laboratory covering all forms of disease and deficit would be unwieldy, expensive, and potentially less effective in developing new methodology. In addition, it was thought that the testing techniques used should be determined in response to a particular research question or goal, and not *ex vacuo*. On the other hand, there was a sense that more special laboratories will be established in the next several years, both for routine patient management and research. The overall conclusion of the workshop was that the age of meaningful neurologic quantitation has begun.

Theodore L. Munsat, M.D.

PART I

Principles and Methodology

Chapter 1

Quantifying the Neurologic Examination: An Introduction

Wallace W. Tourtellotte

Dr. Russell N. DeJong has said[1]:

The classic, or standard, neurologic examination gives essential information enabling the clinician to diagnose and localize a neurologic lesion, identify its pathologic nature, estimate its prognosis, and institute a therapeutic regimen. It does not, however, measure objectively the degree of the patient's neurologic impairment.

Quantitative neurologic testing is a tedious and time-consuming technique but is of utmost value under many circumstances, especially to evaluate objectively and accurately impairment, to establish criteria that can be used to assess the course of spontaneous improvement or worsening, and to assess clinical changes that follow or accompany responses to trials of therapeutic regimens.

Quantitative examination of neurologic function foretells advances in neurologic appraisal which may drastically alter future examination procedures.

In neurology, the term *quantitative examination* implies the use of instrumented devices or ordinal rating scales to evaluate such functions as mental state, vision, brainstem function, strength, reactions, steadiness, sensations, speed and coordination, stance, gait, range of motion, bowel and bladder functions, and activities of daily living. Although the literature on the quantification of neurologic function includes numerous equivocal studies, many sound investigations have also been performed, and several dozen research laboratories have been used to evaluate the functions of patients routinely for a decade or more. These studies, as well as those presented in this volume, have provided convincing evidence that quantitative techniques can reliably document the functions of normal individuals and patients with a variety of sensory and motor disorders when proper tests, procedures, and measures are used.

Potvin and I wrote the first work[1] on quantitative functional assessment because there was no comprehensive sourcebook on the design, development, evaluation, and clinical application of sensory and motor tests, or perceptual-motor tests to which researchers could turn. Even now, there are few literature reviews on quantitative functional assessments that span the pertinent disciplines, so investigators in one discipline are largely unaware of developments in other disciplines. The reports contained in this volume, offered by active and serious investigators several years after the publication of our book, will give the reader a much-needed update on this rapidly developing field.

The science of measurement of human performance draws on the resources and experience of disciplined individuals in the fields of neurology, psychology, biomedical engineering, biostatistics, physical and occupational therapy, and surgery. The large number of available tests has permitted in-depth and wide-ranging studies by providing a selection of tests and procedures for exploring specific disorders and treatments. The general approach has been to identify from a vast literature the available instruments, methods, and procedures; to replicate or modify existing tests and develop new ones; to evaluate tests in normal adults and in patients with disease or injury; to use tests to assess clinical trials; and to make findings available to others in a graphic, statistical style.

Today, hardwired devices and mini- and microcomputer systems for the evaluation of human functions exist in hundreds of clinical and research settings. Increasingly, pharmaceutical and medical-device companies and government agencies are urging investigators to obtain sensitive, objective analyses of changes in functions affected by therapy or assistive devices. The number of clinical trials has increased dramatically, as has the amount of published literature. Although the use of quantitative examinations is not yet a standard procedure, quantitative techniques are becoming important and accepted methods of evaluating clinical trials. With the current availability of low-cost commercial mini- and microcomputers, standardized comprehensive assessments of sensory and motor functions may also become a reality, simplifying current evaluation techniques and eliminating or minimizing less precise procedures. With continued progress, clinicians may soon be able to refer patients to neurofunction laboratories for evaluation, much as they now refer patients to pulmonary-function, cardiac-stress, or evoked-potential laboratories.

The presentations in this book organize and synthesize many segments of human performance. Developments in various disciplines are related, the role of quantitative functional assessment is placed in perspective, and quantitative test batteries useful in particular settings are described. Accordingly, this volume may serve as a guide for neurologists, rehabilitationists, gerontologists, pharmacologists, toxicologists, psychologists, psychiatrists, psychotherapists, industrial and human-factors engineers, and personnel managers, in addition to biomedical engineers who design devices, and biostatisticians who design and analyze studies that evaluate tests and clinical trials.

Some will say that evaluation of neurologic function is not widely performed in medical centers and clinics as it is described in our book[1] and in this volume, and that many of the techniques and ideas discussed and recommended are not widely used. Our justification, if one is needed, is that this book is offered as a forward-looking effort, describing tests and procedures that we believe should be more widely adopted.

We hope that this volume will stimulate advancements in the field rather than simply record current practices in certain laboratories, and that with this sourcebook in hand, serious clinical investigators will start to design, implement, and evaluate quantitative test systems from a base of common knowledge. We are convinced that the quantification of neurologic function is an area in which substantive data will quickly be put to use, and hope that our efforts will encourage others to join in this work.

REFERENCE

1. Potvin AR, Tourtellotte WW, Potvin JH, et al. Quantitative examination of neurologic functions. Vol. I: Scientific Basis and Design of Instrumented Tests; Vol. II: Methodology for Test and Patient Assessments and Design of a Computer-Automated System. Boca Raton, FL: CRC Press, 1985.

Chapter 2

Quantifying the Neurologic Examination: Principles, Constraints, and Opportunities

Wallace W. Tourtellotte and Karl Syndulko

The neurologic examination was the first true imaging methodology for the evaluation of disordered brain function. Careful recording of symptoms and direct observation of a patient's signs are the principal bases for a neurologist's clinical evaluation. This approach, as old as the foundations of our profession, is still based on training, experience, and judgment. In the realm of initial diagnosis, subjective observations, interpretation, and the integrative powers of a curious and investigative mind remain the state of the art. Knowledge-based systems and artificial intelligence will be incorporated into our artful practice, building on what we have developed over the last 100 years.

In a 1985 editorial on the putative obsolescence of the neurologic examination, Ziegler[1] argued that the availability of new imaging technologies "increases the importance of the most sophisticated and meticulous type of neurologic examination, to match the increasing sensitivity of the new machines." The ability to provide technically extraordinary images of the brain has distracted many neurologists from the principal focus of our clinical practice: the patient's ability to negotiate his or her daily life. Directly observing the patient's behavior and questioning the patient about activities of daily living are indispensable methods of evaluating his or her ability to function in the real world.

A primary focus of our own work over the past 25 years[2,3] has been the bridges between technical imaging marvels and our roots in careful observation and questioning of patients. These bridges are based on ever more precise characterizations of patients' behavior and motor, sensory, and intellectual abilities. We have long cham-

This research was supported by funds from Neurology and Research Services, Veterans Administration Medical Center, West Los Angeles, Wadsworth Division.

pioned an approach to behavioral measurement in neurology based on instrumented quantitative assessment, but we have also improved the reliability and validity of ordinal scales.[3] In a world of computerized brain images, we need—more than ever—comparable precision in the behavioral imaging of neurologic function.

This chapter sets the stage for evaluating the new developments in quantitative assessment in clinical neurology. We outline the issues and arguments for objective measurement, the need for precise and repeatable measurement techniques over time and between examiners, and the special aspects of evaluating treatments both in the individual patient and between patients and studies. At this time there are constraints in evaluating neurologic function. We touch on the strengths and weaknesses of ordinal rating scales and on improvements needed. Although the chapter emphasizes general issues and advances in quantitative evaluation, we do refer to a specific application—namely, multiple sclerosis.

Chapter 3 focuses on the characterization of "normal neurologic function, the cornerstone of quantitative evaluations and the benchmark by which instrumented measures make sense for doctors and patients. The concepts of normalization of data and of description relative to age- and gender-matched controls are illustrated and discussed, based on existing measurement systems.

Chapter 4 addresses the state of the art in computerized, instrumented assessment of neurologic function. It presents the expanding range of measurement options, the technical rationale for and description of instrumented testing of specific neurologic functions, the management and display of data for both doctor and patient, the statistical comparisons with the normative data base, and the potential functional imaging of neurologic functions that will emerge from this technology.

Chapters 5 and 6 deal with the use of ordinal rating scales, which are necessary to assess acute change in neurologic function and record episodic disorders. They also provide a type of validity, especially for instrumented tests.

BASIS FOR QUANTIFICATION OF NEUROLOGIC FUNCTION

Are Parametric Data Preferred to Nonparametric Data?

Parametric data are obtained with an instrumented test, such as one that expresses foot-tapping as a number of strokes per minute. When used to evaluate a function or change in function, such data provide more useful information than do non-parametric data—that is, data that result from ordinal rating scales, such as one used by an examiner to grade foot-tapping according to the following categories: (1) super-normal, (2) normal, (3) mildly slow, (4) moderately slow, (5) severely slow, or (6) total loss of function. The reasons that parametric data are preferred are listed in Table 2.1.

Table 2.1 Why are Parametric Data More Useful than Nonparametric Data?

1. Parametric and nonparametric data can both be used to determine whether a change is statistically significant; however, only parametric data can be used to state how much of a change has taken place.
2. Changes in performance can be expressed in terms of ratios with parametric data (e.g., percent of normal function). Changes in performance cannot be expressed in such terms with nonparametric data.
3. More intervals can be compared and finer discriminations can be made with parametric measures.
4. Parametric statistics are more powerful than nonparametric statistics because there is a smaller probability of erroneous rejection of the null hypothesis.

Why Quantify Neurologic Function?

Table 2.2 lists important reasons for quantification of the neurologic examination, beginning with one of the strongest—the need for comparative analyses of various medications for the same disease that are not tested in the same clinical trial. For example, we have shown that compared with no other drugs, amantadine (Symmetrel), benztropine (Cogentin), and cyclobenzaprine (Flexeril) improved manual dexterity by 5, 5, and 10%, respectively, whereas improvement with carbidopa-levodopa (Sinemet) was 15%. Baseline function of Parkinson's disease patients was about 45% of age- and gender-matched normal subjects for the different clinical trials. Though a combination of amantadine and carbidopa-levodopa improved manual dexterity by an additional 3% of normal function, a combination of benztropine and carbidopa-levodopa decreased function by 2%.

Table 2.2 Why Quantify Neurologic Function with Instruments or Ordinal Rating Scales?

1. To improve the evaluation of clinical trials by means of finer discrimination and increased precision, increased reliability and validity, and better reproducibility via standardization at different clinical centers
2. To increase objectivity by employing paramedical personnel, who cannot detect telltale side effects as readily as physicians
3. To follow disease progression more precisely over the long term
4. To detect mild adverse side effects of a treatment
5. To introduce linear scales and relate the patient's performance to the physician's treatment goal of attaining 100% of age- and gender-matched normal function in the patient (applies only to instrumented tests)
6. To measure the relative efficacy of different treatments for the same disease in terms of percent of normal function (applies only to instrumented tests)

How to Quantify?

We have dealt with two types of quantification: ordinal rating scales (nonparametric data) and instrumented examination (parametric data).

Ordinal Rating Scales

Although many investigators in several clinical fields have developed rating scales to assess functions, no rating scale has become a standard, not even within a specific patient population. Our *Coded Examination of Neurologic Function* data sheets,[3] which we have used and modified for over a decade of clinical trials in multiple sclerosis, are also appropriate for use in most other diseases.

Because of our experience and our interpretation of many reports cited in the literature, we fully recognize the dilemma faced by the designer of a coded examination. If the number of rating steps is kept low (e.g., two or three) to aid in obtaining high test-retest reliability, the sensitivity of the test is low, and perceived changes in functions cannot be recorded. Alternatively, if the number of rating steps is made high (e.g., more than four, or certainly more than five) to improve the test's sensitivity and permit the documentation of perceived changes in function, test-retest reliability is poor. Thus, the designer compromises by using a four- or five-point scale that at best provides moderate test-retest reliability and permits modest documentation of perceived changes in functions. Having accepted this compromise, the designer needs to develop a schema for clearly characterizing each rating point of the scale, so that colleagues can understand the absolute value of function associated with each rating point and the amount of change in function that exists between successive rating points. We recommend the approach developed by Williams and associates.[4]

Instrumented Examinations

Although tremendous effort has been expended in developing coded derivatives of the classic neurologic examination (ordinal rating scales), the test-retest reliability and degree of precision of coded examinations are equivocal. As a result, over the past 100 years clinicians have developed a variety of instrumented tests and techniques to measure functions that are affected differentially by various diseases. However, the breadth and sophistication of tests vary widely. Reports often fail to mention such diverse issues as the training of technicians; reliability and validity; and the effects of repeated testing, gender, and age on functions. Normative data bases are seldom established.

Table 2.3 outlines a simplified revision of our Quantitative Examination of Neurologic Function (QENF), which can be performed in 30 minutes by a trained technician. Presented in Volume I of our book,[3] the full battery of tests includes a neuropsychologic examination (p. 118), an instrumented examination of sensory and motor functions (pp. 123–125), and an instrumented examination of activities of daily living (p. 168).

It should be pointed out that the instrumented tests of neuropsychology, vision, and the upper and lower extremities test abilities and thus resemble the classic neurologic examination, whereas the instrumented examination of activities of daily living makes use of abilities in order to test skills. Activities of daily living are included in our QENF test battery because patients want to improve their skills in that area.

Table 2.3 Quantitative Examination of Neurologic Function—Simplified Version[a]

Neuropsychologic examination
Visual acuity
Upper extremity
  Strength (grip, deltoid)
  Speed (finger tapping)
  Speed coordination (reach tapping)
  Dexterity (Purdue pegboard)
  Sensation (2-point discrimination)
Lower extremity
  Strength (dorsiflexion of foot, hip flexion)
  Speed (foot tapping)
  Station (2 legs ⟶ 1 leg with eyes open ⟶ closed)
  Gait (tandem toe-to-toe, touching in parallel bars)
Activities of daily living
  Upper extremities
    Putting on shirt
    Buttoning
    Zippering
    Cutting food
    Dialing telephone
    Speed-writing
  Lower extremities
    Rising from a chair
    Station
    Gait

[a] A 30-minute examination when conducted by a trained technician.

Experimental Evaluation of Instrumented Neurologic Tests

Table 2.4 lists nine areas for investigation in documenting the utility of instrumented tests. Such evaluation has indicated that all parts of our QENF can be used to evaluate

Table 2.4 Experimental Evaluation of Instrumented Neurologic Tests

Reliability (test-retest)
Variability of test measures
Repeated testing (learning)
Gender
Handedness
Age
Motivation
Technician training
Validity

the neurologic function of normal adults and of patients with cognitive, visual, sensory, and motor disabilities. (For details of our investigations, see reference 3, Volume II, pages 3–55.) We recommend that any new test or modification of an existing test be put through this rigorous evaluation.

Technician Training

When evaluation of technician training is included in the design and analysis of a study, unwarranted inferences from instrumental test data are minimized. Adequate training requires experience on the part of the trainer and extensive practice with volunteer subjects on the part of the trainee. Only objective experimental evaluations can assess the adequacy of training.

Our studies have proved that physical therapists can administer instrumented tests as capably as clinicians. Moreover, such technicians add objectivity to a clinical trial, being less likely than clinicians to detect telltale side effects of a treatment.

Ideally, in the future, each neurologist's office will include a trained technician to perform all or part of the QENF to ensure the most objective evaluation of a disability as a basis for long-term follow-up. This would be comparable to a neurologist's quality control of, for instance, electroencephalograms (EEGs) and evoked potentials in an electrophysiology unit. For details on our technician training studies, see reference 3, Volume II, pages 42–47. See Volume I, pages 221–39, for more detail, including instructions for technicians on how to perform each test, a technician-patient dialogue, and data sheets.

Constraints in Evaluating Neurologic Function

A patient's motivation, capability of fulfilling test requirements, and psychological state may all affect the results of neurologic tests. Testing with an instrumented examination of neurologic function should be restricted to cooperative normal individuals and patients who are willing to perform each test to the best of their ability. The patients must be mentally alert, attentive, and capable of following simple instructions. They must have approximately normal corrected hearing in order to understand and follow instructions and, for at least some tests, approximately normal corrected visual acuity in at least one eye.

Our test battery starts with simple tests of mental state, vision, and hearing to assure that patients can carry out other tests in the battery. Such tests should be a part of all instrumented test batteries.

For some individuals, malingering can be an attractive solution to many problems because of its economic, emotional, and social benefits. Individuals often complain of neurologic disorders that are easily confused with psychologic complaints, which can be associated with headaches, memory loss, or sensory and motor disorders. In the early stages of a disease, differences between psychogenic disturbances (e.g., hysteria or malingering) and organic disease often are not apparent during examination or laboratory tests, and those that produce changes in function are difficult for even skilled clinicians, psychologists, and psychiatrists to differentiate. The issue is complicated by patients who may enhance their organic problems with psychogenic problems for personal gain. Such voluntary alteration of neurologic function is identified in clinical practice from evidence of inconsistency in the history or examination, the probability that symptoms and signs fit a reasonable disease pattern, the emotional reactions that accompany the patient's complaints, and the results of tests for specific cognitive and memory defects.

To date, we and others who have designed and used instrumented examinations of neurologic function have used them primarily to evaluate clinical trials. No published data have supported their usefulness as an aid to diagnosis. No investigators claim to have developed tests that can differentiate organic and psychogenic disorders. Although examination of test data for large variances between successive trials or among similar tests that measure related functions could possibly prove useful, considerable research must be done to develop and validate techniques that may differentiate patients with psychogenic or organic disorders.

In their present stage of development, instrumented examinations of neurologic function do not reliably differentiate organic and psychogenic disease. For this reason the results of these tests should not be used for adjudication, except to support findings obtained by other, more traditional clinical techniques.

Occasionally, patients with both organic and psychogenic disease may inadvertently be included in a clinical trial. Such patients do not represent a serious problem in the interpretation of results, because group data analysis is ordinarily used. Experiments that include randomization and double-blind or crossover designs, or both, further minimize the effect of inadvertently including a few psychogenic patients. An unusual data profile may identify such patients.

In summary, it is advisable to have a clinician conduct a preliminary history and physical examination to determine whether a patient should be given an instrumented examination of neurologic function. If a clinician has reason to suspect that a patient is unmotivated to perform as well as possible on tests, is a malingerer, or has hysteria, he or she may wish to screen the individual from testing and refer the patient to a psychiatrist or other trained professional for consultation.

APPLICATION OF QUANTIFICATION OF NEUROLOGIC FUNCTION: DATA DISPLAY

The abundance of data generated by quantitative methods has forced us to develop not only meaningful measures and data reduction techniques but also methods for presenting or displaying data. For example, to evaluate therapy in multiple sclerosis, we have used the concept of percentage of normal function. The multicenter clinical trial conducted in the United States to compare adrenocorticotrophic hormone (ACTH) with placebo for the treatment of multiple sclerosis patients in a stage of acute exacerbation included our Clinical Quantitative Neurologic Examination.[5,6] When the instrumented test data from the study were reevaluated[7] with use of the percentage-of-normal-

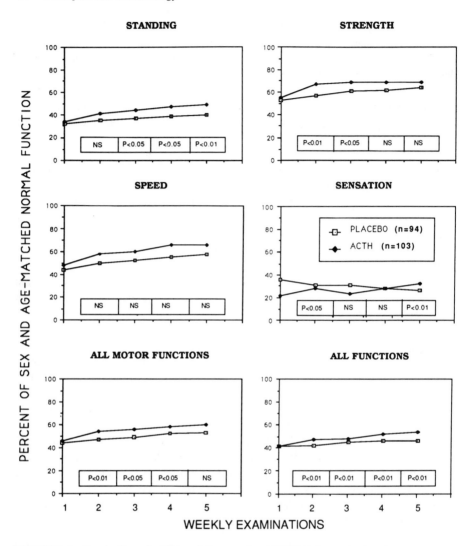

FIGURE 2.1   *Results from the National Cooperative ACTH Trial in multiple sclerosis. Percentage of normal function in the lower extremity, with the same tests combined at each examination period for the placebo (n = 94) and ACTH (n = 103) groups. Statistical significances (P values) are given for the comparisons between the placebo and ACTH groups with respect to mean changes from the pretreatment examination (1) to each of the following examinations (2 through 5). NS denotes not significant. (Reprinted with permission from Henderson et al.[7]).*

function transformation and then reduced into composite neurologic functions versus time (Figure 2.1), remarkable data reduction was accomplished. The original report of the study contained seven full pages of numeric data (three tables with 1,134 numeric entries). Visualization of the overall treatment effect was difficult, exceedingly tedious, and time-consuming. In addition, since data for each test were entered in raw form (e.g., pounds of force for strength or taps per 10 seconds for speed of hand), the maze of numbers made it very difficult to determine whether, for example, a change from 42.5 to 47.0 hand-taps in 10 seconds was clinically important. Further, the numers did not directly relate to the clinician's goal of helping the patient attain 100% function.

The results presented in Figure 2.1 support the positive findings of previous reports[5] without omitting clinically important statistical information. In addition, the methodology and the illustration simplify the task of interpreting results by enabling the clinician to determine how near to normal function the patients came after the treatment trial and to discern the differences between treatment and placebo groups.

CONCLUSION

Although tremendous effort has been expended in developing coded derivatives of the classic neurologic examination (ordinal rating scales), the test-retest reliability and degree of precision of coded examinations are equivocal. For this reason, clinicians have developed a variety of instrumented tests and techniques to measure functions that are affected differentially depending on diseases. With the advent of low-cost microcomputer technology, batteries of tests have been computer automated, greatly simplifying instrument calibration and data collection, analysis, storage, retrieval, and display. Such diverse issues as the training of technicians; reliability and validity; and the effects of repeated testing, gender, and age on functions have to be reported, and normative data bases must be established. As technology for designing instrumented tests improves and as investigators gain experience in conducting evaluation studies, quantification of neurologic functions should evolve to dramatically affect the way in which studies are carried out and the method in which neurology is practiced.

We have described a battery of clinically applicable instrumented tests of neurologic functions and presented the effect of ACTH on multiple sclerosis.

REFERENCES

1. Ziegler DK. Is the neurologic examination becoming obsolete? Neurology 1985; 35:559 (editorial).
2. Tourtellotte WW, Haerer AF, Simpson JF, et al. Quantitative clinical neurological testing. I. A study of a battery of tests designed to evaluate in part the neurologic function of patients with multiple sclerosis and its use in a therapeutic trial. Ann NY Acad Sci 1965; 122: 480–505.
3. Potvin AR. Tourtellotte WW, Potvin JH, et al. Quantitative examination of neurologic functions. Vol I: Scientific basis and design of instrumented tests; Volume II: Methodology for test and patient assessments and design of a computer-automated system. Boca Raton: CRC Press, 1985.
4. Williams RGA, Johnston M, Willis LA, et al. Disability: a model and measurement technique. Br J Prevent Soc Med 1976; 30:71.

5. Rose AS, Kuzma JW, Kurtzke JF, et al. Cooperative study in the evaluation of therapy in multiple sclerosis: ACTH vs placebo in acute exacerbations. Preliminary report. Neurology 1968; 18:1.
6. Rose AS, Kuzma JW, Kurtzke JF, et al. Cooperative study in the evaluation of therapy in multiple sclerosis: ACTH vs placebo in acute exacerbations. Final report. Neurology 1970; 20:1.
7. Henderson WB, Tourtellotte WW, Potvin AR, et al. Methodology for analyzing clinical neurological data: ACTH in multiple sclerosis. Clin Pharmacol Ther 1978; 24:145.

Chapter 3

What Is Neurologically Normal?

Karl Syndulko and Wallace W. Tourtellotte

The issue of what is neurologically normal is really a nonsense issue. The specification of some mythical "normal" being has proven to be a more than formidable task, over and over again, in the many realms of functional measurement in which it has been attempted. Of course, such a mythical being can be conjured statistically. But how meaningful is the concept of normal performance? What are its uses and limitations? How do we approach it in the laboratory and clinic? In this chapter, we address some of these issues in the context of our development and utilization of human performance measurement. In particular, we will discuss the definition of criteria for normal age-related changes in performance, since age has been found to be one of the most critical determinants of performance variability.

WHAT DO WE MEASURE IN NEUROLOGY?

The neuroanatomy, neurochemistry, and neurometabolism of the central nervous system (CNS) represent the basic physiochemical substrata, or "wetware," that underlie all brain functioning. The stream of chemical and electromagnetic communications among the basis elements of the CNS weave a complex set of higher-order, system-level "controlware" that represents the immediate antecedents to thought and behavior. We will call these control circuits *neurofunctional systems*. For the most part, observation and analysis of the wetware through static structural imaging (e.g., computerized axial tomography and magnetic resonance imaging) provide only a hint of the potential integrative complexity of the neurofunctional systems. Currently, direct access to, or functional imaging of, the spatiotemporal stream of neural activity that defines the neurofunctional systems is very limited. Dynamic or neurofunctional

17

imaging technologies include neurometabolic and neurochemical imaging (positron emission tomography, xenon-based regional cerebral blood flow, single-photon emission tomography), neuroelectric imaging (computerized electroencephalographic and event-related potential topographic mapping), and neuromagnetic imaging (spontaneous and event-related magnetoencephalograms). The most basic imaging technology is, of course, the neurologic and neuropsychologic examination. With it, we develop images of CNS function and dysfunction on the basis of observations or measurements of behavioral patterns associated with the activity of a neurofunctional system or set of systems.

Much of our understanding of neurofunctional systems is based on invasive studies in animal brains and inferences drawn from detailed behavioral analyses of (black-box) input-output relationships in both healthy and damaged human brains. This chapter emphasizes three basic principles of organization that such research has delineated: (1) hierarchical organization, (2) multiple specialized neurofunctional systems, and (3) parallel activation. At each level of analysis of the wetware and neurofunctional systems, we can identify a hierarchical organization of elements from simple to complex. In addition, many if not all systems are probably active simultaneously, although input and output at the behavioral level may be partially restricted at any given moment to a limited set of systems and subsystems. These general principles are critical to developing and interpreting behavioral probes of the neurofunctional systems.

As a theoretical foundation for performance measurement in humans, we adopt the general model of neurofunctional systems as relatively autonomous modules, or subsystems. Each has a unique input, output, and integrative circuitry, often including unique neurochemical communication channels, and each has the potential for concurrent and semi- or totally independent operation. The major limitations on the total system are moment-to-moment fluctuations in the accessibility of a given neurofunctional system to any other system, the limited availability of certain species-dependent, dominant output channels (e.g., overt or covert verbal output in humans), and the limited availability of a locally or globally oriented facilitatory system (often called attention). Various versions of this model of human brain function have recently been sketched in popular publications[1-3] and more rigorously developed in the literature of the cognitive sciences.[4,5] The neuro-performance model, which represents a variation of this general model, not only recognizes the hierarchical organizational schema at each of the parallel subsystems but also attempts to incorporate the variable energy underpinnings of the entire system, including cerebral blood (and thus oxygen) flow, blood-borne nutrients, and intracellular molecular production facilities. General energy availability and moment-to-moment regional energy allocation are seen as critical elements of control and maintenance in this model.

HOW DO WE MEASURE BEHAVIOR?

The neuro-performance approach to evaluating the functional integrity and plasticity of the CNS involves delineating and measuring the component elements of neurofunctional systems at the output, or behavioral, level. This involves presenting a series of fixed challenges or tasks to the organism and measuring specific aspects of the speed or accuracy of performance on those tasks. In many applications, the tasks are selected to isolate and challenge major neurofunctional subsystems at each of several levels of the system's hierarchical organization. It is therefore necessary to devise a graded series of challenges, ranging from relatively simple tasks that involve unidimensional inputs and outputs to highly complex tasks that involve the integration of many levels, both within and between multiple subsystems. In other applications, only high-level tasks may be utilized to gauge the overall level of CNS function.

A thorough understanding of the input, output, and integrative and modulative circuitry of a given neurofunction is essential in task development. Our knowledge of CNS circuitry is best defined for the rather simple systems of sensory input or motor output. As is evident in the chapters by Brooke (Chapter 8) and Dyck and O'Brien (Chapter 15), very sensitive analyses of sensory and motor performance can be conducted. The circuitry of more complex neurofunctional systems is considerably less defined. The rigorous and laborious efforts required to define such circuitry and to specify the relevant input-output variables are well illustrated in Chapter 18 by Claman and Zeffiro. Eventually, such effort will produce a battery of behavioral tasks that reflect a thorough understanding of the specific neurofunctional systems they challenge and measure.

The difficulty of developing such tasks is enormous—not only because of the inherent complexity of a given system, but also because relatively minor variations in any aspect of a task may alter the requirements of the system in performing that task, particularly as the complexity of the task increases. The hallmark of cognitive neurofunctional systems is plasticity—the ability to change in the face of new challenges. This inherent plasticity also ensures that system characteristics will change with increasing experience in any given task, even within the evaluation setting. Moreover, each individual represents a unique constellation of neurofunctional abilities that are dependent on genetic potential as well as task history. The dimensions of this unique endowment are not fully known but must be taken into account in establishing the normative limits for any challenge. At present, age, gender, health status, and educational level are generally recognized as critical determinants of system capabilities that must be considered in establishing normative limits.

TYPES OF EVALUATIONS

There are two broad categories of neurofunctional evaluation. The first stems from the medical model of diseases and disorders, in which the emphasis is to discover the nature of an impairment, its pathophysiology, and its etiology—that is, to make a diagnosis. Such questions as, What is abnormal? How severe is the abnormality? and What is the cause? are generally answered in terms of well-defined diseases or syndromes. The critical judgments depend on the detection of abnormal signs, symptoms, or measurement values for specific challenges. Thus, the clinical examination is oriented toward detecting departures of criterion behaviors from normal limits, or the presence of behaviors usually not seen in normal subjects. In this context, the term *normal* is used to describe individuals without suspected disease of or injury to the CNS.

The clinician's ability to detect abnormal signs and symptoms is largely a function of some vaguely defined talent or clinical ability, coupled with a liberal dose of experience with large numbers of patients demonstrating the abnormal signs and symptoms, as well as with a wide range of normal variants.

The use of objective tests is in part an attempt to replace the subjective elements of the clinician as the primary measurement tool with standardized test challenges relevant to the patient's symptoms. Scores for the patient's performance on these tests are compared to a normative data base (i.e., the scores for similar individuals without symptoms); if they show a statistically significant departure, the performance is considered abnormal. The pattern of abnormal performance results can be used to define the disease and disorder or to localize the damage to specific neurofunctional systems. The tests given to the patient are generally those with the most predictability for the disease or disorders initially suspected. The key criteria are the diagnostic sensitivity of a test and its ability to pinpoint the key features of the impairment(s). The diagnostic sensitivity of a test is a strictly empirical issue and need not conform to any particular theoretical framework.

The second major category of evaluation emphasizes the scores and patterns of performance as indicators of the current state of the CNS. The pattern of high and low performance values defines the strengths and weaknesses of various system components, which then can be addressed with training and remediation programs. Although comparisons with normative values are relevant, the primary goal is not to detect abnormalities, but rather to characterize the current level of CNS function, typically as the baseline for future comparison after appropriate intervention. There is an inherent requirement that strengths (relatively high performance scores) as well as weaknesses (relatively low performance scores) be identified. Thus, the absolute score is important, not just whether it is abnormal. The tests selected for the evaluation process tend to reflect some general or specific theoretical framework (e.g., a disease or syndrome). The profile of scores from an evaluation battery can usually be related to inferred conceptual nodes in the theoretical framework. Test development and selection should remain faithful to the underlying conceptual structure.

In many diagnostic and evaluation settings, neither approach is followed strictly. Rather, tests are often selected on the basis of availability, training, experience, and other expedient criteria. In addition, evaluative tests developed under one theoretical umbrella are often incorporated under another, sometimes with a poor practical and conceptual fit.

HOW DOES BEHAVIOR CHANGE WITH AGE?

In the evaluation of behavior—whether by inquiry, physical examination (i.e., unaided or minimally assisted observation), or instrumented measurement—there is always an implicit or explicit range of acceptable values. The specification of this normal range is critical and complicated, as a number of human characteristics have been strongly related to changes in individual performance, independent of specific diseases or disorders. The acceptable range of "normal" values on a particular behavioral test may change systematically with age, gender, and education level, as well as other variables extrinsic to clinical variables of interest.

Age is perhaps the most ubiquitous variable, and the objective specification of normal behavior across the life span is a highly empirical undertaking. However, implicit assumptions about the nature of aging are critical to the way data are collected in any study of normal aging. These assumptions follow directly from one's a priori theoretical views on aging. The two major theoretical views are the uniform decrement model[6] and the programmed deterioration model.[7] The first postulates that a system wears down by genetic design, because of accumulated genetic errors or accumulated intrinsic or extrinsic damage, or as the result of combinations of these factors. In this model, the brain's senescence parallels, or even leads, the general deterioration of all organ systems, from skin to hair to muscles to heart, lung, kidneys, etc. No particular hypothesis is offered regarding the rate of decline of the various component systems. In contrast, the programmed deterioration model postulates that the ultimate deterioration (i.e., death) is indeed inevitable and probably genetically determined, but that most of the body's component systems can continue to function at or near optimal levels (defined as those of the late teens or twenties) in the absence of disease or insults related to life-style. Major proponents of this view, such as Fries and Crapo[7] point to the longer life spans and generally improving quality of functioning in later life (up to the terminal drop at death) over the past few thousand years of recorded history and particularly over the last 100 years, which have seen improved medical and social care in our society. These proponents believe that self-control of major life-style determinants of body and brain injury play an important role in helping to ensure continued well-being. They believe that multiple environmental and life-style risk factors can be manipulated so as to mitigate performance changes associated with advancing age.

What implications do these contrasting views of the aging process have for the definition of *normal* at each stage of adult development? The uniform decrement model predicts failures of organ systems and the general deterioration of function. Such failures are de facto typical and, by definition, normal. The selection of subjects for studies of any body-brain function over time must therefore include individuals with disease and any known risk factor. Stricter criteria would presumably bias the results by providing for study only highly selected, possibly exceptional individuals who have a unique genetic endowment for long, healthy life and who have been lucky enough not to contract any serious disease by the time of study. Such individuals may be of scientific interest as representatives of a unique genetic variant, but they are probably not normal.

Studies not using explicit exclusion criteria for disease and life-style risk factors have generally supported the decrement theory.[8-10] But when thoroughly analyzed in order to spread the variability of changes over the lifespan, such studies have revealed that decrements are definitely greater in individuals who have a variety of systemic diseases. The performance of such individuals may overlap with that of specific CNS disease-defined subgroups. For example, reaction time shows greater age-related decrements in individuals with diagnosed cardiovascular disease, those with definite signs of cerebrovascular disease, and those with progressive degenerative diseases of all types.[3] The finding that many systemic diseases and disorders may have CNS consequences indicates that performance measures can probably be affected by many different medical factors. This sensitivity to health variables may make these measures nonspecific for diagnostic purposes but may make them particularly sensitive for longitudinal evaluations of treatment.

The issues surrounding the course of normal age-related changes in the CNS remain hotly debated and will not be solved by any one study. The definition of normal aging is undoubtedly changing with the increase of the population of adults over the age of 65, especially those over age 75. The limits of aging cannot be fully tested until the effects of extrinsic factors known to affect longevity and functional ability have been tested extensively. A generation of older adults who have controlled bad life-style habits throughout their lives and engaged in what we now consider optimal behaviors (e.g., longstanding aerobic exercise, better diet, better stress control, more lifelong functional stimulation, and better medical care) may completely revise our concepts of the limits of aging. Intervention studies in adults over 55 years old have already demonstrated that performance improvements of 20 to 80% can be achieved through aerobic exercise programs,[11] specific motor-task training (e.g., video games or divided attention tasks)[12,13] and specific information-processing strategy training, particularly memory-enhancement techniques.[14] Adults who have engaged in aerobic exercise training programs for 10 to 20 years do not show the "typical" decline in reaction time between the ages of 60 and 70.[15]

In future definitions of normal performance, it may be more accurate to partition normal age-related variability along dimensions related to interventions such as those mentioned above. In designing their Human Performance Measurement System, Kondraske and colleagues (Chapter 4) have taken the approach that extensive norms are needed for each measurement variable. In this view, only by testing large numbers of individuals can one control for the relevant dimensions of normal variability. A unique control group must be assembled for each individual, based on life-style characteristics and risk factors that may include the following.

1.   Current exercise frequency and number of years sustained, to control for cardiovascular and general fitness level. A more generic and objective measure for defining a range of normal limits in this domain might be maximum oxygen consumption, resting heart rate, or resting blood pressure.

2.   Sensory, motor, and cognitive skill levels, to control for specially developed abilities. The issue is how much talent and training a patient has had in a particular measurement realm, which relates to the more general issue of the premorbid level of functioning. Individuals with very high skill levels may show substantial performance decrements because of a disease or disorder, yet may still perform within normal limits. This is particularly true in the cognitive testing domain but may also be relevant to certain sensory and motor skills. This problem arises infrequently in diagnostic evaluations but is often ignored when it does occur, because individual-specific normal limits are not available at more than one level of normal functioning. Of course the

problem concerns not only very high but also very low level of functioning relative to the general population.[16] In cognitive testing, education level is sometimes invoked to control for this general factor. A particularly ingenious approach promoted by Corkin et al. (Chapter 22) involves the use of healthy family members (spouses or similar-age siblings). The assumption is that family members of the same household or neighborhood are very likely to be matched along a variety of life-style characteristics. However, it remains to be proven that this approach will control for such dimensions as age, education, or health. Appropriate statistical comparisons must be made along such dimensions to demonstrate that the control population does not differ significantly from that of the patients.

3. Habitual behaviors, such as smoking, drug, or alcohol intake. These habits have increasingly been associated with cumulative damage to the CNS, and a patient with a long history (e.g., of smoking) may show behavioral performance decrements related solely to damage done by the habit and not specifically related to any suspected CNS diseases or disorders. Are the appropriate normal controls therefore persons with a similar history of habitual behavior who have suffered no CNS damage? For alcohol and drug use, general guidelines relate only to the upper limits of habitual abuse (i.e., drug dependency and alcoholism).

4. General health. This being a widely accepted criterion for normal individuals with acute medical conditions or a history of certain major disorders (e.g., cancer, heart disease, other organ diseases or disorders, and any CNS disease) are generally excluded from the ranks of normal controls. The problem of health in older individuals is more difficult because of the greatly increased frequency of health problems with age. The cumulative effects of many subclinical health problems may be very common in older adults.

Arrival at the ultimate definition of true aging changes may take generations. The question of how to define normal performance on instrumented testing cannot wait. Researchers using typical aged subjects (who may have all the same extrinsic risk factors as the patient at hand but no sign of the disease at issue) cannot be far wrong in determining the relative standing of the patient to his peers. However, it would seem that this approach lends itself to a general decrease in sensitivity by inflating the variability of performance data for older adults, who are more susceptible to extrinsic risk factors. Many studies, covering virtually all realms of cognitive and psychomotor performance, have shown increased variability of performance in older, unselected, or minimally selected populations. The threshold for the detection of abnormalities is, of course, highly dependent on the variability of the criterion data base. The higher the variability, the higher the threshold.

The threshold problem is an issue only when the measures of interest are to be used for diagnosis. Thus far, instrumented testing of motor and cognitive functions has not yielded definite diagnostic tools for any neurologic disorder. This is due in part to the considerable overlap between the earliest expressions of any given neurologic disorder and normal function, particularly in older subjects. Typically, a wide spectrum of tests is given, and the pattern of results—even if no single test is abnormal—seems to provide much more definite information than any single test or small set of tests. The test-battery approach provides multiple windows on each of many functional systems, and the astute interpreter comes to relate specific pattern types with particular clinical states. These considerations take us full circle, back to the issue of what is normal. The question may be, What is a normal pattern of results? rather than, What is an abnormal result on any one test? Diagnostic issues certainly reflect this concern.

For longitudinal evaluations, the emphasis on what is normal changes considerably. The overriding issue becomes how much session-to-session variability a test may demonstrate, and thus how sensitive it is to intraindividual changes. The performance of the individual from session to session becomes the standard by which to make inferences regarding the progression of a disease process or the efficacy of a treatment. It is in this realm that instru. ented testing currently has the most to offer the neurologist. The availability of a standardized testing protocol and sensitive and reliable tests can potentially free the clinician from the grossly subjective task of assessing his memory of what a patient was doing or not doing during previous visits. Munsat and colleagues (see Chapter 7) have demonstrated that normal control records are not even essential in longitudinal evaluations of disease progression. Their use of standard scores based on the entire severity range of disease expression permits sensitive assessment of the course of the disease and its response to treatment. However, the relative assessment of change does not answer the question of how the patient's current performance relates to that of his undiseased peers.

Longitudinal testing is not without problems, however, particularly when measurement error or other sources of intraindividual variability are high.[17] When intraindividual variability equals or exceeds interindividual variability, the tests in question may be totally insensitive to sequential changes in function.[11]

The general problem of developing extensive normative data is the enormous cost of screening, selecting, testing, and analyzing large numbers of normal control subjects for each performance measure. This must be undertaken for every modification of a procedure and (though this is seldom done) for repeated uses of a measure over weekly or monthly intervals, as in clinical trials or other longitudinal investigations. The cost has greatly limited the number of adequately normed test batteries and ensured that conceptually outdated or inappropriate test batteries are used all too frequently. Resolution of this problem will require a concerted effort from professional groups to create evaluation and funding mechanisms specifically for the collection of adequate data on normal control groups for human-performance test batteries.

DEFINITION OF NORMAL NEUROLOGIC
FUNCTION ACROSS THE AGE SPAN

Our group has published a number of papers addressing the definition of normal neurologic function across the age span.[18-21] Our studies have defined as normal those individuals without obvious signs or symptoms of neurologic or major systemic disease as indicated by history or screening examinations conducted prior to testing. The design and results of our last study of normal aging[19,20] are briefly summarized below.

Subjects were recruited primarily from community sources, such as veteran's organizations, churches, service clubs, and senior citizens' groups. We selected 61 healthy subjects, attempting to recruit one of each age in the 20- to 80-year range, or five subjects per half-decade. With a few exceptions, we were able to do so. All subject declared themselves to be right-handed.

As part of the recruitment process, each prospective subject was interviewed by telephone according to a structured questionnaire.[18,21] We excluded subjects who smoked heavily (more than half a pack daily), who were alcoholics or recovered alcoholics, who drank caffeinated liquids excessively (i.e., more than the equivalent of one cup of coffee per day), or who had used amphetamines, LSD, marijuana, tran-quilizers, stimulants, or depressants regularly within the previous two months or at all within the previous few weeks. We also excluded artistic subjects and others with highly developed sensori-motor or physical proficiency skills. Subjects who passed the screening examination were brought into the hospital and given a structured neuromedical examination. We eliminated those with a history or direct evidence of serious head injury or any neurosurgery; those who had experienced complications with anesthetics or surgery; and those with contractures, clinically abnormal tremor or joint disease, any disabling dysfunction of the limbs, evidence of cardiovascular or other systemic disease, or any serious uncorrected visual, auditory, or tactile-sensory deficit. We considered the definition and selection of normal, healthy subjects to be a critical issue in the study. Some of our exclusion criteria (e.g., those related to smok-ing and caffeine) may seem too stringent, but we believe that only subjects without symptoms or signs of physical, neurologic, or psychiatric disorders can be considered normal. Complete details regarding our recruitment and selection of normal subjects are reported elsewhere.[18,21]

On two occasions seven to ten days apart, each subject underwent 138 tests in a neurofunction laboratory. The testing sessions lasted from three and a half to four hours, including breaks. The second session provided data with which to assess test-retest reliability and learning or practice effects. The wide age span of 20 to 80 years was amenable to data analysis by polynomial best-fit equations. Where appropriate, right and left body sides were tested to evaluate dominance effects.

Three principal statistical analyses were conducted: a two- or three-way analysis of variance on each measure to assess the main effects of age, examination (first or second), and extremity (dominance), as well as their interactions; analysis using polynomial best-fit equations for degrees of one to three, to determine whether age-related changes are best described by linear, quadratic, or cubic relationships; and fac-tor analysis to assess relationships among measures that may be related to aging. For measures showing significant age effects, the percent decline in neurologic function from 20 to 80 years was calculated on the basis of the expected test values at 20 and 80 years as determined with the polynomial best-fit equation.

The results of the analysis of variance and polynomial analysis of the normal aging study data are detailed elsewhere.[19,20] Figures 3.1 through 3.4 show composite results from the various measurement domains that were evaluated. Most measures showed evidence of declining performance with age. All tests that showed significant declines with increasing age were best described statistically by polynomials of degree one (i.e., linear relationships).

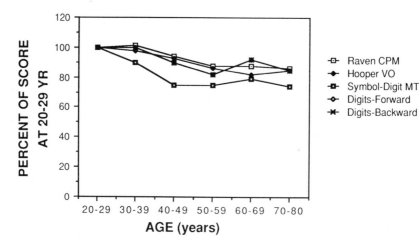

FIGURE 3.1   *Decreases in normal functions with age for five neuropsychologic test measures, based on data from Potvin et al.[19,20] The 20- to 29-year-old subjects served as the standard (100%). Percent differences in functions were averaged over decades from 20 to 80 years. The five neuropsychologic measures are the Raven colored progressive matrices (Raven CPM), Hooper visual organization test (Hooper VO), symbol-digit modalities test (symbol-digit MT), digit span forward (digits—forward), and digit span backward (digits—backward). Note that digits forward and backward overlap.*

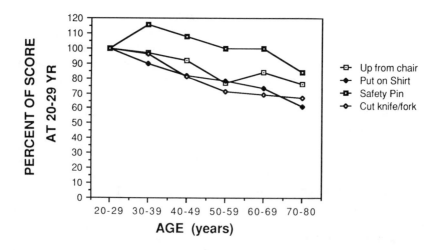

FIGURE 3.2   *Decreases in normal functions with age for four selected simulated activities of daily living (ADL) measures, based on data from Potvin et al.[19,20] The 20 to 29-year-old subjects served as the standard (100%). Percent differences were averaged over decades from 20 to 80 years. The four timed measures were rising up from a chair with support, putting on a shirt, manipulating a safety pin, and cutting with a knife and fork.*

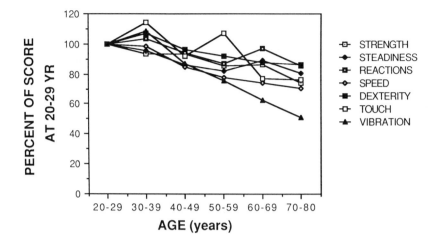

FIGURE 3.3   *Decreases in normal functions with age for six composite upper extremity perfor-mance measures, based on data from Potvin et al.[19,20] The 20- to 29-year-old subjects served as the standard (100%). Percent differences were averaged over decades from 20 to 80 years. Each composite is the average of all patients for that decade for the several components of the composite. The strength composite score included averaged data from six tests: grip strength, right and left hands; hand dorsiflexion strength, right and left hands; and extended-arm abduc-tion strength, right and left arms. The steadiness composite included averaged data from eight tests; hand resting tremor, right and left; arm-sustention tremor, right and left; hand force con-trol, right and left; and arm force control, right and left. The reactions composite included averaged data from six tests: simple hand reaction time, right and left; and step-tracking reaction time for flexion reactions, right and left, and extension reactions, right and left. The speed com-posite included averaged data from six tests: hand-tapping speed, right and left; and step-tracking movement time for flexion movements, right and left, and extension movements, right and left. The dexterity composite included averaged data from four tests: finger grasping and placing, right and left (the Purdue Pegboard), and interfinger manipulation, right and left (pencil rotation). The touch sensation composite included averaged data from two tests: distal touch threshold of the right and left forefinger and the palmar surface. The vibration threshold com-posite included averaged data from twelve tests: vibration threshold of the finger pad, wrist, elbow, shoulder, rib, and collarbone, all for both right and left.*

The data strongly support and supplement previous studies that have shown signifi-cant cross-sectional declines in many sensory functions and most speeded motor perfor-mance tasks (see reference 22 and Chapter 15 of this volume for extensive reviews). The data strongly support the need to take age into account in establishing a normative data base for sensory assessments and motor performance tasks, even in normal con-trols well screened for medical and neurologic problems. The degree of screening for life-style factors that put persons at risk for such problems (e.g., smoking, drug or alcohol use history, poor diet, sedentary habits) remains an open research issue. An overly restrictive definition of normal may exclude too many members of the popula-tion available for study, but it probably provides a more accurate estimate of the normal level of human performance on any given test.

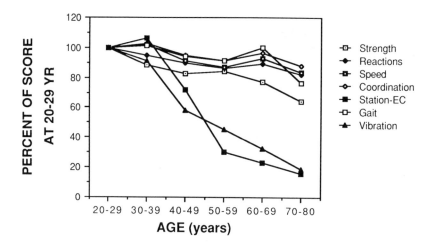

FIGURE 3.4   *Decreases in normal functions with age for six composite lower-extremity perfor-mance measures, based on data from Potvin et al.[19,20] The 20- to 29-year-old subjects served as the standard (100%). Percent differences were averaged over decades from 20 to 80 years. Each composite is the average of all patients for that decade for the several components of the composite. The strength composite score included averaged data from four tests: foot dorsiflexion strength, right and left, and extended leg flexion, right and left. The reactions composite included averaged data from two tests: simple foot reaction time, right and left. The speed composite included averaged data from two tests: foot tapping speed, right and left. The coordination com-posite included averaged data from two tests: lateral reaching and tapping, right and left. The station-EC composite (one-legged standing with eyes closed) included averaged data from stand-ing with right and left legs. The gait test included data from the test of tandem stepping with hand-arm aid. The vibration composite included averaged data from eight tests: vibration threshold of the toe, ankle, tibia, and hip, all for both right and left.*

THE USE OF NORMAL DATA WITH PATIENTS

Once a normal range of values is established for any test measure, the issue becomes how to relate a given patient's data to that range. We have argued for the use of percent of normal function,[15] in which ratio of the patient's score to the appropriate normative score times 100 is obtained. The normative score depends on the sensitivity of the measure to age-related differences. The normal value may reflect any value, from the mean of all patients (regardless of age when no age-related differences are noted) to the mean value at a particular age or within a small age range (e.g., 5 or 10 years) for measures with large age-related changes. The decision regarding the precision of age-related differences should reflect an adequate sampling of performance across the entire age range of interest. In our study of normal aging,[20] we found that percent of change varied from no significant change to significant declines of 80 to 90% by age 80 relative to age 20. Most were linear changes, but this cannot be assumed before an appropriate analysis is performed.

Other investigators in this volume (e.g., Kondraske) have argued strongly against the use of percent of normal function because it does not take into account the inherent

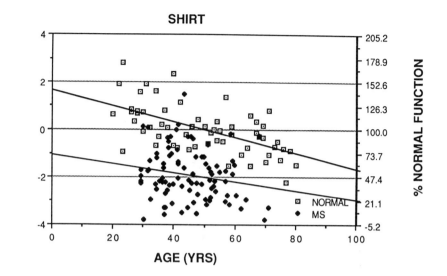

FIGURE 3.5 *Data from the simulated activity of daily living (ADL) measure of putting on a shirt for 61 normal subjects, taken from the study of Potvin et al.*[19,20] *and from the base-line records of 94 multiple sclerosis (MS) patients participating in the UCLA Azathioprine Clinical Trial (unpublished data). The z-score values for both the normal subjects and MS patients were calculated with use of the mean and standard deviation of the normal control values: z = [(data value) − (normal mean)]/(normal standard deviation). The percent normal function axis was determined by putting 100 at the mean of the normal values (corresponding to a z-score of 0) and then adding (or subtracting) the normal standard deviation for each z-score unit.*

variability of a measure. Thus, in a measure with a large standard deviation, percent of normal values in the range of 50 to 100% may all fall within normal limits (i.e., within 2 SD of the mean). Figure 3.5 shows data in normal controls and multiple sclerosis patients for the simulated activity of daily living task of putting on a shirt. The data are plotted as a function of age, using both z-scores and percent of normal function scores calculated relative to the mean of all normal control data for the data in both the normal subjects and multiple sclerosis patients. At a z-score of −2 units, the corresponding percent of normal function value is 47.4%, so that the normal range is over 50% of the mean normal value. In contrast, in a measure with a smaller standard deviation (such as hand speed of the right hand, shown in Figure 3.6), a value of 75.6% of normal function is within 2 SD of the normal mean, making the normal range for this measure 25% of the mean normal value.

The use of a z-score metric, as in Figures 3.5 and 3.6, inherently takes variability into account. However, while z-scores are perhaps strongly defensible on statistical grounds, they may not be easy to interpret by clinicians, patients, and other nonstatisticians. A possible compromise might be to include both the percent of normal function and z-score metrics on the same printouts to aid understanding (e.g., Figs. 3.5 and 3.6) while using the z-score alone in the creation of composites and performance of statistical analyses.

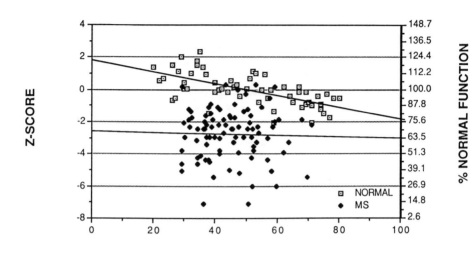

FIGURE 3.6   *The hand-tapping speed test data for the right hand only. Data sources and calculations are the same as those described for Figure 3.5.*

SOME CONCLUSIONS AND FUTURE PERSPECTIVES

Where does this leave us in attempting to determine what is normal? Where would the ideal future lead in this regard? First, we need a full taxonomy of functional abilities, one that directly relates extrinsic performance to specific sets of neuro-functional systems in the CNS and, in turn, to specific physiochemical structures. In short, we need nothing less than a more complete understanding of brain-behavior relationships. Kondraske (Chapter 4) addresses these issues in a technically elegant manner with regard to human performance measurement. At present, of course, we utilize our most recent understanding of such relationships to develop appropriate performance challenges. The availability of a multi-dimensional testing system is essential in this endeavor, to reflect the emerging models of highly complex, multidimensional neurochemical substructures that generate any given performance element. Normative issues should not be of concern. More important is the elucidation of natural developmental sequences of each human performance measure and the specification of the variety of intrinsic and extrinsic modifying factors of those sequences. Each individual could represent his own control if served by institutions that catered to life-long monitoring, early detection, and preventive actions. There is no better control than the performance of an individual before disease onset or before an acute insult to the CNS. This condition can currently be attained in clinical trials (see Chapter 2) but is almost entirely absent in routine medical evaluation and care.

REFERENCES

1. Minsky M. The society of mind. New York: Simon & Schuster, 1986.
2. Ornstein, R. Multimind. Boston: Houghton Mifflin, 1986.
3. Gazzaniga MS. The social brain. New York: Basic Books, 1985.
4. Rumelhart DE, McClelland JL, the PDP Research Group. Parallel distributed processing. Explorations in the microstructure of cognition. Vol. 1: Foundations. Cambridge, MA: MIT Press, 1986.
5. McClelland JE, Rumelhart DE, the PDP Research Group. Parallel distributed processing. Explorations in the microstructure of cognition. Vol. 2: Psychological and biological models. Cambridge, MA: MIT Press, 1986.
6. Strehler BL, Mildvan AS. General theory of mortality and aging. Science, 1960;132: 14–21.
7. Fries JF, Crapo LM. Vitality and aging. San Francisco: W.H. Freeman, 1981.
8. Birren JE, Spieth W. Age, response speed and cardiovascular functions. J Gerontol 1962;17:390–1.
9. Heron A, Chown S. Age and function. London: J & A Churchill, 1967.
10. Jalavisto E, Lindquist C, Makkonen T. Assessment of biological age. III. Mental and neural factors in longevity. Ann Acad Sci Fenn 1964;106:3–20.
11. Dustman RE, Ruhling RO, Russell EM, et al. Aerobic exercise training and improved neuropsychological function of older individuals. Neurobiol Aging 1984;5:35–42.
12. Clark JE, Lanphear AK, Riddick CC. The effects of videogame playing on the response selection processing of elderly adults. J Gerontol 1987;42:82–5.
13. McDowd JM. The effects of age and extended practice on divided attention performance. J Gerontol 1986;41:764–9.
14. Sheikh JI, Hill RD, Yesavage JA. Long-term efficacy of cognitive training for age-associated memory impairment: A six-month follow-up study. Dev Neuropsychol 1986; 2:413–21.
15. Spirduso WW, Clifford P. Replication of age and physical activity effects on reaction and movement time. J Gerontol 1978;33:26–30.
16. Ryan CM, Morrow LA, Bromet EJ, et al. Assessment of neuropsychological dysfunction in the workplace: Normative data from the Pittsburg Occupational Exposures Test Battery. J Clin Exp Neuropsychol 1987;9:665–79.
17. Salthouse T, Kausler DH, Saults JS. Groups versus individuals as the comparison unit in cognitive aging research. Dev Neuropsychol 1986;2:363–72.
18. Potvin, JH, Potvin AR, Tourtellotte WW, et al. Methods and procedures for recruiting and selecting individuals to serve as normal subjects in the neurofunction laboratory. VA Technical Report WT/AP IX. Los Angeles: VA Wadsworth Medical Center Press, 1977.
19. Potvin AR, Syndulko K, Tourtellotte WW, et al. Human neurologic function and the aging process. J Am Geriatr Soc 1980;28:1–8.
20. Potvin AR, Syndulko K, Tourtellotte WW, et al. Quantitative evaluation of normal age-related changes in neurologic function. In: Pirozzolo FJ, Maletta GJ, eds. Advances in neurogerontology. Vol. 2: Behavioral assessment and psychopharmacology. New York: Praeger, 1981, 13–57.
21. Potvin AR, Tourtellotte WW. Quantitative examination of neurologic function. Boca Raton, FL: CRC Press, 1985;2:60–8.
22. Katzman R, Terry RD. The neurology of aging. Philadelphia: F.A. Davis, 1981.

Chapter 4

Measurement Science Concepts and Computerized Methodology in the Assessment of Human Performance

George V. Kondraske

Quantification of parameters that reflect a human's ability to execute daily tasks or that document clinical factors of interest has been the focus of many individual and often diffuse interdisciplinary research efforts. Very few exacting tools have been available to practitioners in health care (e.g., neurologists, orthopedists, therapists), practitioners in personnel selection and screening (e.g., for airline pilots, police, firefighters) or those concerned with the human factors of engineering design—all of whom need objective and quantitative data in order to make critical decisions. Typically, such data concern central processing, strength, handedness, range of motion, muscle tone, speed, dexterity, coordination, and sensory perception. Subjective rating scales (1 = good, 2 = average, 3 = poor) have been the most widely used methods of obtaining discriminating documentation of such performance aspects, and are still considered by many to represent the state of the art.

The relatively few research efforts that have recognized the need for a more sensitive and comprehensive array of measurement tools have lacked either sufficient scope or the coordination and follow-up necessary to gain widespread acceptance. Perhaps even more significant, there has been a notable absence of an organized structure on which to build a measurement science for human performance. This may be due to a lack of sufficient quantitative methods of measurement with which to obtain data that could yield the knowledge required to fuel the development of such an evaluation system.

As a result of our past and continuing research, an expandable systematic structure and philosophy of human performance measurement has been established. A broad quantitative measurement system, performance data base, and ten cooperating data-collection centers (using identical devices and methodology based on our concepts) have been developed and put into operation. It is now feasible to draw from a broad "toolbox" of noninvasive measurements of strength, speed, reaction, coordination, body stability, and other functions, with initial results computed, recorded, and added to the data base automatically. In turn, an appropriate result report can be selected from an array designed to address the wide range of clinical needs.

The array of standardized measurements, together forming what has come to be called a human performance profile, represents the blueprint of an individual's capacity to perform tasks of daily life. While directly addressing the apparent immediate clinical needs for measurement, the system provides the opportunity to study the process of integrating basic or primitive elements of performance into higher-level activities. Consequently, through the use of individually designed analysis software packages and emerging theoretical concepts of human performance, one can now expect to obtain objective interpretations of the human performance profile for specific applications, such as diagnostic assistance, treatment plan determination, and objective documentation of patient status. The profile can also be used to predict the probability of a person's success in athletics or professions that maximally stress the human system, such as piloting complex aircraft.

This chapter outlines the measurement system as well as its background and basic underlying concepts. A primary purpose is to draw attention to the idea of a human performance measurement science and to provide a brief, preliminary foundation for future work in this area.

NEED AND CONCEPTS FOR A MEASUREMENT SCIENCE

A fundamental component of any science is a well-defined language to facilitate communication. In this respect, there is no greater need than in the field addressed here, nor has there been any greater impediment to progress. For example, it is assumed that the type of quantitative information desired is essentially the same across several related clinical disciplines: neurology, orthopedics, physical therapy, and physical medicine. A review of several recent texts of relevance is informative. The following titles can be found: *Functional Assessment in Rehabilitation Medicine,*[1] *Functional Assessment in Rehabilitation,*[2] *Measurement in Physical Therapy,*[3] and *The Quantitative Examination of Neurologic Function.*[4]

In addition to assessment, measurement, and quantitative examination, we must also deal with terms such as *disability determination, functional capacity, functional status,* and *impairment.* Each of the above-referenced texts has attempted to define some of these terms, and some agreement has been achieved. However, the fundamental delineation between the distinguishing features of **measurement** and **assessment** has yet to be widely recognized. These words are often used (or misused) interchangeably. For example, Halpern and Fuhrer offer the following definition:

Functional assessment is the measurement of purposeful behavior in interaction with the environment, which is interpreted according to the assessment's intended uses.[2]

Such worthwhile efforts at definition can be more confusing than clarifying. *Measurement* refers to the use of a standard (such as a metric ruler) to quantify an observation (such as length). In contrast, *assessment* is the process of determining the meaning of a measurement or collective set of measurements in a specific context or the result of such a process. The specific assessment process employed depends on the application. For example, we may subjectively examine a patient and determine that he is too weak to transfer from a wheelchair to a bed yet strong enough to dress himself. Assessments can be made (as many frequently are) by subconscious or rudimentary subjective methods, without the aid of standard measurements. Assessments are often based on intuition. Whereas measurements are facts, assessments can generally be viewed as conclusions. Measurements are tools of assessment that can contribute to increased objectivity and accuracy. While assessment represents the ultimate clinical need, measurement offers a means to improve the assessment process.

Based on the foregoing, one should be concerned first with measurement. A fundamental decision must be made in determining what to measure. Many disability rating or assessment scales include components that may or may not be directly measured in the true sense of the word, though they can be assessed. Arguments continually rage over the content of a particular scale, providing further evidence of the difficulty of determining what should be quantified. A possible source of this great confusion is that in many cases, we have been attempting to measure things that should be assessed by comparing a set of measurements to established criteria.

To clarify this last statement, it seems plausible to view a human as a defined architectural structure composed of a finite set of interconnected functional units capable of operating along specific dimensions of performance (e.g., strength, endurance, range of motion, speed).[5] Consideration of all the functional units results in the realization of a finite set of distinct basic elements of performance (BEP). Human functional units are either a single or collective set of anatomic structures (as described by the terminology of human anatomy—e.g., elbow flexors, knee extensors, visual information processor) that work together (function) to realize the respective dimensions of performance. Each functional unit maps into its own performance space (defined by dimensions of performance; see Figure 4.1) and is responsible for contributing a fraction to the totality of human BEPs. Thus, to specify a single BEP, one must delineate both the functional unit and the dimension of performance.

It is also useful, and perhaps essential, as a modeling construct to view performance in terms of resources (used to accomplish various tasks) available to the human system. A subtle but distinct and important implication for measurement results from this model. When resources are to be measured, it is natural to define measurands that range from zero (no resources) to some positive value. Currently, there is no consistent definition of performance measures. The definition of measures or scales often seems to be arbitrary; that is, for certain standards, sometimes a smaller number indicates

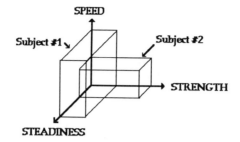

FIGURE 4.1   *An example of a multi-dimensional (three dimensions in this example) performance space associated with a system. Measures are defined such that dimension labels represent unique (with respect to each other) and desirable qualities, and the measurement scales are defined consistently so that a larger number always represents better performance. Note that a performance space of this type can be applied to describe either basic functional units (such as an elbow flexor) or to a coalition of basic units that work together in higher level tasks (such as the speech production system). When applied at the basic functional unit level as in the elemental resource model (see text), the name of the system (e.g., elbow flexor) and the name of a single dimension (e.g., strength) combine to identify a single basic element of performance. Idealized performance regions are illustrated for two different subjects. The volume of each box represents the performance capacity of the selected system or subsystem for the subject. This implies that a product relationship should be used to combine such measures if composite scores are desired.*

better performance (e.g., timed activities, manual muscle test scales) and other times a larger number denotes better (e.g., a grip strength test with a dynamometer). This can create confusion and requires extra thought to determine which rule applies for a given measurement. However, a more serious result is that generalizable laws important for measurement interpretation cannot be defined. With consistency in definition required by the resource construct, we achieve not only simplicity in communication but also the ability to apply the basic law of ***resource economics*** to all aspects of human performance. This law simply states that the amount of resource(s) available must be greater than the amount required for the desired task.

Use of the resource construct in human performance implies that attention should be restricted to the desired resources (i.e., those useful for accomplishing tasks). It is natural to focus on measures of speed (in contrast to measures of the lack of it; e.g., bradykinesia), strength (in contrast to weakness), steadiness (in contrast to tremor), and so on. To determine if bradykinesia is present, a speed resource measurement is obtained and compared with some established criteria (e.g., speed of the average normal subject of the same age and gender). This represents assessment. For clinical purposes, criteria can be set for individual resources to determine the presence of a problem. A particular pattern of resource deficits may be indicative of a particular disease or disorder. Performance resources can be the focus of rehabilitation (as some are now, such as strength and range of motion for specific functional units). The same measurements may be used to track progress or effectiveness of interventions as well as to make assessments of broader scope related to a patient's quality of life, such as independent living, etc.

Thus, each BEP is a unique performance resource. The combination of elemental and resource constructs provides the basis for an elemental resource model that describes human performance. The elemental model assumes that humans draw on these BEPs to varying degrees in order to accomplish a virtually infinite number and variety of tasks. The amount of a specific performance resource required is determined by the task. The multidimensionality of high-level tasks (for example, how fast, steady, and long can one walk) precludes a valid single measurement of performance. A set of measurements at the task level representing the multiple dimensions of the task and a set of comparison criteria can be used as a basis for assessment if one merely desires to know how well the task is performed. However, if one desires to know why performance at a high level is below an established target, the resources at the basic element level must be considered. Thus, assessment requires consideration of the higher level applications. (e.g., grooming, driving, feeding) of basic elements of performance; measurement does not. Rating scales for high-level activities can be interpreted as an intuitive integration of subconsciously made measurements to assess the level of competence in a defined application of multidimensional performance resources. Additional discussion and application of these concepts can be found in references 5 through 9, along with references to relevant additional literature.

The need for such a conceptual framework, or scientific construct, has been articulated by Cappozzo.[10] Although his comments were made with respect to gait, they seem appropriate in a more general sense as well:

> What is really missing is a conceptual background. The approaches to clinical gait analysis and evaluation are not supported by general theories. The best concrete achievements have their foundation in theory, in abstraction, and gait analysis, in this sense, is no exception. We biomechanicians have been working hard, during the last decades, designing new instruments and experimental methodologies, applying old analytical techniques to our new problems. We have been gathering a great deal of numbers regarding the various aspects of human locomotion. Now, I think, more efforts should be devoted to speculation. We should try to interpret the phenomena we have observed, we should try to identify, through the generalization of single observations, the laws that govern them. In other words, we should go back to a more genuine scientific operation.

With the exception of a few components, the human performance measurement system described here is based on the concept that the measurement of human performance (i.e., the collection of all basic elements of performance) be oriented toward a finite number of **application-independent** (in terms of their definition) performance resources, as opposed to a nearly unlimited number of applications of human system resources (e.g., specific high-level tasks such as lifting or putting on a shirt). Given this approach, basic elements of performance (functional units and performance dimensions) must be identified. Measurement methods are employed that stress the individual functional units along each of the dimensions of performance (one dimension at a time) to determine the amount of performance resources available. Some tests that evaluate the coordination of multiple functional units are also necessary and are therefore also included.

COMPUTERIZED MEASUREMENT SYSTEM

Building on previous work in the quantification of neurologic function by Tourtellotte and colleagues,[4] we expanded the scope of quantification to include additional measures important in physical therapy, occupational therapy, and orthopedics. We also now use the above-described concept of human performance to help refine tests and provide a context for interpretation of measures. The first computerized system was developed to serve as the framework of the overall system we envisioned.[11,12] Since 1983, research toward the realization of a comprehensive system has been conducted under funding from the National Institute on Disability and Rehabilitation Research through a rehabilitation engineering center. The Center for Advanced Rehabilitation Engineering is a consortium involving the University of Texas at Arlington (College of Engineering), the University of Texas Health Science Center at Dallas (Departments of Physical Therapy, Neurology, and Orthopedic Surgery), and the Dallas Rehabilitation Institute (coordinated by the Dallas Rehabilitation Foundation). New measures, test scenarios, and concepts have been developed, investigated, and applied.[13-27]

System Overview

The human performance measurement system can best be understood in terms of three basic components: (1) an application-independent measurement laboratory, (2) a human performance data base, and (3) application-dependent software for measurement presentation and interpretation (Figure 4.2). Application-independent measurement, in keeping with the philosophy and goals behind in-test designs, is a contrast to the quantification of higher-level tasks that represent the activities humans perform in daily life. These types of tasks are viewed as applications of more intrinsic performance resources. Therefore, any parameters quantified in these tasks are application dependent.

Procedures once carried out manually (e.g., by recording scores and filing results) or subjectively (e.g., by rating performance or determining the degree of functional loss) are now computerized. The integrated nature of the system required the development of special devices (e.g., transducers, stimulators) and test scenarios to facilitate this process.

Measurement Laboratory

In designing the measurement laboratory, we considered that (1) the capability to measure a broad range of human performance is essential; (2) the battery of tests must be applicable both as a whole and as selected subsets of tests; (3) scenarios used for tests of individual dimensions of performance should resemble those used in traditional evaluative methods; (4) a test result should document the level of a measured basic element of performance, and the result should be simple (ideally, a single number) and quantitative; (5) aspects subject to the influence of human error or opinion should be

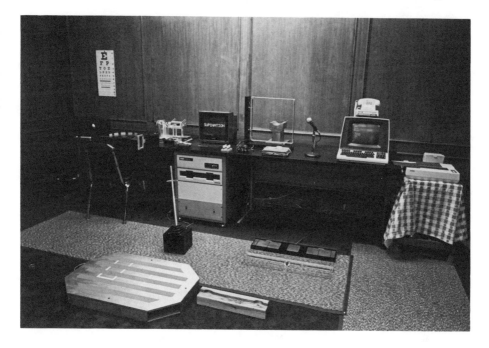

FIGURE 4.2 *The human performance measurement system at the University of Texas Health Science Center at Dallas.*

minimized to achieve increased objectivity; and (6) the tests should be designed in such a way that they can be administered by a trained technician (e.g., a physical therapist assistant).

The measurement laboratory is illustrated in Figures 4.3 and 4.4. Its physical components include a microcomputer system base unit (LSI–11/23, Digital Equipment Corp.) connected to 14 modular peripheral test devices through special interface modules. Thus, a laboratory can be fully equipped or more modestly configured, containing only the modules required to implement the desired set of tests. When fully configured, the battery is capable of obtaining nearly 500 different human performance measures (Table 4.1).

A given test consists of a 5- to 60-second scenario, during which the subject responds to instructions given immediately before administration or to stimuli presented during the scenario. The scenario consists of a task selected to stress a specific dimension of performance at a given body site(s). The computer is used to control the administration protocol, data acquisition, and recording of results. Special software is used to record time-series data and extract defined features (performance resource measurands) via specific parameterization schemes to yield single-number results. For example, during sensory tests (e.g., touch, vibration, temperature, two-point discrimination), the subject is presented with computer-controlled, precisely generated stimuli. The threshold level at which the subject can correctly identify

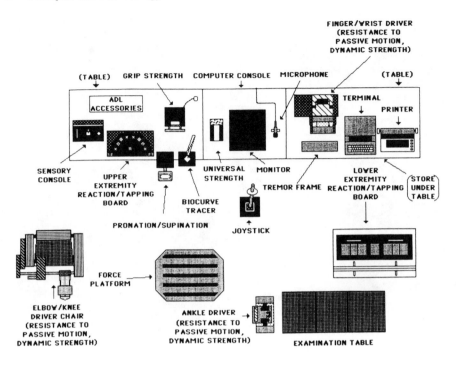

FIGURE 4.3   *A typical floor plan for the human performance measurement system. ADL denotes activities of daily living.*

the presence or absence of a stimulus 50% of the time is determined with the two-alternative, forced-choice method.[28]

The anthropometric features category includes the measurement of the length of body segments of diagnostic interest in the evaluation of orthopedic problems (e.g., differences in leg lengths). Measurements are made with a special three-dimensional digitizer, the Biocurve Tracer, which is also employed with special software to measure range of motion and anatomic contours.[18,19] Strength measurements are acquired with test protocols modeled after manual muscle tests (isometric) and a transducer mounted to the test administrator's hand,[11,12] as well as with motorized devices (dynamic). The latter do not place demands on the strength of the technician. The dynamic instruments are also used to measure muscle tone[15] (the general term we use to encompass differences among normal subjects in this aspect of muscle function) as well as pathologic conditions, such as rigidity and spasticity.

Upper extremity, lower extremity, and head tremor measures are included in the steadiness category. Sustention and resting modes are available for use when applicable and therefore result in separate measurands. A noncontacting capacitive displacement transducer[14] is used to measure average vertical and horizontal displacement during a 15-second timed trial in which the subject attempts to achieve perfect steadiness. Body balance includes both one- and two-leg stability measures, executed with the patient's eyes either open or closed. An instrumented force platform is used to measure average

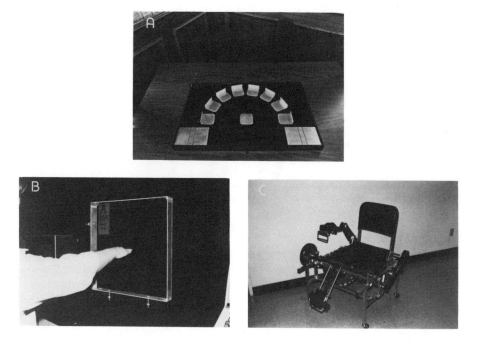

FIGURE 4.4 *Selected devices used in the human performance measurement system. (A) Upper-extremity reaction/speed/coordination board, in which touch-sensitive plates and light-emitting diode stimulators interface with the computer. Special protocols are used for simple and multichoice visual reaction time, movement speed measures, finger- and hand-tapping speed, and arm lateral reaching and tapping coordination (similar to finger-to-nose) tests. (B) Hand/arm tremor frame, a device with a noncontacting sensor that determines average vertical and horizontal tremor amplitude. (C) Elbow/knee driver chair, a computer-controlled, motor-driven apparatus used to measure muscle tone (resistance to passive motion) of selected upper- and lower-extremity body sites from recorded torque and angular position of the limb segment.*

lateral (sagittal) and fore-aft anteroposterior stability on the basis of movement of the center of pressure on the platform.[22] Special devices for the upper and lower extremities are used in protocols that stress central response speed (reactions), movement speed, and coordination.

Gait is a special category, much like speech. We consider it to represent a high-level activity dependent on lower-level performance resources, which are measured independently. Its extreme importance in daily life also makes it worthy of special consideration. A robotic video system is being developed to permit the quick measurement of critical gait parameters that have been shown to be sensitive clinical indicators. As for speech, a complete acoustically based sub-battery is under development.[20] The subject is required to perform specific speech tasks that stress different components of the articulatory and central processing systems with respect to selected dimensions of performance.

Activities of daily living and manual dexterity are also viewed as combinations

Table 4.1 Major Function Categories and Number of Measures in Each

Mental status (4)	Muscular endurance (12)
Vision (2)	Muscular tone (24)
Audition (4)	Coordination (15)
Tactile sensation (20)	Speech (78[a])
Anthropometric features (27)	Manual dexterity (6)
Range of motion (132)	Body stability (12)
Strength (85)	Gait (10[a])
Speed (33)	Activities of daily living (8)
Reactions (response speed) (21)	Steadiness (12)

[a]Under active development; not yet implemented.

of many basic performance resources applied simultaneously. Measurement of the time of execution of specific tasks within these broad categories is currently employed.

For muscle endurance measurement, myoelectric techniques are being investigated[29] since they offer the potential of a technique that is independent of subject motivation. This is the only dimension of performance measurement in which electrode-based tests are employed.

With regard to the clinical use of a broad measurement system, a "toolbox" concept is emphasized. It can be applied either comprehensively, semicomprehensively (utilizing subsystems of tests), or in smaller, very selective subgroups (i.e., utilizing only a few "tools"). The selection of specific tools or measurements is determined by the clinical application or task at hand. In neurology, the clinician's knowledge of signs associated with common disorders (i.e., which performance resources are likely to be impaired) serves to guide test selection.

Human Performance Database

Along with basic methods of measurement, standardized and simplified methods of interpretation are needed. Performance is measured in physical units (e.g., milliseconds, kilograms), and interpretation is often difficult because (1) several hundred measures of function may appear on a single printout; (2) raw test results contain many different physical units; (3) in order to identify normal and abnormal findings, the clinician must have some knowledge of normal results for each test; and (4) normal function changes with age and is different in males and females. We therefore developed a database approach to relieve the clinician's burden of memorizing a host of normal test result values and to present results in a format that is immediately interpretable. The system was not designed to merely store masses of data but to facilitate the interpretation of test results and simplify the execution of systematic studies based on the data base.[30]

With the Human Performance Data-Base Management System, data collection and some report-printing are performed with the on-site measurement laboratory computers. A central research data base is maintained on a mainframe computer (VAX

11/780, Digital Equipment Corp.) and can be accessed by telephone with use of a terminal and modem. This system permits networked access from multiple test sites.

Test Result Reports

Test result reports offer the simplest example of application-dependent software. The philosophy used to define basic elements of performance is also used to structure these reports. Individual measures are organized as subcategories of the appropriate major function categories based on dimensions of performance or selected high-level tasks (e.g., gait, speech). For example, the major category of speed includes measures acquired during finger-tapping, forearm supination and pronation, arm movement, and weight-shifting in standing tasks. Five types of computerized reports are currently available: (1) standard comparison report—a comparison of the subject's data with appropriate norms; (2) composite standard report—individual test results within major functional categories, averaged after comparison with norms; (3) trend report—selected individual measures or composite changes in functions over time; (4) measurement report—raw scores and norms; and (5) abnormal findings report—results below a specified threshold.

Test results can be obtained for single test dates or in a merged format for multiple selected test dates. A report can be tailored to include only data on selected major categories (e.g., sensation, coordination, strength) or specific body sites (e.g., trunk, lower right extremity). Part of a standard comparison report is shown in Figure 4.5.

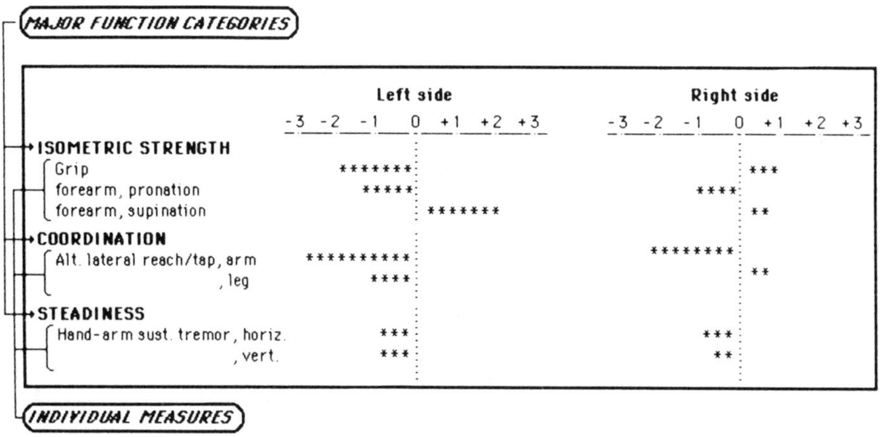

FIGURE 4.5   *A portion of a standard comparison report. This report compares patient data with appropriate age- and gender-matched norms, reported as standard deviations above or below the population mean.*

Clinical Evaluation and Research Studies

Most measures in the test system have been evaluated for reliability and the effects of test repetition (learning), age, and handedness.[4] For previously used tests, the results of computerized and noncomputerized versions compare favorably.[4] A more comprehensive evaluation of reliability and learning has recently been completed.[23,31] In addition, short-term changes in function, a constantly continuing process, are being studied with a five-day protocol in which a representative subset of tests is repeated each day. Long-term changes in function are being studied with annual retests of both normal and pathologic subjects.

Several patient group studies have been conducted. Early performance changes in subjects at risk for Huntington's disease[24] have been measured, as have changes in normal neurologic function brought about through hypnosis.[4] Other reported studies have characterized the functional status of parkinsonian[4,11] and head-injured patients.[25] Research using the system to investigate spasmodic dysphonia, thought to be exclusively a speech disorder, has shown that it may be a more widespread motor disorder.[26] Studies are underway to document functional deficits in patients with postoperative low back pain and to increase our understanding of postpolio sequelae.

Applications

The system's broad, flexible measurement protocols and automated data-management features facilitate the execution of clinical trials. During research and development, we also placed great emphasis on the system's capabilities for documenting the performance status of individual patients. For example, Figure 4.6 shows a test-retest comparison report for a head-injured subject undergoing rehabilitation. Results may also serve as the basis for determining the extent of a disability relevant to reimbursement for services and injury claims settlements. With the success of current research and development activities, the system may eventually suggest vocational options for patients and evaluate their capacity for driving and other activities. Screening applications of the system may permit the early detection of disease or predisposition to injury (e.g., in a potential employee) and the determination of functional age (e.g., in a potential retiree).

Future plans call for enhancement of the scope and quality of measurements that define the human performance profile. Pursuit of applications research targets involving the use of computerized *expert systems* to process the measurement profile and provide more assessments or bottom-line results (e.g., the site and extent of a lesion or the percent disability for an individual or extremity) will help define the work to be done.

For example, in an effort referred to as function-oriented identification of neuromuscular anatomic abnormalities,[27] nervous system structures, innervations, and muscles responsible for given actions have been mapped to body sites (functional units) and actions (e.g., flexion, extension) stressed by various tasks. Based on a complex computerized tracing scheme and measurements of specific dimensions of performance at various sites in a given individual, the system is being designed to identify and print the names of muscles functioning abnormally, along with their innervations.

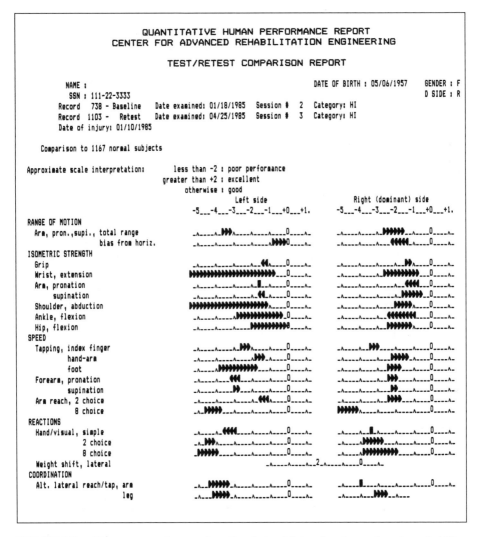

FIGURE 4.6   *Test-retest result report for a female head-injured patient undergoing rehabilitation. Two separate test dates approximately three months apart are shown to indicate changes in function. The directions of the arrowheads indicate the directions of changes on a scale of standard deviation units after comparison with a normal subject population.*

Work is planned to identify lesions in higher-level brain structures, taking into account such characteristics of actions as steadiness, positioning accuracy, speed, and coordination. All results will contribute to attempts to formulate a systems-level, quantitative model of human performance, providing a framework with which to gauge developments and understand complex functional interactions. Education, via demonstration projects, will be a high priority as our group attempts to promote an understanding of quantitative methods and their clinical use.

CONCLUSION

A scientific approach is urged in the measurement of human performance and its constituent components, such as neurologic and musculoskeletal function. Although the complexity at the component level approaches that seen biochemically, there has been a tendency to oversimplify human function, especially with respect to its measurement. Scientists have been concerned with the structure and functions of individual physiologic systems and have investigated these internal components in great detail. They should now apply equal efforts and resources to studying the whole from an external point of view—i.e., human performance. Although high-level tasks will remain of interest, it is suggested that the study of tasks at an intermediate "stepping-stone" level may be more fruitful.

An integrated system of measuring selected aspects of human performance, consisting of a computerized measurement laboratory, a data-base system and result-presentation software, is described. Measurements are classified according to major function categories, and the system's methods emphasize the application-independent measurement of basic performance resources. A microcomputer coordinates the acquisition of measurements with a series of short-duration tests. To facilitate interpretation, the normal data base permits the immediate comparison of patient data to data for an appropriately matched subgroup. Most measures in the system have been evaluated for reliability, and several patient group studies are underway or already completed. The system permits the measurement of selected sensorimotor functions for use in quantifying individual patient performance, justifying reimbursement of medical expenses, screening employees and athletes, and improving the scientific bases of clinical practice, and facilitates the execution of clinical trials with large groups of subjects.

REFERENCES

1. Granger CV, Gresham GE. Functional assessment in rehabilitation medicine. Baltimore: Williams and Wilkins, 1984.
2. Halpern AS, and Fuhrer MJ. Functional assessment in rehabilitation. Baltimore: P. H. Brookes, 1984.
3. Michels E. Foreword. In: Rothstein JM, ed. Measurement in physical therapy. New York: Churchill Livingstone, 1985.
4. Potvin AR, Tourtellotte WW, Potvin JH, et al. The quantitative examination of neurologic function. Boca Raton, FL: CRC Press, 1985.
5. Kondraske GV. Human performance: science or art? In: Proceedings: thirteenth annual northeast bioengineering conference. Philadelphia: March 1987.
6. Kondraske GV. Looking at the study of human performance. SOMA: Engineering for the Human Body. American Society of Mechanical Engineering 1987; 2(2):50–4.
7. Kondraske GV. Human performance measurement: Some perspectives. IEEE Eng in Med and Biol Society Mag 1988; 7(1):11–16.
8. Kondraske GV. Workplace design: An elemental resource approach to task analysis and human performance measurements. International Conference of the Association for the Advancement of Rehabilitation Technology. In: Proceedings. Montreal: 1988;608–11.
9. Kondraske GV. Computation of functional capacity: Strategy and example for shoulder. Ninth annual IEEE Engineering in Medicine and Biology Society conference. In: Proceedings. Boston: 1987;477–78.

10. Cappozzo. Considerations on clinical gait evaluations. Biomechanics 14:33–45.
11. Kondraske GV. Design, construction, and evaluation of an automated computer-based system for quantification of neurologic function. Doctoral dissertation, the University of Texas at Arlington and the University of Texas Health Science Center at Dallas (joint program), 1982.
12. Kondraske GV, Potvin AR, Tourtellotte WW, et al. A computer-based system for automated quantification of neurologic function. IEEE Trans Biomed Eng 1984; 31: 401–14.
13. Smith SS, Kondraske GV. A computerized system for quantitative measurement of sensorimotor aspects of human performance. Phys Ther, December 1987.
14. Kondraske GV. A non-contacting human tremor sensor and measurement system. IEEE Trans Instr Meas 1986; IM–35:201–6.
15. Chan HC, Manry MT, and Kondraske GV. Classification of resistance to passive motion using minimum probability of error criterion. Annals of Biomed Eng 1987; 15:579–90.
16. Kondraske GV. Quantitative assessment of speech function. In: Proceedings of the seventh annual Engineering in Medicine and Biology Society conference. Chicago: 1985; 671–4.
17. Smith SS, Kondraske GV. A clinical test for quantifying forearm pronation and supination function. In: Proceedings of the eighth annual conference on rehabilitation engineering. Memphis: 1985; 174–6.
18. von Maltzahn WW, Kondraske GV. An instrument to measure range of motion. In: Proceedings of the eighth annual conference on rehabilitation engineering. Memphis: 1985; 165–7.
19. von Maltzahn WW, and Kondraske GV. Computer assisted characterization of the human spine. In: Proceedings of the seventh annual Engineering in Medicine and Biology Society conference. Chicago: 1985; 689–91.
20. Jafari M, Kondraske GV. Computerized quantitative speech profile. In: Proceedings of the eighth annual Engineering in Medicine and Biology Society conference. Fort Worth, TX: 1986; 1880–2.
21. Bhargava R, Behbehani K, Kondraske GV. Phase plane analysis of the upper extremity step response. In: Proceedings of the eighth annual Engineering in Medicine and Biology Society conference. Fort Worth, TX: 1986; 1596–8.
22. Kondraske GV. Toward a standard clinical measure of postural stability. In: Proceedings of the eighth annual Engineering in Medicine and Biology Society conference. Fort Worth, TX: 1986; 1579–82.
23. Richmond JR, Kondraske GV, Smith SS. Reliability in quantitative measures of sensorimotor function: results for a broad computerized test battery and methodologic issues. Arch Phys Med Rehabil (submitted 1988).
24. Steward RM, Levy F, Kondraske GV, et al. Computer-based quantitative assessment of sensory and motor functions in Huntington's disease (HD). Neurology 1983; 33(suppl.2): 243.
25. Wise M, Kondraske GV. Quantitative functional assessment and characterization of head injured patients. In: Proceedings of the eighth annual conference on rehabilitation engineering. Memphis: 1985; 168–70.
26. Cannito MP. Extralaryngeal functions in spasmodic dysphonia: vocal tract and upper extremity control. Doctoral dissertation, University of Texas at Dallas, Callier Center for Communicative Disorders, 1986.
27. Chwialkowski M, Kondraske GV. Function oriented identification of anatomic abnormalities. In: Proceedings of the eighth annual Engineering in Medicine and Biology Society conference. Fort Worth, TX: 1986; 781–4.
28. Sekular R, Nash D, Armstrong R. Sensitive, objective procedure for evaluating response to light touch. Neurology 1973; 23:1282–91.
29. Kondraske GV et al. Myoelectric spectral analysis and strategies for quantifying trunk musculature fatigue. Arch Phys Med Rehabil 1987; 68(2):103–10.
30. Richmond JR, Kondraske GV. Establishing and using normal values in a clinical data-

base. In: Proceedings of the eighth annual Engineering in Medicine and Biology Society conference. Fort Worth, TX: 1986; 866–8.

31.   Pape ES, Richmond JR, Kondraske GV. Age and gender effects on measures of sensorimotor function. In: Proceedings of the eighth annual Engineering in Medicine and Biology Society conference. Fort Worth, TX: 1986; 1883–5.

GLOSSARY OF TERMS

The following terms and definitions are suggested to help clarify issues in quantification.

Structure   Anatomic building block of a system.

Function   A system's purpose (e.g., motion, flexion, integration, cognition, perception, transduction). Function cannot be measured; it either exists or it does not.

Performance   *How well* a system accomplishes its intended function. Usually multidimensional (e.g., speed accuracy, strength), performance can be both measured and assessed.

Functional unit   The simplest system capable of achieving a specific function. A system or subsystem that has only one basic function within the context of the task being analyzed (e.g., elbow flexor, tongue dorsum elevator, etc.).

Dimension of performance   A category of performance measurement representing a unique, desirable quality of performance such as speed, accuracy, endurance, steadiness, etc. It can be thought of as representing a principle axis in a multidimensional performance space defined for a specific functional unit.

Performance resource: The generic term associated with a functional unit's dimension of performance to characterize quantitative information in a conceptually useful manner; i.e., one that facilitates the use of resource economic principles. Thus, elbow flexion speed is a performance resource and either the available or required amount can be quantified.

Task   Goal directed (criteria oriented) activity requiring allocation of specific amounts of performance resources via specific functional units. Precise definition is required for meaningful use in performance quantification contexts (e.g., "draw a line" vs. "draw a straight line" vs. "draw a straight line 6 cm long in 2 seconds").

Basic element of performance (BEP)   One of the set of items uniquely identified by specifying a single human functional unit (e.g., elbow flexor) *and* a single dimension of performance (e.g., speed). The collective set of BEPs represents a common ground between a human system and tasks. BEPs are the natural choice for a standardized set of quantification targets because they result from a generalized definition approach based on fundamental knowledge of the human system's structure and function independent of a specific disease, injury, etc., and they can reflect quantitatively any performance profile traditionally characterized with disease, disorder, or injury-specific impairment and/or disability scales.

Chapter 5

Statistical and Methodologic Considerations in Scale Construction

Nicholas G. LaRocca

The neurology literature is replete with methods of measuring a dazzling spectrum of human attributes. From natural killer cell activity to the quality of life, neurologic science is full of optimism concerning the measurability of every sort of phenomenon. This chapter presents a brief introduction to the topic of measurement, focusing mainly on the construction and testing of new scales. Scales enter the world naked and unprepared for the difficult tasks that lie ahead. Investigators often seem determined to push the fledglings out of the nest before they have really tried their wings. It is hoped that this chapter will encourage investigators to allow a longer childhood for newborn scales so that they can undergo adequate trials and hone the qualities they will need to survive and flourish. The chapter concludes with a sample protocol for scale evaluation.

Stevens[1] provided an oft-cited definition of *measurement:* "the assignment of numerals to objects or events according to rules." This definition is most applicable to directly observable phenomena such as length and volume. In measuring human attributes, however, the object is often something quite abstract, such as praxis. Most of the objects of measurement in neurology are not directly observable. Rather, the investigator constructs an abstract concept (e.g., praxis) and attempts to specify a number of observable indicators of the abstraction. Numerals are then assigned to these indicators. For instance, the indicators could be several items on a rating instrument that together form a scale that attempts to measure praxis. Polite debates often appear in the literature concerning investigators' conceptualizations of constructs. Because constructs are not directly observable, they exist in the realm of theory and are thus subject to differing interpretations. In scale construction, the starting point is the

Preparation of this manuscript was supported in part by grants from the National Institute on Disability and Rehabilitation Research (H133B80018 and G0085C3504) and the National Multiple Sclerosis Society (RG 1459-A-7).

delineation in theory of the theoretical construct to be measured. In this chapter, the term *construct* will be used to refer to this theoretical, abstract, unobservable object of measurement. Several formats are utilized for measurement in neurology.

1. *Biologic assays.* Assays such as IgG synthesis or P100 components offer an attractive format, since we tend to think of the biologic assay as a sort of immutable visitor from the platonic world of ideas—as somehow more real than our more abstract constructs. After all, one can actually see and feel spinal fluid and electricity. However, like all methods of measurement, biologic assays require theoretical delineation of a construct, followed by intensive study of reliability and validity. For example, creatinine is often used as an observable indicator of the abstract construct "renal function." However, creatinine may remain within normal limits when the glomerular filtration rate is reduced by 50%.

2. *Performance measures (noninferential).* These entail a standardized procedure for testing a human function in which scores are not dependent on the judgment of the examiner. For instance, the tests making up the Quantitative Examination of Neurologic Function[2] are noninferential performance tests. This format obviates a potential source of unreliability: variations in human judgment. However, in order to eliminate inference, complex human functions must be broken down into a very large number of extremely simple, discrete segments. The potential loss of sophistication and insensitivity to nuance may be justified by the gain in standardization. The cost of tests of this type tends to be high, since performance in many tasks must be evaluated and equipment is generally necessary.

3. *Rating scales.* Ordinal rating scales requiring human inference are probably the most common type of measuring instrument in neurology. The Kurtzke system,[3] the standard neurologic examination, the Glasgow coma scale,[4] the Toronto stroke scale, and countless other familiar instruments are rating scales based on observation and inference. Their reliability can be quite high if the scale grades are clearly defined and the raters well trained. However, success with these measures is much affected by the skill of the examiner. Although rating scales may break function down into very small segments, one advantage of these instruments is that they permit the grading of more global functions whose individual components are difficult to identify and analyze. While many such scales can be rated quickly, the need for a trained clinician raises the cost of these methods.

4. *Self-report measures.* More common in psychiatry and the social sciences, self-report measures may take the form of a structured interview or a questionnaire. In a structured interview, the self-report is often combined with extensive clinical observation and inference. The Incapacity Status Scale[5] is a self-report measure of disability in multiple sclerosis. Such instruments are subject to errors arising from response sets, inattention, cognitive problems, and other factors. Nevertheless, when carefully constructed with multiple items that act as indicators of each construct, such scales can provide the most cost-effective approach to measurement. Their reliability and validity can equal or exceed those of the more expensive approaches described above. Moreover, they can be used in situations in which other scales cannot (e.g., mail surveys).

LEVELS OF MEASUREMENT

The rules for assigning numbers to observable indicators fall into four broad categories: nominal, ordinal, interval, and ratio.[1] These are often referred to as *scales of measurement* or *levels of measurement.* Each level of measurement implies certain basic empirical operations vis-à-vis the observable aspects of the construct under study: (1) nominal—determining equality of class membership, (2) ordinal—rank ordering, (3) interval—determining equality of differences, (4) ratio—determining equality of ratios. The level of measurement is determined by the nature of the observable indicators being measured and by the procedures followed by the investigator in assigning numbers. In turn, the level of measurement achieved determines which operations (e.g., addition, multiplication) are permissible with a given scale and the appropriate interpretation of scores. Permissible operations are those that do not alter the relationships between the objects described by the scale. Each level of measurement, with its appropriate interpretation and permissible operations, will be described.

Nominal (Categorical)

In a nominal scale, the unit of measurement is a category or classification. The identifiers used to designate different categories are merely labels and have no quantitative significance. For example, race is measured on a nominal scale. People may be classified as white, black, oriental, and so on; however, no one can be described as having "more race" than another person.

The basic relationships described by a nominal scale are equality and difference. Two individuals belong to either the same class or different classes. The only permissible operation is one-to-one substitution—i.e., substitution of a new set of labels for the old. Medical diagnosis exemplifies the use of the nominal level of measurement. Neurologic patients may be classified according to such categories as stroke, epilepsy, multiple sclerosis, amyotrophic lateral sclerosis, and Parkinson's disease.

Ordinal

An ordinal scale classifies an attribute according to its rank order on a scale (e.g., from low to high). However, the steps in the scale are not presumed to be equal. For instance, in the United States, the quality of beef is rated as "commercial," "good," "choice," or "prime." "Prime" beef is of a higher quality than "choice," but we cannot say by how much.

The basic relationship described by an ordinal scale is greater or less. On an ordinal scale, either two individuals are equal in a given respect or one is ranked higher than the other. Permissible operations include transformation by any monotonic (order-preserving) function. For instance, as long as the rank ordering among objects is preserved, the actual numbers assigned do not matter. Thus, the rank ordering 1,2,3,4 is equivalent to 1,5,7,23. Conversely, it makes no sense to add ranks, since the sum has little or no quantitative meaning. The disability status scale of Kurtzke[3] is an ordinal scale. Patients rated 9 are more disabled than patients rated 8. However, the difference between 7 and 8 may not be of the same magnitude as that between 8 and 9. Most of the rating scales used in neurology are ordinal. Virtually all the measurements in the standard neurologic examination are made with ordinal scales (e.g., items rated "mild," "moderate," or "severe").

Interval

An interval scale also orders things. However, all the steps in the scale are presumed to be equal. On a centrigrade scale, for instance, the difference between 20 and 25 is the same as the difference between 90 and 95.

The basic relationships described by an interval scale are equality of intervals and difference of intervals. The magnitude of the difference between any two individuals is a meaningful quantity and may be compared with the magnitude of the difference between any other two individuals. Permissible operations include any linear transformation—i.e., one that preserves the equality of the intervals. An example of such a transformation is multiplication by and addition of a constant: $X' = aX + b$. Scale points may legitimately be added together, as when the mean is calculated. True equal-interval scales are rare in neurology. Appropriately constructed composite or summative scales, consisting of several ordinally rated items, are often treated as if they have equal intervals. This practice is justified by the theoretical model for composite scales, which is described later in this chapter.

Ratio

Like interval scales, ratio scales have equal intervals, but in addition they have a true (nonarbitrary) zero. The centigrade and Fahrenheit scales are not ratio scales, since their zeros are arbitrary. On the other hand, the Kelvin scale is a ratio scale, since it is based on absolute zero.

The basic relationship described by a ratio scale is the equality of ratios. This means, for instance, that the ratio of 9 units to 3 units at one part of the scale is the same as the ratio of 9 units to 3 units at any other part of the scale. This can only be the case if there are equal intervals and a true zero. Permissible operations include only those transformations involving multiplication by a constant—i.e., those that preserve the true zero point. An example would be $X' = aX$. In contrast to interval scales, points on a ratio scale can legitimately be multiplied or divided by one another. Thus, only when using a ratio scale is one justified in making statements such as "A is twice as large as B" or "B is 50% of A." For instance, 100 K is twice as warm as 50 K. However, 100 °C is not twice as warm as 50 °C. Simple enumeration can constitute a ratio scale, as in cell counts, length of stay, or dollars. In addition, many physical measurements, such as height, weight, length and age, are ratio scales; so are many derived functions, such as density.

Implications of Level of Measurement

Level of measurement is more than just a quaint theoretical classification. Level of measurement carries broad ramifications concerning the statistics, mathematical operations, and interpretations appropriate to a given measure. Table 5.1 lists some of the more common statistics that convention dictates to be appropriate with each level of measurement. Here, the term *convention* is used loosely, since the issue is not without controversy, especially regarding when it is permissible to utilize parametric techniques such as the *t* test or the Pearson product moment correlation coefficient. Many authorities believe that parametric methods can be used only with interval or ratio-level data, never with ordinal data. Others accept the use of parametric methods with ordinal data under certain conditions. Biostatisticians and epidemiologists seem more likely to take the restricted view. On the other hand, social scientists seem more likely to take the broader view, in part because the measures they use can rarely be described as interval measures with absolute certainty.

Since this topic bears on the choice of statistical methods, at least a brief discussion of some of the important issues is necessary. The notion that choice of statistic must be determined by level of measurement is debatable. Zar put it most succinctly:

> It is sometimes declared that only nonparametric testing may be employed when dealing with ordinal scale data . . . but this is not so. There is nothing in the theoretical basis of parametric hypothesis testing that requires interval or ratio scale data.[6]

Often the argument is advanced that since ordinal data is not additive, it makes no sense to use methods, such as the *t* test, that entail basic arithmetic operations. How-

Table 5.1 Quantitative Methods Generally Utilized with Different Levels of Measurement

Level of Measurement	Group Description	Group Comparison	Correlation/ Reliability	Inter-Rater Agreement
Nominal	Frequencies Proportions Mode	Chi-square test Fisher's exact test Normal test for proportions Odds ratio	Phi Tetrachoric R Contingency coefficient	Kappa Weighted kappa
Ordinal	Median Range	Mann-Whitney U test Wilcoxon test Kruskal-Wallis- Friedman test	Spearman rho Kendall tau	Kappa Weighted kappa
Interval	Arithmetic mean Variance	*t* test Analysis of variance	Pearson R	Intraclass R
Ratio	Geometric mean Coefficient of variation	*t* test Analysis of variance	Pearson R	Intraclass R

ever, the issue is far more complex and has been the subject of considerable research and debate. As Zar points out,[6] violations of the theoretical assumptions underlying parametric tests need to be considered as well. Numerous Monte Carlo simulation studies have examined the effects of using parametric methods with data that are ordinal or that violate theoretical assumptions such as normality and homogeneity of variances.[7,8] Most such studies have found parametric methods to be robust in the face of violation of assumptions. Compared to nonparametric methods, parametric methods generally show the most favorable balance between power (probability of detecting a true effect if one is present) and alpha (probability of incorrectly concluding that there is an effect when none is present). The debate over this issue will no doubt continue for years to come. Many scales used in neurology are ambiguous as to level of measurement. How radically they deviate from equal-interval scales may be less than crystal clear. For the present, one must either adopt the safe but restricted view or proceed on the basis of reasonable assumptions. The latter course necessitates the thorough delineation of constructs, the careful definition of observable indicators, and extensive knowledge of the data being measured. Even Stevens,[1] one of the chief proponents of the restricted view, said that "outlawing" the use of parametric methods with ordinal data "would probably serve no good purpose." He pointed out that it is a matter of degree—i.e., that parametric statistics will be in error to the extent that the successive intervals are not equal. As Kim and Mueller put it:

> [A]s long as one can assume that the distortions introduced by assigning numeric values to ordinal categories are believed to be *not* very substantial, treating ordinal variables as if they are metric variables can be justified.[9]

In conclusion, the selection of statistical methods is an important step in scale construction and should not be based on simple rules of thumb, whether restrictive or broad. Instead, it should rest on careful consideration of theory, data, assumptions, and interpretation.

RELIABILITY

Rules for assigning scores to the observable indicators of a construct are of little use if they lead to inconsistent results. Reliability is the extent to which a measure yields the same results on repeated trials.[10] Concern about the reliability of measurements dates back at least to the eighteenth century and Johann K.F. Gauss, a German physicist. When Gauss and other early scientists compared physical measurements of the heavens and other natural phenomena, they often arrived at different figures; errors were obviously being made. Gauss found that these errors were distributed in a specific way: large errors had a low frequency, whereas small errors were more common. When the frequency of errors was plotted against the magnitude of errors, a bell-shaped curve resulted that to this day is called a gaussian distribution.

Whether derived from a physical measurement or clinical rating, any score may be thought of as consisting of two parts: true variation and error. Reliability is the proportion of variation in scores due to true variation. Error variation may be divided into random error and systematic error. Random error is that which is attributable to fluctuations in scores due to irrelevant chance factors. Since it is based on chance, random error is equally likely to occur in both directions (i.e., above and below true scores) and so has an approximately Gaussian distribution. In contrast, systematic error occurs as the result of some consistently biasing factor. The resulting effect is therefore likely to be directional—i.e., a consistent overestimation or underestimation of true scores. Systematic error is an important issue in considering inter-rater agreement, response sets, practice effects, fatigue, and validity. For instance, one neurologist might consistently rate a ten-point scale one point lower than another; this is systematic error. The usual reliability coefficients (e.g., Pearson) are insensitive to systematic bias. For this reason, this chapter describes some alternatives that are useful in assessing systematic error. However, the major concern in evaluating the reliability of a measure is usually random error. Several methods of assessing reliability have been developed.

Test-Retest Reliability (Coefficient of Stability)

Test-retest reliability is the correlation between measurements taken on different occasions in the same persons with identical instruments. It measures random error introduced by any factor intervening between assessments. Although the test-retest paradigm may seem to be the most straightforward measure of reliability, it is not necessarily the most desirable. Its greatest drawback is the generally untenable assumption that the phenomenon under study does not change between assessments. For instance, in many neurologic conditions, muscle strength can fluctuate. A measure of muscle strength may appear to be unreliable when it is actually recording true fluctuations in muscle strength reliably. If either self-report measures or clinical ratings are involved, memory can inflate reliability. In performance tests, practice effects that are not uniformly distributed can confound the measurement of reliability. On the other hand, evenly distributed systematic effects may be missed by the correlational techniques ordinarily used with the test-retest paradigm.

An improved approach to the evaluation of test-retest reliability is the analysis of the components of variance in a replication study.[11] In such a study, the parameter of interest is measured two or more times in several subjects. The resulting data are subjected to an analysis of variance (ANOVA). Several useful statistics can be derived from the ANOVA, including the intraclass correlation coefficient, interpretable as the proportion of true variance in the scores. This coefficient is sensitive to both random and systematic error, making it particularly suitable for studies of inter-rater agreement.

Alternate-Form Reliability (Coefficient of Equivalence)

Alternate-form reliability is the correlation between two forms of the same measure. As in the evaluation of test-retest reliability, random error introduced by any factor intervening between evaluations is assessed. In addition, alternate-form reliability is affected by differences in content between the two forms of the measure in question. Differences due to actual changes in the phenomenon under study can be reduced by minimizing the time between assessments. This approach is most suitable for performance tests (e.g., list learning), for which alternate sets of items can readily be developed.

Internal Consistency and Composite Scales

Internal consistency is an important issue when multiple items are summed to form a composite scale. A brief description of the theoretical model underlying composite scales will be presented first, followed by a discussion of methods of assessing internal consistency. In the medical literature, it is not unusual to encounter ad hoc composite measures. These are untested summative scores created by arbitrarily adding a number of separate items together. Usually the items appear to be related to one another on the basis of "clinical experience." However, such composites are completely unjustified in the absence of empirical support regarding the intercorrelation of the items.

Whereas untested ad hoc summative scales are to be avoided, appropriately constructed composite scales do have many advantages over the use of single items.[12] First, an individual item generally represents only one of many facets of a complex construct. For instance, if one wanted to arrive at a global measure of pyramidal function, one would need to use many different tests. Second, individual items can have only a few grades and often have just two. As a result, individual items lack the precision to distinguish finer differences. An item with five grades can discriminate among five levels of a construct. A scale consisting of ten such items can discriminate among fifty levels. Third, multi-item scales are generally more reliable than individual items. Every item has some random error associated with it. When items that correlate are combined, these random errors, which are not correlated, tend to average out. For instance, if the average correlation among the items in a scale is 0.40, that scale will have an alpha reliability of 0.57 with two items but 0.87 with 10 items—a significant improvement in reliability.

Although many composite scaling models exist, the linear composite, summative, or Likert model[13] is the one most frequently encountered. It is known as a probability monotone model because it assumes that the probability of obtaining a higher score on any given item is a monotonic function of the underlying construct being measured. A monotonic function is one that is either always increasing or always decreasing. Individual items may be ordinal, and each would tend to have a slightly different monotonic curve or trace line when plotted against the construct. However, a second assumption of the model is that when the items are summed, the trace line plotting total scores against the construct being measured will approximate a straight line.[14] This is one reason why composite scores are treated as equal-interval scales—i.e., a linear trace line can occur only if the scale intervals are equal. A final assumption of the Likert model is that the sum of the items measures one and only one construct—i.e., the scale has internal consistency. Later in this chapter we will discuss the fact that summative scales at times measure more than one dimension and need to be divided into separate subscales.

The term *linear* is applied to this model for two reasons. First, the total score is assumed to have a linear, or straight-line, relationship to the construct being measured. Second, the total score is a linear combination of the individual items, obtained by simple addition.[12]

The theory behind the linear composite model illustrates why it makes no sense to sum unrelated items. Uncorrelated items violate all three assumptions of the model: uncorrelated items are not related to the construct of interest in a monotonic fashion; the trace lines of individual items do not combine to form a straight line; and, most important, the summed score does not measure a single construct and thus lacks internal consistency. Several methods are available to evaluate the internal consistency or reliability of linear composite scales. These will be discussed next.

Internal consistency is a concept rather than a specific procedure. There are several ways to assess internal consistency. The investigator examines all the evidence and then arrives at a judgment concerning internal consistency. Viewed as a form of reliability, internal consistency is sensitive to unreliability attributable to content sampling. Thus, the two components of internal consistency are (1) selecting items that all measure the same construct and (2) measuring a construct that is itself homogeneous. Internal consistency will be low if the items mainly reflect random fluctuations (error variance) rather than actual differences (true variance) in the construct under study, or if the items are unrelated to each other.

1. *Item-total correlation.* One way to assess internal consistency was suggested by Likert[13] as part of the item analysis of a scale.[14] Each item is correlated with the sum of the remaining items. Items that have relatively low correlations with the total score may be dropped from the scale or combined with other similar items to form a different scale. Items with low item-total correlations appear to measure something other than what is measured by the summative score.

2. *Discriminatory power.* A second approach used by Likert[13] for item analysis involves dividing subjects into those with high and low overall scores. The average scores on each item in the high and low groups are then compared to determine which items discriminate best between the two groups. Items that do not discriminate are suspect.

3. *Split-half reliability.* This method of estimating reliability is similar to alternate-form reliability. It is the correlation between two halves of the same test (usually the test's odd- and even-numbered items). It assesses unreliability attributable to differences in content between the two halves. It is somewhat preferable to the two-session, alternate-form paradigm, since it eliminates error due to the passage of time. Because two half-length versions of the test are employed, the Spearman-Brown prophecy formula[15] is used to estimate the reliability of the full-length test. A short-coming of the split-half method is that there are many ways to divide a set of items into two groups, and each such split may produce a different reliability coefficient.[12]

4. *Inter-item consistency (coefficient of internal consistency).* The inherent indeterminacy of the split-half method is avoided with coefficient alpha. Also known

as Cronbach's alpha, it was first introduced by Guttman[16] as an extension of the Kuder and Richardson[17] formula 20 and later described by Cronbach.[18] Alpha is the most widely used method of assessing internal consistency. It may be interpreted as the average correlation between two halves of a test when the test is split into all possible combinations of two half-tests. As the average correlation between the items increases and the length of the scale increases, alpha also increases.

A high alpha indicates that there is at least one homogeneous dimension underlying the summed score and that at least some of the items correlate substantially with one another. The methods for item analysis described above can be used to eliminate weak items and thereby increase alpha. Other methods, to be described below, can be used to determine whether more than one dimension exists in the scale and whether the construction of subscales is justified. Perfect reliability would result in an alpha of 1.00. In real life, alpha is always lower. An acceptable size for alpha will depend on the context of a given use of the scale. Nunnally[12] has suggested some guidelines. In research settings, where the main implication of unreliability is the attenuation of correlation coefficients and the accuracy of group means is of primary importance, a minimum acceptable alpha might be 0.70. However, in applied settings—especially when clinical decisions must be made—measurement error on the individual level is the main consideration. In such settings, an alpha of 0.90 or higher ought to be the goal. With an alpha between 0.80 and 0.90, group statistics are little affected by unreliability, but the accuracy of individual scores is only fair. Of course, these are very rough guidelines; each situation must be judged separately.

5. *Reliability of factor scores (theta and omega).* Alpha is an appropriate statistic for assessing the internal consistency of linear composite scales in which the items are unweighted. Alpha assumes that the items are parallel—i.e., that each item measures the construct equally.[10] However, composite scales that do not meet the unidimensional assumption may also be constructed with use of factor-analytic techniques. Item weights can be calculated that reflect the fact that certain items are more highly correlated with the composite score than others. The internal consistency of factor-based scales can be assessed using theta (principal-components model) or omega (common factor-analytic model). When applied to the same scale, theta and omega will be higher than alpha,[10] rendering a more accurate estimate of reliability. However, the difference is generally so small that little is gained from using factor-based weighting of items instead of simply adding items together.

DIMENSIONALITY

Measures of internal consistency such as alpha will indicate whether or not there is at least one fairly homogeneous dimension (such as disability) underlying an unweighted additive scale. However, they are relatively insensitive to the presence of more than one dimension (e.g., mobility and self-care). It is often the goal of the investigator to construct a scale that measures several subdomains of a particular construct. At other times, however, it is discovered—after the scale has been developed—that what was thought to be a homogeneous construct actually harbors two or more dimensions. At yet other times, the investigator may be unsure whether a construct is unidimensional or multifaceted; the goal may then be to reduce a large set of loosely related indicators into their most parsimonious multidimensional representation.

Factor Analysis

Factor analysis encompasses a variety of multivariate techniques used to identify clusters of variables. In general, the clustering of variables is based on the pattern of their correlation with one another. Factor-analytic techniques make it possible to represent a set of interrelated variables in terms of a smaller number of factors.[9] Factor analysis assumes that such factors are weighted linear combinations of the variables.

Generally, factor-analytic research is either exploratory or confirmatory. Exploratory factor analysis is used to reduce data and to determine the minimum number of dimensions needed to explain the interrelationships in a set of data. In contrast, confirmatory factor analysis is used to test specific hypotheses concerning the number and types of dimensions in a set of variables and the interrelationships between the variables and the factors.[12] In scale construction, exploratory factor analysis can reveal whether there is more than one dimension within a scale. Confirmatory factor analysis can assist the investigator in the construction of subscales and the selection and deletion of items.

A discussion of the various theoretical models, computational algorithms, and options used in performing factor analysis is beyond the scope of this chapter. Readable presentations can be found in Kim and Mueller[9,19] and Nunnally.[12] The basic steps involved are as follows:

1. A group of subjects is evaluated with use of a number of items having an interval or ratio level of measurement.
2. All or some of these items are selected for analysis. Items may be selected because they are thought to be related to one another on theoretical grounds or because they intercorrelate. Any items in the set that do not correlate with any other item should probably be dropped.
3. Factors are "extracted" using one of many methods, such as principal components, principal axis, alpha, or image analysis.
4. The resulting factors may then be "rotated" to improve the interpretability of the solution. Rotation methods may be orthogonal (preserving the independence of the factors) or oblique (allowing for some correlation between the factors).
5. If the factors are to be used as subscales, then the internal consistency of each subscale is evaluated. This may be done with use of alpha, theta, or omega. Alpha is used if the items making up the factor will be added together without weighting. Theta and omega are used if factor weights will be used. Although theta and omega generally yield higher reliabilities than alpha, the difference is often too small to justify the inconvenience of working with weighted items in a clinical setting.

In conclusion, factor analysis provides a powerful tool revealing important information concerning the constructs under study and the relationships among the observable indicators of those constructs.

Multidimensional Scaling

Multidimensional scaling is a multivariate technique related to factor analysis. In general, multidimensional scaling is used to discover the natural dimensions underlying similarities and differences among objects.[12] Similarities and differences can be generated by human judges, or correlation coefficients can be used. These similarities and differences are represented numerically and translated into distances in euclidean space (i.e., our everyday notion of space).[20] By examining the configuration of points and the characteristics of more- and less-distant objects, the investigator can ascertain which parameters best explain the observed similarities and differences.

Item Response Theory

Item response theory is a multivariate scaling model that represents one application of latent trait theory to scale development.[21] As Osterlind pointed out,

> Simply put, latent traits are examinee characteristics that cause a consistent performance on a test of any given cognitive skill or achievement or ability. A trait is not a hypothetical construct; rather, it may be thought of as an intervening variable between what is there and what can be measured. It causes a test performance.[22]

Scales developed within this model may be thought of as estimating the value of the latent trait by using information derived from the several items comprising the scale. A practical advantage of item response theory is that it allows subjects to be scored on the same scale even if their scores are based on different sets of items. In addition, item response models make better use of the information inherent in individual items than do other scaling models. Several different item response models and computational algorithms exist.[23,24] Effective use of item response theory requires specialized statistical expertise, ample computer resources, and large samples (in some cases, thousands of subjects). However, given the many theoretical and practical advantages of item response theory, its use is likely to increase dramatically in coming years.

IDENTIFICATION OF SUBGROUPS

In the previous section, the focus was on the identification of dimensions among items. However, there are instances in scale construction when the investigator needs to identify subgroups of persons. Some of the techniques for identifying subgroups are briefly described in this section.

Cluster Analysis

Cluster analysis is a set of several multivariate techniques used to identify subgroups of persons on the basis of the interrelationships among a set of several variables. Like factor analysis, cluster analysis can be used to discover subgroups or to confirm the existence of predicted subgroups. Many algorithms and options are available, and cluster-analytic solutions are thus somewhat arbitrary and indeterminate. Many investigators use cluster analysis with inappropriately small samples (e.g., 50 subjects) and fail to cross-validate the subgroupings with a new sample.

Cluster analysis may be used in the following way. An investigator devises a battery of tests to evaluate traumatic brain injury and wants to determine if there are distinct subgroups of patients. Analysis reveals three clusters: (1) patients with extensive language and memory deficits but few other problems, (2) patients with extensive motor deficits but without cognitive problems, and (3) patients with seizures and affective disturbances.

Discriminant Analysis

Also a multivariate technique, discriminant analysis is useful in identifying the variables that best discriminate between two or more previously identified groups. For example, a psychologist might wish to identify the items on a test battery that best discriminate between patients with Alzheimer's disease and those with multi-infarct dementia. Once a differential diagnosis has been established, samples of each of the two types of patients can be tested with the battery. Analysis will reveal the extent to which each item in the battery discriminates between the criterion groups, controlling for all the other items. In addition, a "discriminant function" will be calculated, yielding the weighted combination of variables that best differentiates the groups. Percent correctly classified by the function can also be calculated. If it is sufficiently accurate, this discriminant function can be cross-validated with a new sample and then used in the future to classify new patients.

INTER-RATER AGREEMENT

In medicine, observer rating scales are widely used. Thus, the issue of inter-rater agreement is important. In evaluating inter-rater agreement, several methodologic pitfalls must be avoided. The topic of reproducibility across raters is often subsumed under that of reliability. However, while random error is the main focus of reliability studies, systematic error (bias) assumes much more importance in the study of raters. Disagreement between two observers rating the same phenomenon may arise because of chance errors or systematic observer bias. For instance, one of two neurologists examining flexor spasms may consistently rate spasticity higher than the other; this is a systematic bias. Correlation coefficients, the statistics generally used in reliability studies, are sensitive to random error but insensitive to systematic bias. For instance, if there were no random error in the ratings described above, but one of the two neurologists rated every patient 2 points higher than did the other, the correlation coefficient would be 1.00, indicating perfect correlation; however, the inter-rater agreement would be poor. Another pitfall is failure to take into account the level of agreement likely to occur on the basis of chance. For instance, it is common to see reports of the "percent of agreement" between raters. However, a certain proportion of agreement is to be expected on the basis of chance. If a large proportion of patients fall into one category on a rating scale, the amount of agreement to be expected on the basis of chance will increase. Thus, in studying observer reliability, standard correlational methods should generally be avoided in favor of methods specifically designed for studies of inter-rater agreement.

There are specialized methods of assessing inter-rater agreement that avoid the pitfalls described. In rating scales with a nominal or ordinal level of measurement, Cohen's kappa[25] or weighted kappa[26] can be used. Both yield the proportion of agreement corrected for chance, but weighted kappa also takes into account the "seriousness" of disagreement.[27] When an interval or ratio level of measurement is used, the intraclass correlation coefficient provides a measure of agreement sensitive to both random and systematic error.[28] Fleiss and Cohen[27] have shown that the interpretations of kappa and the intraclass correlation coefficient are equivalent. These two statistics therefore permit the comparison of extent of agreement across different levels of measurement.

A brief word should be said about the design of studies of inter-rater agreement. Raters should be well trained and experienced with the testing instrument they use. Administration procedures should be standardized. Conditions should approximate those that will prevail when the scale is put into general use. Sources of variation unrelated to observers should be minimized; thus, multiple observers should examine or rate the patient in close temporal proximity, simultaneously if possible. The same room, lighting, and instruments should be used by all observers. Ratings to be compared should be arrived at independently, with no discussion or consultation between observers. In addition, observers should not discuss their ratings with each other until the study has been completed. The patient sample should be representative of the target population and of sufficient size and distribution to allow the analysis of agreement in the observers' ratings of various subgroups.

VALIDITY

Validity is generally defined as the extent to which an instrument measures what it is designed to measure.[10] However, viewed more broadly, validity is the degree to which an instrument does what it is intended to do—i.e., how scientifically useful it is.[12] Thus, validity concerns not only the relationship between an instrument and the construct it purports to measure, but also whether the relationships between the instrument and other variables are consistent with the theory and intended purpose of the instrument. For instance, a screening scale for brainstem function should (1) relate well to some established measure of brainstem function and (2) relate to measures of other neurologic systems in a way that makes anatomical and functional sense. There are several strategies for evaluating the various facets of validity that cumulatively help the investigator to arrive at a sound conclusion concerning a given measure.

   1. *Face validity:* the extent to which an instrument gives the user the subjective impression that it measures what it purports to measure. All too often, this is the only

form of validity many new scales can claim to achieve. The term *face validity* is perhaps a misnomer, since face validity is theoretically unnecessary in an instrument. For instance, if measuring fingernail thickness provided a valid measure of nerve conduction in a given digit, it would matter little that such a test lacks face validity. From a strategic point of view, however, face validity is important. Users generally remain skeptical of instruments that, although empirically valid, subjectively appear to bear little relevance to the target construct.

2. *Ecologic validity:* this concept has generated considerable interest in recent years. If a measure satisfies all the conventional requirements for validity and reliability but is inappropriate or impractical in actual use, it is said to lack ecologic validity—i.e., there is a poor fit between the measure and its context. Whether or not they have any predictive validity, written examinations for police officers may be doomed as a result of litigation instituted by groups who feel that such tests discriminate against them. Those examinations may be said to lack ecologic validity.

3. *Content validity:* the extent to which a scale includes a representative sample of items from the domain to be measured. The major issue is whether or not one is justified in generalizing from a sample of scale items to the universe of items germane to a given construct.[12] All major aspects of the domain should be included and, if possible, in the correct proportions. For instance, a global scale of depression should include items measuring not only dysphoric mood but also such variables as low self-esteem, hopelessness, lassitude, and vegetative symptoms. Content validity should be thought of as one of the earliest steps in sound scale construction rather than something to be evaluated after the fact. Content validity can be maximized by fully delineating the construct to be measured, consulting with colleagues, reviewing previous research, interviewing patients, and performing pilot studies. Since there is no simple empirical technique for testing content validity, the investigator must judge its adequacy.

4. *Criterion-related validity:* the assessment of this type of validity involves the comparison of the results on one measure with the results in the same individuals on another, independent measure. The independent measure is the criterion, since the scale under investigation is thought to predict the results on the criterion. An obvious assumption of this paradigm is that the validity of the criterion has already been established beyond question. For instance, the Blessed test[29] was validated in part by its comparison with postmortem verification of Alzheimer's disease. The term *prediction* is used here in the statistical sense, since the measure under study may follow (postdictive validity), precede (predictive validity), or be contemporaneous with (concurrent validity) the criterion.[12] Independence of measure and criterion are crucial. For instance, it makes little sense to compare two measures rated by the same individual, since rater bias may account for much of the association between them. Simple correlational techniques are generally used to evaluate criterion-related validity. However, evaluation of an instrument's ability to discriminate criterion groups is another strategy (e.g., by comparing scores on a test of praxis in brain-damaged patients and in normal healthy adults). Increasingly, multivariate techniques, such as multiple regression analysis and discriminant analysis, are being employed in validity studies.

Screening scales are frequently used in medicine, and special techniques are available to evaluate their validity. Screening is designed to be an economic method of identifying, in a large group of patients, a smaller subgroup likely to have a given condition. A specific cutoff score on the screening scale is established, and a definitive criterion for the condition is selected. Patients with scores above the cutoff are called positives, and those whose scores do not exceed the cutoff are called negatives. True positives are patients who are screened as having the condition and actually do have it; false positives are screened as having the condition but do not. True negatives are patients who are screened as not having the condition and indeed do not have it; false negatives are screened as not having the condition but do have it. Sensitivity is the ability to identify correctly those who have the condition. Specificity is the ability to identify correctly those who do not have the condition.[30] Setting the cutoff score to maximize sensitivity will lower specificity, and vice versa. The investigator must establish a cutoff point that will result in the most favorable balance between sensitivity and specificity, depending on the condition in question and the context of the screening. One method of evaluating the usefulness of screening scales involves the application of Bayes theorem. With this method it is possible to estimate the probability of obtaining a false positive and false negative result, given the sensitivity and specificity of the test and the base rate of the target condition in the population.

Correlation with a criterion does not necessarily have to be very high for a measure to be useful. For example, the use of a screening test with a correlation of 0.30 or higher with actual performance can substantially improve the average performance of the group as compared with what it was without screening.[12] Thus, in some situations criterion validity must be viewed in light of the improvement in prediction over existing methods.

5. *Construct validity:* the extent to which a scale adequately measures a theoretical construct. Most parameters of interest (e.g., brainstem function) are not directly observable. Instead, the scientist constructs an abstract concept of brainstem function and attempts to specify a number of observable indicators thought to be related to the abstraction. If they are adequately measuring the construct, the observables should produce results that are consistent with accepted theoretical propositions concerning the construct.[12] The construct and its relationship to other parameters must be carefully delineated, and the hypothesized relationships tested.[10]

Construct validation involves a long series of inter-related steps. The process may include the assessment of content validity, criterion-related validity, and internal consistency, and involve factor analysis. Both convergent and discriminant validity should be achieved[31]; that is, predicted relationships should be consistent across raters, formats, and items. A measure should be related to other similar measures of the same construct. In addition, the measure should be independent of parameters that in theory are independent of the construct. Discriminant validation is of particular importance in the development of new scales that purport to measure a new construct or improve on an old one. Construct validation involves the gradual accumulation and interpretation of multiple pieces of theoretical and empirical information.

APPLICABILITY ACROSS POPULATIONS

Scales are often implemented in settings quite dissimilar to those in which they were developed. An instrument developed and tested in a large urban teaching hospital may later be used in an outpatient clinic for the rural poor. A scale constructed in the United States may be translated into Danish. Measures validated in patients with late chronic progressive multiple sclerosis may be used to evaluate patients with early relapsing-remitting disease.

In translating a rating scale into a new language, care must be taken to preserve the originally intended meaning. Even if linguistic equivalence is achieved, cultural differences affecting both raters and patients can dramatically alter results. There is no guarantee that findings on validity and reliability will remain the same across target populations. In particular, the predictive validity and factor structure of a scale are likely to vary when the scale is applied in more than one population. Thus, the applicability of an instrument must be established through field testing whenever the investigator contemplates its implementation in a population that differs substantially from that originally studied.

CONCLUSION: A SAMPLE PROTOCOL FOR SCALE EVALUATION

This chapter has briefly reviewed some of the major methodologic issues that must be considered in the construction and testing of a new scale. The sample protocol that follows, drawn from a variety of sources,[6,9-14,19,32] provides a plan for the development and evaluation of a scale, from initial conceptualization through testing and revision. It will serve both as a summary of this chapter and as a suggested design for projects having the primary goal of scale construction.

1. Develop a theoretical construct that defines in abstract terms what the scale will measure.
2. Review the literature and existing scales.
3. Define the various subdomains that make up the construct.
4. Operationalize the construct in terms of several observables (i.e., items to which numbers can readily be assigned). Design a format and an algorithm for assigning numbers to items using one of the four levels of measurement.
5. Develop predictions concerning the relationship of the construct and its observable indicators vis-à-vis other parameters.
6. Determine the users and uses of the scale.
7. Decide what the target population of patients will be.
8. Establish a concise format and standardized administration procedures for the scale.
9. Pilot the scale in a small sample of patients to smooth out the roughest of the rough edges.
10. Field-test the scale in a sample of adequate size (depending on the nature of the scale).
11. Evaluate the scale's reliability by using one of the many techniques available, preferably coefficient alpha.
12. Assess the dimensionality of the scale. Does the scale have internal consistency? Are all the items correlated with the overall score? Does the scale measure more than one dimension?

13. Test the reproducibility of the scale across raters by using an appropriate measure of agreement, such as coefficient kappa, weighted kappa, or the intraclass correlation coefficient.
14. Evaluate the convergent and discriminant validity of the measure. Are relationships between this measure and others consistent with theory? Is this measure uncorrelated with parameters that theoretically should be independent?
15. Revise the scale based on the results of field testing, and repeat steps 11 through 14.
16. Conduct a standardization study in which norms appropriate to age and sex (and possibly other strata) are established in a sample representative of the target population.

REFERENCES

1. Stevens SS. On the theory of scales of measurement. Science 1946; 103:677–80.
2. Potvin A, Tourtellotte W. Quantitative examination of neurologic functions. Vol. I: Scientific basis and design of instrumented tests. Boca Raton, FL: CRC Press, 1985.
3. Kurtzke J. Rating neurological impairment in multiple sclerosis: an expanded disability status scale (EDSS). Neurology 1983; 33:1444–52.
4. Teasdale G, Jennett B. Assessment of coma and impaired consciousness. Lancet 1974; 2: 81–4.
5. Haber A, LaRocca N, eds. Minimal record of disability for multiple sclerosis. New York: The National Multiple Sclerosis Society, 1985.
6. Zar J. Biostatistical analysis. Englewood Cliffs, NJ: Prentice-Hall, 1985.
7. Boneau C. The effects of violations of assumptions underlying the *t*-test. Psychol Bull 1960; 57:49–64.
8. Woodward J, Overall J. The significance of treatment effects in ordered category data. Psychiatr Res 1977; 13:169–77.
9. Kim J, Mueller C. Introduction to factor analysis: what it is and how to do it. Beverly Hills, CA: Sage Publications, 1978.
10. Carmines E, Zeller R. Reliability and validity assessment. Beverly Hills, CA: Sage Publications, 1979.
11. Fleiss J. The design and analysis of clinical experiments. New York: John Wiley, 1986.
12. Nunnally JC. Psychometric theory. New York: McGraw-Hill, 1978.
13. Likert R. A method of constructing an attitude scale. In: Maranell G, ed. Scaling: a sourcebook for behavioral scientists. Chicago: Aldine, 1974.
14. McIver J, Carmines E. Unidimensional scaling. Beverly Hills, CA: Sage Publications, 1981.
15. Spearman C. Correlation calculated from faulty data. Br J Psychol 1910; 3:271–95.
16. Guttman L. A basis for analyzing test-retest reliability. Psychometrika 1945; 10:255–82.
17. Kuder G, Richardson M. The theory of estimation of test reliability. Psychometrika 1937; 2:151–60.
18. Cronbach L. Coefficient alpha and the internal structure of tests. Psychometrika 1951; 16:297–334.
19. Kim J, Mueller C. Factor analysis: Statistical methods and practical issues. Beverly Hills, CA: Sage Publications, 1978.
20. Kruskal J, Wish M. Multidimensional scaling. Beverly Hills, CA: Sage Publications, 1978.
21. Warm TA. A primer of item response theory. Technical report 941078. Oklahoma City: U.S. Coast Guard Institute, Department of Transportation (NTIS AD A063072), 1978.
22. Osterlind S. Test item bias. Beverly Hills, CA: Sage Publications, 1983.

23. Birnbaum A. Some latent trait models and their use in inferring an examinee's ability. In: Lord FM, Novik MR, eds. Statistical theories of mental test scores. Reading, MA: Addison-Wesley, 1968.
24. Thissen D, Steinberg L. A taxonomy of item response models. Psychometrika 1986; 51: 567–77.
25. Cohen J. A coefficient of agreement for nominal scales. Ed Psychol Meas 1960; 20:37–46.
26. Spitzer R, Cohen J, Fleiss J, et al. Quantification of agreement in psychiatric diagnosis. Arch Gen Psychiatry 1967; 17:83–87.
27. Fleiss J, Cohen J. The equivalence of weighted kappa and the intraclass correlation coefficient as measures of reliability. Ed. Psychol Meas 1973; 33:613–619.
28. Shrout P, Fleiss J. Intraclass correlations: uses in assessing rater reliability. Psychol Bull 1979; 86:420–8.
29. Blessed G, Tomlinson B, Roth M. The association between quantitative measures of dementia and of senile changes in the cerebral grey matter of elderly subjects. Br J Psychiatry 1968; 114:797–811.
30. Morton R, Hebel J. A study guide to epidemiology and biostatistics. Baltimore: University Park Press, 1979.
31. Campbell D, Fiske D. Convergent and discriminant validation by the multitrait-multimethod matrix. Psychol Bull 1959; 56:81–105.
32. Struening EL, Guttentag M, eds. Handbook of evaluation research. Beverly Hills, CA: Sage Publications, 1975.

Chapter 6

Statistical Considerations for Quantitative Techniques in Clinical Neurology

J. Philip Miller

One of the primary reasons for quantification in clinical neurology is its utility in the evaluation of the efficacy of interventions. Of particular interest is its use in randomized controlled trials of pharmacologic agents, which is the primary focus of this chapter. Many of the issues considered here relate as well to quantitative measures that differentiate normal from diseased subjects, but such studies require a great deal of attention to issues of sampling from relevant normal and diseased populations. Although clinical trials need to utilize patients characteristic of a given diseased population so that results may be generalized, the costs of formal sampling schemes are rarely justifiable.

Normally, investigators must study the natural history of a disease with quantified measures before initiating a trial, in order to understand the measurement properties and ensure that the proposed trial will have sufficient power to provide a definitive evaluation of the intervention. Natural history studies are also useful in generating more precise statements about an individual patient's prognosis and uncovering clues about a disease's etiology.

In some cases, what is discussed in this chapter is more an ideal to strive for than a description of how research is actually done. The ideal may inspire us to strive for better approaches. It is important for the clinical researcher to recognize that applied biostatistics is itself a clinical activity. Although it rests on precise mathematical foundations, it is the application of these principles to concrete situations that is required in a research program. These applications are implemented with use of a statistical model as an abstraction for a physical reality. Of course, the model is not the reality and will be deficient in one or more facets. It is the role of the biostatistician, in collaboration with clinical investigators, to judge the adequacy of the chosen statistical

Supported in part by a grant from the Muscular Dystrophy Association and grants (AG05681 and AG03911) from the National Institute on Aging, National Institutes of Health.

model to reflect the reality as it is currently understood and to communicate the results to the scientific community with clarity. Frequently, the choice among models is not clear-cut, and it is the practice of many investigators to apply several statistical models that approximate the phenomenon at hand. If they all lead to the same conclusion, then that conclusion appears to be fairly robust with respect to the underlying assumptions, and the analysis that is the most powerful or most illuminating is reported. If the conclusions differ according to the assumptions made, the choice of assumptions and the reasons for the discrepancies must be carefully reviewed.

TYPES OF SCALES

A primary concern in our choice of statistical models relates to the measurement properties of a scale. A taxonomy of scales (originally proposed by Stevens some 35 years ago[1]) has developed in the literature of the social sciences. It includes the nominal, ordinal, interval, and ratio scales. LaRocca describes these scales in Chapter 5; my discussion will be restricted to statistical considerations in their use.

In biomedical studies, diagnoses and symptoms are the most common examples of variables that are nominal in nature; other examples are the defined pathognomic endpoints or milestones of a disease. Considering the time and thought expended to construct a decent research definition of a diagnosis, it is clear that more complex scales require even more effort—yet such effort is not often made. Careful attention to the precise definition of what and how we are measuring is, however, basic to all quantification. In most large-scale clinical trials, such definition is codified as a manual of operations—an exercise that can benefit any study.

Frequently, a ranking procedure is applicable to the categories of a scale—e.g., muscle strength may be graded on a scale of weak to strong. The traditional clinical gradings of +, ++, and +++ represent this ordinal type of scale. Descriptive statistics based on percentiles (e.g., medians) are appropriate for ordinal scales, but common statistics (e.g., means or standard deviations) are not. Many statistical methods have been developed for testing of hypothetical group differences with ordinal scales. Such methods are often used with variables that are derived from numeric measurements but do not lend themselves to an interval or ratio scale.

Most important from the standpoint of quantitative techniques is the interval scale, on which the difference between 1 and 2 is assumed to be the same as the difference between 9 and 10. Only when we can make this assumption can we perform standard statistical operations, such as computing a mean value or doing a regression.

It is helpful to distinguish between the scale used for making the measurements and the underlying biologically relevant dimension that is the focus of interest. For neuromuscular disease, muscle strength is measured, but it is then used as an index of the degree of muscular dystrophy, which cannot easily be measured directly. Quantification of the force a muscle can exert in kilograms clearly calls for an interval scale. When the measurement is used as an index of the degree of muscular dystrophy, however, it may not be clear that a change from 1.0 to 1.5 kg is the same as a change from 20.0 to 20.5 kg.

Investigators frequently utilize scales that represent the number of positive symptoms observed in a particular patient. In such cases, there is no question that an interval scale is needed. If the scale is to be used as an index of severity, the symptoms must be equivalent—i.e., having symptoms A, B, and C is the same as having symptoms B, D, and F. It would then meet the assumptions of an ordinal scale. Adding the assumption that going from no symptoms to two symptoms is the equivalent of going from four to six symptoms would make it an interval scale.

The relationship between the physical measurement and the underlying dimension is rarely well understood. Even if one is quite comfortable making assumptions about the scale of actual measurements, one cannot assume that a linear change in one scale is reflected by a linear change in the other unless one also assumes that the scale of measurement has a linear relationship to the underlying biologic dimension. Information about such relationships can frequently be inferred from natural history studies.

Ratio scales meet our assumptions for interval scales and also have a definite zero point. With ratio scales, it is possible to talk about one value being twice as great as another. Most physical measurements (e.g., length, weight, duration) are made with ratio scales. Except for some sophisticated biologic modeling, however, few statistical methods commonly utilized in clinical trials require assumptions about ratio scales. This is partly because most popular statistical techniques are based on linear models. When multiplicative models hold, logarithms of the scale scores are taken, transforming the multiplicative model into an additive one.

LESSONS FROM NATURAL HISTORY STUDIES

One approach to developing a scale for use in studies evaluating intervention strategies is to require that the scale scores change in a linear fashion over time. Figure 6.1 shows an example of scores in a cohort of boys with Duchenne muscular dystrophy (DMD). The natural history of the disease has been described in an earlier report,[2] and the data presented here are augmented by data from negative therapeutic trials.[3-6] Plotted on the graph are the empirical percentile points for average muscle strength at each age. The average muscle strength score was derived by rating 34 different muscles on a modified Medical Research Council (MRC) scale and converting each rating to a numerical value between 10 (for a muscle of normal strength for a boy of the patient's age) and 0 (for a muscle incapable of voluntary movement). The numerical scores for the 34 muscles were then averaged. The data represent 3,394 examinations of 189 boys, each of whom was followed for up to eight years. At each age, the empirical percentiles were computed, and a spline function was fitted to provide the smoothed curves shown.[7] Between the ages of 5 and 13 years, the patients' median score (50th percentile) remained quite linear, with a change of about −0.4 units per year. We have found this type of presentation useful because of its combination of longitudinal and cross-sectional data, though one must avoid uncritically ascribing group behavior to individuals.

Figure 6.2 is an example of what we usually term a *spaghetti plot*. Each individual point is shown, and the points for an individual patient are connected. These spaghetti

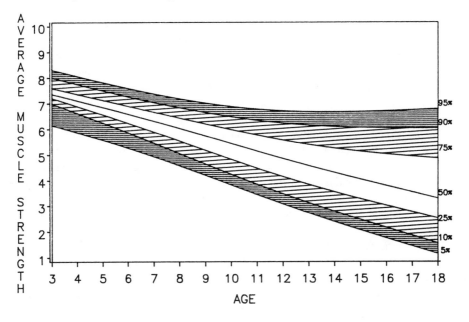

FIGURE 6.1 *Empirical 5th, 10th, 25th, 50th, 75th, 90th and 95th percentiles computed for each age, and individual values joined by a smoothed spline fit. Average muscle strength is a mean of the strengths of 34 muscles, each graded on a scale of normal strength (10 points) to unable to move (0 points). See text for more details.*

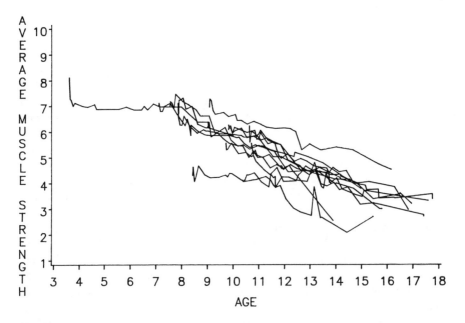

FIGURE 6.2 *Average muscle strength as in Figure 6.1, representing a subset of 13 patients from a single clinic. The average muscle strength scores of each patient are shown, connected by solid lines.*

plots and the regression lines fitted to each patient's longitudinal data support a linear relationship with age for each patient. Plotting the change in average muscle strength (or the slopes of the individual regression lines) with age and other measures of disease status (e.g., functional grade) has indicated that average muscle strength is a good index of the severity of the disease. That it is linear in time implies that we can use the same measure in boys of differing ages and expect that the change will average the same for all boys over a fixed period (e.g., a 12-month trial). If changes are nonlinear, then we can expect differing amounts of change in boys of differing ages over the duration of a study. The increased variance in the expected amount of change will adversely affect the power of the study.

The formal natural history study, in which data are gathered in a prospective protocol in a manner similar to that employed in an actual trial, is the most desirable method of determining rates of change. Alternatively, quantitative techniques may be incorporated into the routine clinical care of patients, and the information obtained may be incorporated into a registry.[8]

MEASUREMENT REPRODUCIBILITY

A manual of operations for a study helps to assure that measurements are made in the same manner in different patients and at different times in the same patient. Such a manual is an absolute necessity for a multicenter trial.[9] Training sessions for the evaluators, and even formal certification procedures, aid in producing highly reproducible measurements. Attention to such details as the time of day of the examination, its surroundings, and prior activity of the patient help to reduce measurement variability. Such considerations serve to reduce measurement error and make measurements more easily replicated. Interestingly, many investigators have discovered that nonphysicians are more likely than physicians to adhere strictly to a specified protocol.

As they commit to the quantification of measurements, investigators must also commit to the quantification of the reproducibility of their measurement protocol. Only by developing a protocol that ensures the availability of measurements appropriate for reproducibility studies can actual quantification of the measurements' reproducibility be achieved. The protocol can be a special reliability study or the byproduct of a protocol that involves multiple evaluations of patients within a period short enough that the disease status can be assumed to be unchanged.

In our studies of boys with DMD, portions of the protocol require examination of the boys twice within a two-week period, during which it is reasonable to assume that the disease status has not changed. The resulting data permit the examination of measurement reproducibility across the entire history of the study. Figure 6.3 shows a histogram of the differences in total muscle strength between all such visits. We have previously reported that the reproducibility improved during the first few months of the protocol's implementation.[10] Subsequent investigation has revealed improvement as patients gained experience with the protocol. Thus, the first two examinations of a new patient are less reproducible than later examinations.

Although it is conventional to report reproducibility as a specific correlation, the degree of a measurement's reproducibility must be considered with respect to the

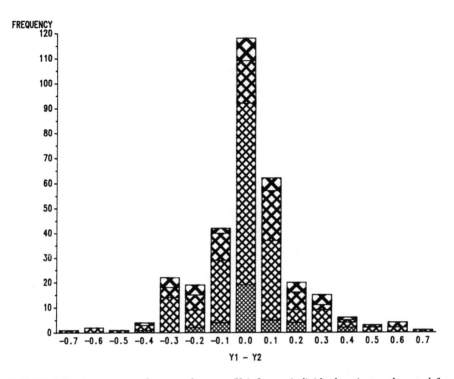

FIGURE 6.3 *Average muscle strength score (Y₂) for an individual patient, subtracted from that obtained within the previous two weeks (Y₁). The bars are hatched to indicate which of four clinics the patient was attending. The data summarized represent 320 pairs of visits, at which muscle strength was graded by the same evaluator in the same clinic. The average was 0.01, and the standard deviation was 0.19.*

questions that are to be addressed with that measurement. A simple model can permit the numerical examination of the consequences of various trial designs. A very simplistic model for variables that may be measured on an interval scale might be represented by the following equation:

$$Y = X + S + E \qquad (6.1)$$

Y is the measured score, X represents the current status of the disease, S represents the day-to-day fluctuations in the status, and E is the measurement error. Assuming that the various components are independent, we can postulate that the total variance of Y can be partitioned into three components: that due to the variance of X across the differing patients in the population, that due to the variation of S across time, and that due to variance of E (the technical error variance). For purposes of modeling, we usually consider S and E to be independent random variables with means of 0.0.

If we consider Y an index of the severity of the disease, then the variances of both S and E are considered errors for the analysis. If Y_1 represents the measured score at the first visit and Y_2 the score on the second visit, then

$$Y_1 - Y_2 = X_1 - X_2 + S_1 - S_2 + E_1 - E_2 \tag{6.2}$$

Since we assume that there is no change in disease status, $X_1 - X_2 = 0$, and that term drops out. If we assume that the time between visits has been sufficiently long that whatever factors influence S have changed and that S_1 and S_2 are therefore uncorrelated,

$$\text{Var}(Y_1 - Y_2) = 2\,\text{Var}(S) + 2\,\text{Var}(E) \tag{6.3}$$

This allows for the computation of a reliability coefficient or, traditionally, the intraclass correlation coefficient:

$$r^2 \frac{\text{Var}(X)}{\text{Var}(Y)} \tag{6.4}$$

$\text{Var}(Y)$ can be directly estimated from the data, and $\text{Var}(X)$ can be estimated by subtraction from algebraic manipulations of equation 6.3. Fleiss[11] describes a similar but more extensive development of this type of model. Its calculations are frequently carried out with use of computer software that handles random-effect analysis of variance models.[12,13]

Of interest to the reader of a study reporting such reliability coefficients is the population used for the calculation of r. For the same amount of absolute error, $\text{Var}(S) + \text{Var}(E)$, r increases as the heterogeneity of the population, $\text{Var}(X)$, increases. Thus, coefficients computed on a mixture of normal and diseased subjects are likely to be higher than those computed on one type of subject.

Of importance in the further manipulation of such quantitative scale scores are assumptions that the distribution of $Y_1 - Y_2$ is approximately normal and that the magnitude of the differences does not change as the scale values themselves change. The former assumption can be examined with a histogram of the type shown in Figure 6.3, or with a cumulative distribution function, such as that shown in Figure 6.4. The latter is usually preferred by statisticians, since it is unaffected by the choice of intervals for construction of the bars of the histogram and can be plotted so that the cumulative distribution of a normal is a straight line. The assumption that the errors do not increase as the range of scores changes can readily be examined by plotting the difference between two scores against their average.

Departures from these assumptions are frequent rationales for applying transformations of the underlying scales. Although statisticians are occasionally guilty of simply transforming variables so that simpler statistical models will suffice, it is important to consider the implication of the change in metric for our reasoning about the variable. Frequently, these transformations do correspond to our conceptualization of the underlying biologic scale. For example, the utilization of a logarithmic transformation on light intensity roughly corresponds to the perception of intensity.

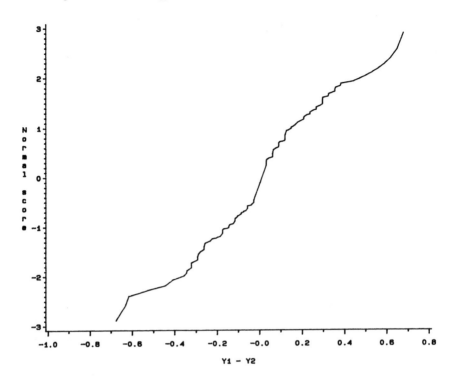

FIGURE 6.4 *Cumulative distribution of differences in average muscle strength within a two-week period. The data are the same as those shown in Figure 6.3. The normal score is an approximation of the expected-order statistics for a normally distributed random variable with a mean of 0.0, standard deviation of 1.0, and sample size of 320. A straight line indicates a distribution that is approximately normal.*

COMPUTATION OF THE POWER OF A STUDY

Information about changes in measurements is critical in the planning of an intervention study. For most neuromuscular diseases, practical studies involve the recruitment of individuals with differing stages of disease. Even when we study only patients with newly diagnosed disease, they frequently represent various stages of the disease. Therefore, the most efficient measure of outcome will generally be a change score—i.e., the score given at the end of the trial minus that given at the beginning. Change scores in the treated group are compared with those in the placebo (untreated) group. Statistical models that incorporate the baseline measure as a covariate rather than compute the difference score are possible but are not discussed here because of the complexity of the power calculations. However, these covariate models usually have slightly greater power than do the simple differences described here.

The power of a study is the probability that it will demonstrate a significant difference between the treated and untreated groups. In recent years, consideration of a study's power has become a required part of the planning of any study. A trial planned without such consideration is unethical. If the power is too low, subjects are being placed at risk without any reasonable hope of answering the question asked by the study. If the power is too high, more patients are being placed at risk than is necessary to answer the question. The emphasis on designing a trial with high power is based on the assumption that if no significant difference is observed at the end of the trial, and if the trial was carried out according to the assumptions made for the power calculations, then it can reasonably be concluded that no difference of the magnitude postulated is actually present. Such negative trials are often required to counter enthusiastic reports from small, uncontrolled series of patients treated with new agents.

To calculate the power of a study, one must specify not only the particular statistical model to be utilized in testing a given treatment, but also the magnitude of the difference to be detected between the treated and untreated groups, the significance level to be used for the test, the size of each study group, and the power desired. Given any three of these quantities, the fourth is uniquely determined. Although precise computational formulas are not presented here, approximations can be found in most bio-statistical texts,[14,15] and many books present selected results in tabular form.[16] During the planning of most clinical trials, the magnitude of the expected difference and the sample size are the primary quantities varied. The magnitude of the difference is usually standardized. For example for a simple t test of the difference in change scores:

$$d = \frac{(M_T - M_P)}{SD(Y_E - Y_B)} \tag{6.5}$$

M_T is the expected mean change score in the treated group, M_P is the expected mean change score in the placebo group, and $SD(Y_E - Y_B)$ is the standard deviation of the differences between the scores given at the end of the study and those given at baseline (the latter is assumed to be the same in both the treated and placebo groups). M_P can be estimated from natural history studies if the disease is of a progressive nature, or can be assumed to be 0.0 if the study subjects are at a nonprogressive stage of the disease. Choosing a value for M_T is usually more problematic. Utilizing a specified percentage of M_P is often a clinically useful method—e.g., when seeking to detect a difference between the two groups when the placebo group progresses at the rate projected during the natural history studies and the treated group progresses at a rate of only 50% of that observed in the natural history studies. Figure 6.5 shows a histogram of the amount of change in average muscle strength over a 12-month period in the natural history data base of the boys with DMD described earlier. Figure 6.6 shows power curves for a one-year study of patients with DMD, with M_P estimated at -0.39, and the standard deviation of $Y_E - Y_B$ of 0.37 based on the 1,032 differences shown in Figure 6.5. Curves are drawn for 25, 50, 75, and 100% reductions in the rate of disease progression, the last curve representing complete arrest of progression. When M_P is assumed to be near zero, the selected value for M_T may be chosen as a percentage of the distance back toward mean values for normals.

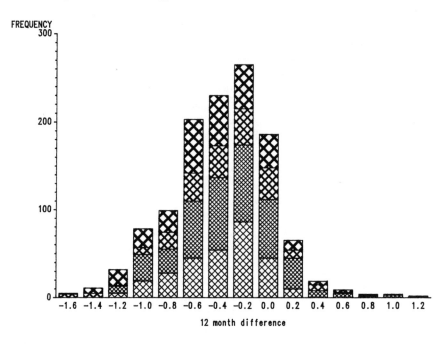

FIGURE 6.5 *Distribution of differences in average muscle strength between two examinations performed 12 months apart. The data represent 1,212 such differences. The average time was 364 days, and average difference −0.37, with a standard deviation of 0.39. The units are the same as in Figure 6.3.*

The efficacy of the use of the change from baseline can be seen by noting that in the same group of boys, the average muscle strength is 5.0, with a standard deviation of 1.6. If one compares two groups—one with the disease totally arrested and the other following the expected natural history of decreasing 0.37 units—then $d = (-0.37 - 0.0) \div 1.6 = -0.23$, and the power is about the same as that shown in Figure 6.6 for the 25% reduction ($d = [-0.37 - (-0.37 * 0.75)] \div 0.39 = -0.24$). Thus, the same sample size required to detect complete arrest of the disease when measuring only at the end of the trial could reveal a 25% reduction in the rate of disease progression if a change from baseline design were used. Note, however, that the change design requires that measurements be made on an interval scale, whereas statistical comparisons can be made for ordinal or nominal scales only with measurements made at the end of the trial (although such tests generally have less power than those based on interval scales). Obviously, the magnitude of the difference will change, depending on the disease and the measurement scales, but such quantified comparison between competing designs is the type of calculation that can be made with use of carefully collected natural history data.

If the power calculations for a study protocol have been completed and the resulting sample size or power appears economically unattractive, it is appropriate to

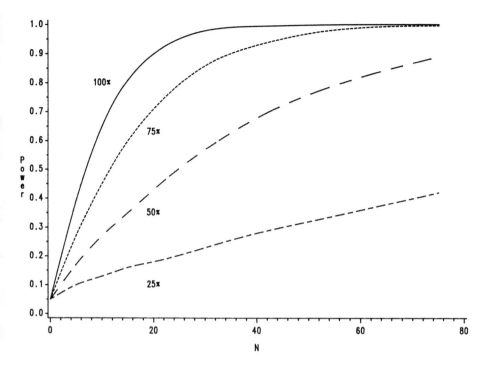

FIGURE 6.6 *Power curves for one-tailed* t *tests at P = 0.05 for the difference in change scores in an untreated (placebo) group versus a treated group. The expected change in the placebo group is based on the data in Figure 6.5. Curves are drawn for reductions in the rate of progression of the disease by 100% (complete arrest of the disease, mean change of 0.0), 75% (mean change of 0.0925), 50% (mean change of 0.185) and 25% (mean change of 0.2775). N represents the size of each group.*

consider alterations in the protocol. Since it is much more expensive to recruit patients for many studies than it is to follow or treat them, changes in the number of examinations or the duration of the trial are often attractive alternatives. Increasing the number of visits at the beginning and end of the trial will reduce the magnitude of the measurement variance. If the visits are spaced far enough apart that S_1 and S_2 of equation 6.1 can be considered independent, the variance of the mean of Y_1 and Y_2 for a particular individual is $[\text{Var}(S) + \text{Var}(E)] \div 2$. Then the difference from the baseline to the end of the study will be

$$\text{Var}(Y_E - Y_B) = \text{Var}(X_E - X_B) + \text{Var}(S) + \text{Var}(E) \tag{6.7}$$

rather than

$$\text{Var}(Y_E - Y_B) = \text{Var}(X_E - X_B) + 2\text{Var}(S) + 2\text{Var}(E) \tag{6.8}$$

Using the data from Figures 6.3 and 6.4 to estimate $\text{Var}(S) + \text{Var}(E)$—and using the observed one-year variance, $0.39^2 = 0.15$, and the estimated $\text{Var}(S) + \text{Var}(E)$ of $0.19^2 \div 2 = 0.018$ from the data of Figure 6.3—we see that the one-year difference scores have a standard deviation of 0.37, only slightly smaller than that observed with a single visit. Obviously, for other measures, the differences between the total variance and the technical error variance, $\text{Var}(E)$, may be quite different. When the error variance is a large proportion of the total, multiple measurements provide a large increase in the power of a study.

MISSING DATA

Since many of the measures included in neurologic assessment batteries are functional in nature, it is not uncommon for a patient's condition to progress to a point that particular tasks cannot be performed at all. Such measures are therefore inadequate to evaluate the efficacy of a proposed treatment. The data they provide must be viewed with caution. Trials in young children can present difficulties if the measured tasks are beyond the ability of even normal children at a given age (e.g., time to walk 30 feet, measured in an infant). If the missing values are simply ignored and summary statistics are computed only for patients measured at both time points, the progression of the disease will generally be underestimated. An alternative is to treat the missing values as censored values. Although statistical techniques are available to determine whether the values at the end of a trial are different in the treated and nontreated groups, standard techniques are not available to both incorporate the censored values and utilize changes from baseline. Thus, measurements obtained in only a subset of the patient pool for a trial are generally uninformative, except for measurements in the subset evaluable at both the beginning and end of the trial.

For example, consider data obtained from a cohort of 43 individuals[17] classified as having senile dementia of the Alzheimer type. They were recruited at a mild stage of the disease (clinical dementia rating of 1) and had been given no other diagnoses that might have confused the dementia diagnosis at entry (e.g., depression, Parkinson's disease, psychosis). Figure 6.7 shows a plot of their scores on the Pfeiffer test at baseline and approximately fifteen months later. In the 33 patients with values at both points, the scores averaged 5.63 at baseline and 6.85 at 15 months. Scores above the identity line indicate improvement in measured performance after one year, but the averaged measured changes indicate a decreased performance of 1.61, with a standard deviation of the change score of 2.28. Note the difference between this average change score and that of 1.22, obtained by subtracting the differences in the means of those tested at each point.

In choosing the primary efficacy measure for an intervention trial, then, the number of patients who will be evaluable at both the beginning and end of the trial is an important consideration. Table 6.1 shows how many of the 43 patients with mild dementia described above were evaluable at 15 months for each of six different dementia-related scales. Since the "box score" required for computing scores on the Blessed dementia scale and cognitive subscale can be obtained from a collateral source,

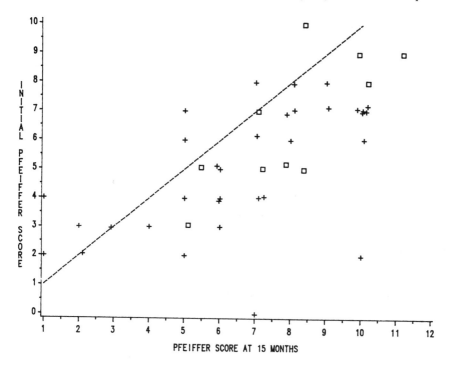

FIGURE 6.7 *Score on the Pfeiffer test of cognitive impairment at baseline and at 15 months' follow-up. Plusses represent actual measurements at both points, and squares represent actual measurements at baseline and an imputed value calculated from a regression model fitted on the 33 patients with values at both points. The regressors were the Pfeiffer test score, the face-hand test score, the sum of the box scores, and the score on an aphasia battery. The r^2 value for the model was 0.62. The line represents the same score at both points. Scores above the line indicate that tested performance was better at 15 months than at baseline.*

more individuals were evaluable with those instruments than with instruments that require patient interaction, such as the Pfeiffer test, the aphasia battery, and the face-hand test. The mean and standard deviation of the change scores were computed for patients who could be evaluated at 15 months, and d (equation 6.5) was computed for a complete arrest of the course of the disease. According to these criteria, the Blessed cognitive subscale would be a good choice, and the power of a study could be roughly estimated from the data in Figure 6.6 for a 100% reduction in the rate of progression. The sample size could be augmented by about 20% to allow for those who could not be tested at the end of 15 months. For a test such as the Pfeiffer, the power could be estimated by the 75% reduction curve in Figure 6.6, and the sample could be augmented by about 30% to account for the untestable patients. Of course, additional patients may be required for any contemplated trial because of treatment-related withdrawals during the study.

Of particular interest are the ten individuals without values at 15 months. Imputed values for these individuals are based on a regression analysis of an ensemble of clinical

Table 6.1   Change Scores in Senile Dementia of the Alzheimer Type

Variable	N	Mean	SD	d
Sum of box scores	38	3.52	3.66	0.96
Blessed dementia scale	36	3.64	4.77	0.76
Blessed cognitive subscale	36	2.75	2.81	0.98
Pfeiffer test	33	1.58	2.03	0.78
Face-hand test	31	3.10	6.30	0.49
Aphasia battery	31	3.79	6.12	0.62

items measured at baseline, including the Pfeiffer test, and identified by squares in Figure 6.7. Note that several of these ten patients had the worst scores at baseline. Our imputed values for them are also poor; in fact, several are over 10.0, the worst possible score. If we include these ten imputed values, the estimated mean score at 15 months would be 7.15. If we use an endpoint-only design, these values can be considered censored and most of the rank-order tests will be able to utilize the information, but it is difficult to know what type of "change score" to employ.

One approach to this problem is to combine individual measurements into a battery with an overall "megascore." The first step in the construction of such a single score is the standardization of the individual scales so they can be measured on a common scale. Two methods are discussed in this volume. Munsat and his group (Chapter 10) standardize measurements in their patients with amyotrophic lateral sclerosis by reference to a historical data base of past ALS patients seen in their clinic. Each measure is then standardized by subtracting the mean and dividing by the standard deviation to produce a z-score. Tourtellotte and his group (Chapter 2) have standardized by reference to a normal group. As their battery has been used to evaluate multiple sclerosis, which affects patients of many ages, they have corrected for age in their standardization procedure. Age correction is very important, especially in dealing with diseases in childhood, when normal growth and development produce changes opposite to the deterioration caused by the disease—particularly when the rates of those changes differ among patients of various ages. Similar concerns are now being recognized in diseases of the elderly, because changes in patients can take the same direction as those in nonpatients who are simply aging. Since age corrections are usually estimated from rather small samples of normal subjects, they can cause more errors than they remove when used in the standardization process.

After the standardization of individual scores to a common metric, the scores are averaged across several measures that are conceptually related to form the megascores. Only measures that are appropriate for a particular patient's stage of disease are included. A slightly more complex method of computing the megascore is to use imputation techniques to generate the missing values and then include those values in the computation of the overall score. This may lead to fewer distortions of overall scores due to changing tasks, but the risk of introducing additional error remains.

SOPHISTICATED STATISTICAL MODELING

As a statistician, I would be remiss if I did not mention various more complex statistical techniques that may be considered for use in quantitative clinical neurology. In each case, however, application requires significant collaboration between the statistician and clinician. Most familiar to many neurologic researchers will be the techniques of test construction developed by the psychometricians; LaRocca (chapter 5) covers many of these. The megascore concept is similar to the concept of tests to be used over a wide developmental range, such as standardized IQ tests. Techniques such as factor analysis and more complex linear modeling often provide insights into a battery of measurements.

The utilization of the growth curve models developed by biometricians is frequently insightful because of their designers' significant experience in studying the natural histories of diseases. We have developed one type of statistical model[18] that takes advantage of observations of the progression of an individual's clinical condition over an extended baseline in order to increase the power of a trial. We have recently initiated open trials of postulated therapeutic agents against historical controls based on our extensive natural history database of DMD patients. Although such trials cannot adequately control for a number of biases, most of these biases would be expected to be toward efficacy. A negative trial could therefore be used to exclude an agent that failed to demonstrate a change from the natural history.

REFERENCES

1. Stevens SS. Mathematics, measurement, and psychophysics. In: Stevens SS, ed. Handbook of experimental psychology. New York: John Wiley, 1951.
2. Brooke MH, Fenichel GM, Griggs RC, et al. Clinical investigation in Duchenne dystrophy. 2. Determination of the "power" of therapeutic trials based on the natural history. Muscle Nerve 1983; 6:91–103.
3. Mendell JR, Griggs RC, Moxley R, et al. A double-blind controlled trial of leucine in Duchenne muscular dystrophy. Ann Neurol 1982; 12:78.
4. Mendell JR, Griggs RC, Moxley RT, et al. Clinical trials in Duchenne dystrophy. IV. Double-blind trial of leucine. Muscle Nerve 1984; 7:535–41.
5. Moxley RT, Brooke MH, Fenichel GM, et al. Clinical investigation in Duchenne dystrophy. VI. Double-blind controlled trial of nifedipine. Muscle Nerve 1987; 10:22–33.
6. Fenichel GM et al. Clinical investigation of Duchenne dystrophy. VII. Double-blind controlled trial of penacillamine and vitamin E. Muscle Nerve 1988; 1164–1168.
7. SAS Institute. PROC GPLOT, SAS/GRAPH user's guide: version 5 edition. Cary, NC: SAS Institute, 1985; 279–306.
8. Miller JP. Use of diagnostic registries and data bases. In: Wolf S, Lewis JN, eds. Clinical trials in chronic neuromuscular diseases: Proceedings of a colloquium at Totts Gap Institute, Bangor, PA. Muscle Nerve, July/August 1985.
9. Meinert CL. Clinical trials: design, conduct, and analysis. New York: Oxford University Press, 1986.
10. Florence JM, Pandya S, Robinson J, et al. Clinical trials in Duchenne muscular dystrophy. 3. Standardization of and reliability of evaluation procedures. Phys Ther 1985; 64:41–5.

11. Fleiss JL. The design and analysis of clinical experiments. New York: John Wiley, 1986.
12. SAS Institute. The VARCOMP procedure. In: SAS Institute. SAS user's guide: statistics, version 5 edition. Cary, NC: SAS Institute, 1985; 817–23.
13. Jennrich R, Sampson P. P8V general mixed model analysis of variance—equal cell sizes. In: Dixon WJ, ed. BMDP statistical software. Berkeley: University of California Press, 1981.
14. Rosner B. Fundamentals of biostatistics. Boston: Duxbury Press, 1986.
15. Snedecor GW, Cochran WG. Statistical methods. Ames: Iowa State University Press, 1980.
16. Cohen J. Statistical power analysis for the behavioral sciences. San Diego: Academic Press, 1977.
17. Berg L, Hughes CP, Coben LA, et al. Mild senile dementia of the Alzheimer type: research diagnostic criteria, recruitment and description of a study population. J Neurol Neurosurg Psychiatry 1982; 45:962–8.
18. Madsen KS, Miller JP, Province MA, the CIDD Group. The use of an extended baseline period in the evaluation of treatment in a Duchenne muscular dystrophy trial. Statistics in Medicine 1986; 5:231–41.

PART II

Clinical Applications

Chapter 7

Measurement of Strength in Neuromuscular Diseases

Patricia L. Andres, Linda M. Skerry, and Theodore L. Munsat

There is an increasing need for accurate and reliable measurement of deficit in neuromuscular disease. In clinical research, precise and sensitive quantification is needed in order to judge therapeutic interventions, especially when their effects may be modest. Accurate measurement of disease severity can also promote better understanding of the natural history of neuromuscular diseases. The changing nature of reimbursement, with diagnosis-related groups and stiffer Medicare regulations, requires that physicians carefully document patients' progress in measurable, standardized terms.

Although interest in quantification has increased recently, current techniques to measure neuromuscular deficit remain quite primitive. The validity of data resulting from clinical investigations hinges on the ability of test items to describe events accurately in numerical terms. Yet millions of dollars are spent each year on clinical research whose results rely on poorly constructed, insensitive grading scales.

Unfortunately, there are no currently available chemical or electrophysiologic techniques to measure the loss of motor units or muscle viability precisely. Thus, we must rely on less direct measurements to judge disease progression, and close attention must be given to assessing the clinical components specific to each disease.

The neuromuscular diseases, by definition, are limited to the voluntary motor system, without cerebellar, intellectual, or sensory impairment. Except for amyotrophic lateral sclerosis (ALS), which has upper motor neuron involvement, these diseases are confined to the motor unit. The hallmark clinical manifestation is weakness. Therefore, assessment of strength is the most direct measure of neuromuscular deficit[1] (Figure 7.1).

Strength is a vague term used to describe various components of motor perfor-

Supported by grants from the Muscular Dystrophy Association and National Institutes of Health General Clinical Research Center (M01RR000054 and RO1NS24623).

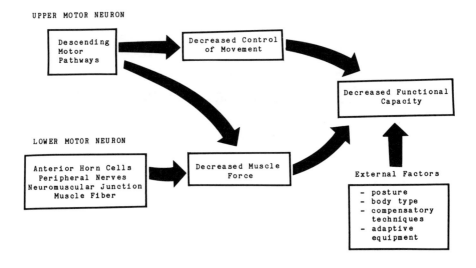

FIGURE 7.1   *Clinical manifestations of neuromuscular disease.*

mance. It is dependent on many factors, including type of contraction (isometric, isotonic, isokinetic), speed of contraction, length-tension relationship, pattern of neuronal discharge, cross-sectional area of muscle, and motivation.[2] It is influenced by factors operating at many different levels of the nervous system, from the cerebral cortex to the muscle fiber itself. Lesions affecting the central nervous system (e.g., the cortex, cerebellum, or extrapyramidal tracts) can affect the quality of motor output. One broad definition of strength is the capacity of a muscle or muscle group to produce the tension necessary to maintain posture, initiate movement, or control movement during conditions of loading on the musculoskeletal system.[2] For the purposes of this chapter, however, since neuromuscular disease affects the motor unit rather than the central control mechanisms, we will define strength as the force-generating capacity of muscle.

Several studies support the validity of strength measurement as an indicator of motor loss in neuromuscular disease. In ALS patients, muscle strength measured two to six months prior to death correlated closely with the number of motor units at autopsy.[3] In addition, motor unit counts determined by electrophysiologic techniques showed a close correlation with isometric muscle strength.[4] Similarly, in patients with muscular dystrophy, muscle force and cross-sectional area of the muscle were found to be highly correlated.[5] In addition, patients with neuromuscular disease can perform a maximal voluntary contraction with the same force as when electrically stimulated.[1,6] Also, the metabolic demand of muscle during maximal voluntary contraction, as determined by magnetic resonance spectroscopy, is similar to that produced by electrical stimulation.[7] Thus, when assessing the muscle force of a patient with neuromuscular disease, maximal voluntary contraction is a valid measurement of disease severity. Motivation does not significantly alter the force generated.

In light of this evidence and our own experience, we agree with Edwards et al.[8] that "the measurement of force production in a single muscle or muscle group is therefore the only way of identifying that component of the patient's symptoms due solely to impaired muscle function per se."

SUMMARY OF TRADITIONAL METHODS USED TO MEASURE STRENGTH

Since weakness and loss of functional capacity are the most prominent symptoms of neuromuscular disease, assessment of strength and functional loss are important components of the clinical evaluation. Muscle strength assessed at the bedside using manual resistance is often subjectively graded as normal, mild, moderate, or severe. This approach is unstandardized and is useful only to screen for deficit, as it reflects the subjective perception of a single examiner. In addition, strength is commonly assessed at the bedside by functional strength tests such as deep knee bends, heel-and-toe walking, and holding arms over head. These tasks merely screen for possible motor impairment but cannot measure the extent of a deficit.

When standardized grading of strength is needed, the manual muscle test (MMT) is the most commonly used method. MMT was originally developed by Lovett to evaluate isolated weakness associated with poliomyelitis.[9] It is a grading system in which strength is subjectively rated on a scale of 0 to 5 according to the patient's ability to move against gravity and hold against the examiner's manual resistance. Several groups, including the Medical Research Council,[10] Kendall et al.,[11] and Daniels and Worthingham,[12] have devised variations on the MMT technique.

MMT can screen for muscle weakness and provide a quick estimate of whether the patient is better or worse. It is well standardized and is cost- and time-efficient, as no equipment is required. Also, it can yield highly reproducible results when standard test positions are used by trained examiners.[13,14]

The quantitative capacity of MMT, however, is limited, because although the data is ranked, the intervals between ranks are not equal. The force generated by muscles in the same MMT grade can vary as much as 40%.[15] The biceps brachii requires only 3% of its expected maximal force to move against gravity (fair grade, or 3).[16] In this situation, the two grades of good (4) and normal (5) represent 97% of the muscle's capacity to contract (Figure 7.2). It is important to recognize that a change of 40% of expected strength could go undetected by MMT because the stronger end of the scale is very insensitive. In addition, MMT grading is subjective and can be greatly influenced by the examiner's strength and the weight of the patient's limb.[16]

The MMT produces ordinal data. For research purposes, standard statistical analyses utilizing means are not properly applied to ordinal data. Ordinal data appropriately permit only the analysis of frequencies.[17] For example, Bohannon[19] found that although MMT and objective strength measurements were highly correlated, they were significantly different when MMT scores and objective force measurements were converted to percent of normal, due to the relative differences in the breadth of the

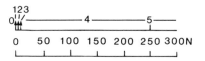

FIGURE 7.2   *An analog MMT scale compared with actual dynametric force measurement of the biceps brachii muscle. Note that only 3% of normal expected force corresponds to an MMT grade of 3. Modified from van der Ploeg.*[16]

various MMT grades. MMT may provide a general indication of improvement or worsening, but it is quite deficient in measuring degrees of change over time.

The Clinical Investigation of Duchenne Dystrophy group,[18] organized by the Muscular Dystrophy Association, has developed a test protocol to track disease progression in Duchenne dystrophy. It consists of MMT of 34 muscle groups, measurement of contractures, and functional testing. The protocol is comprehensive and has been extensively tested to assure high reproducibility.[13] However, emphasis is placed on the mean muscle score determined by averaging the 34 raw MMT scores. This is disadvantageous because MMT is relatively insensitive and because parametric techniques are applied to ordinal data.

MEASUREMENT OF FUNCTIONAL CAPACITY

Clinical measurement of disease severity can be performed on two different levels. The first, which most directly reflects the disease process, includes manifestations of the disease or impairments in strength, speed of movement, or coordination. The second is the reduced functional capacity, or disability, of the patient. The disability that results from the disease is influenced by external factors such as posture, pain, compensatory movements, and adaptive equipment. Therefore, the measurement of functional outcome or disability is a less direct measure of the disease itself (Figure 7.1).

Functional scales are subjective ratings of performance and are widely used in assessing neuromuscular deficit.[18,20,21] They are easily performed in the office setting and broadly reflect clinically relevant functional disturbances. However, they are insensitive to the degree of motor unit loss, and they produce ordinal data. Functional scales are less sensitive in reflecting disease progression than isometric force testing (Figure 7.3). Functional scale can determine how many patients improve or worsen, but not how much or how fast improvement or deterioration takes place. They can answer questions about functional performance but not about changes in the motor neuron pool.

Functional capacity is often measured with use of timed tasks.[18,22] Recording the time needed to rise from a chair, walk 6 meters, or dial a telephone number produces interval data and is therefore more objective, reducing examiner bias. However, the values generated may not accurately reflect the disease process. Certain tasks may require a critical number of motor units, and the time required for performance may not change until this threshold is reached (Figure 7.4).

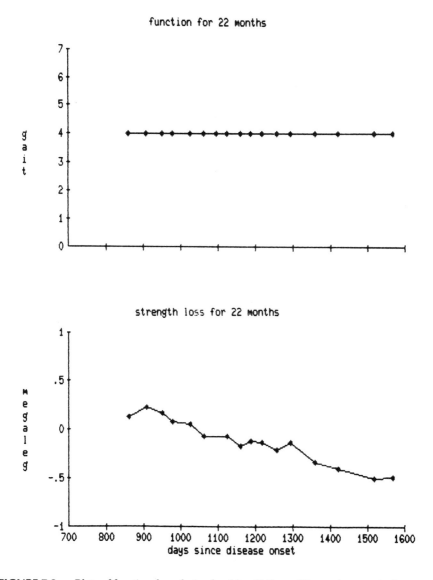

FIGURE 7.3 *Plots of functional grade (scale of 1 to 7) for walking and composite leg strength (megaleg) over 22 months in the same patient with ALS. Note the prominent progressive loss of strength without change in functional grade.*

In addition, timed activities may be influenced by environmental or other factors external to the disease process, such as adaptive equipment or compensatory movements. Timed ambulation, for instance, may actually improve dramatically when the type of assistance is changed (Figure 7.5). Though obviously important, functional outcomes may be indicators of the disease process itself.

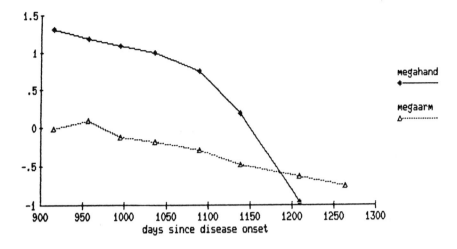

FIGURE 7.4   *Composite MVIC testing of arm (mega-arm) demonstrates a linear decline in strength, whereas timed hand function shows a rapid drop-off after approximately day 1,100. It is clear that the loss of a relatively small number of motor units can lead to prominent functional change.*

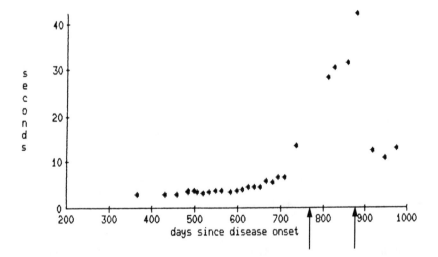

FIGURE 7.5   *Timed walking tests of a single ALS patient. The patient ambulated independently until day 760 (first arrow), when he started using a rolling walker. After day 900 (second arrow) he could no longer use the walker and depended on physical assistance to ambulate. This illustrates the remarkable effect that assistive devices can have on timed performance.*

INSTRUMENTED STRENGTH MEASUREMENT

In an attempt to provide data that are more objective and sensitive, quantitative methods utilizing either isokinetic or isometric testing have recently been developed. Isokinetic dynamometers (e.g., CybexII [Lumex, Ronkonkoma, NY], Kin-Com [Chattex, Chattanooga, TN]) contain a preset speed-controlling mechanism that offers resistance proportional to the dynamic tension developed by the exercising limb.[23] Interval printouts of torque are generated throughout the entire range of motion as the limb moves at a constant velocity. Isokinetic testing can provide information about the pattern of force generation, effect of speed on force development, and work performed. It is useful not only in adults but also in children. High test-retest reliability in children has been demonstrated in tests of ten large-muscle groups.[24]

Isokinetic dynamometers have several disadvantages, however. Their cost may be prohibitive at $25,000 to $35,000. The Cybex device is time-consuming to adjust, and the measurement of several different muscle groups is laborious. Also, muscles with less than Fair+ (3+) strength cannot be tested through the full arc of motion, as the limb is too weak to exert force against the machine's moving lever arm against gravity.

Several other instruments are available for quantitating maximal voluntary isometric contractions (MVIC). These include spring balances, cable tensiometers, hydraulic myometers, and various types of strain gauges.[25] Isometric testing has the advantage of eliminating velocity and muscle length as variables.[16,26-28] However, the examiner must be carefully trained to assure that limb position and stabilization are standard.[27-29]

Hand-held myometers have been increasingly used in studies to measure MVIC, and they have excellent test-retest reliability.[16,29] Their pocket size and portability make them extremely practical for office use. A major disadvantage is that the maximum force recorded is limited by the strength of the examiner, who must be able to break the patient's resistance. The device is therefore not suitable for detecting minor degrees of weakness in large adults. Also, it does not produce a hard copy of results.

Several investigators have used electronic strain gauges to measure isometric force.[26-28] Nonportable strain gauges offer certain advantages over myometers. Force is measured in standard units (kilograms), and a hard copy of the measurement is produced. The subjects pull against an immovable strap rather than against the force of the examiner (Figure 7.6).

This system requires office space and about $2,000 of customized equipment to accommodate the testing of 20 muscle groups. Once the strain-gauge system is set up and a carefully standardized testing procedure is established, precise monitoring of the patient's disease progression is possible. About 30 minutes is required to test 20 muscle groups.

QUANTITATION OF SPACTICITY

Because ALS is manifested in both upper and lower motor neuron damage, quantitating motor performance becomes more complex. Lower motor neuron damage is directly

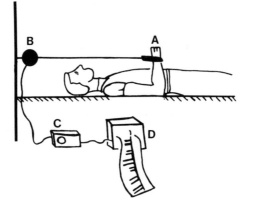

FIGURE 7.6   *The testing set-up used for force measurement. MVIC is measured with the patient in a standard position. Force exerted on the strap (A) is transduced by the amount of distortion within the strain gauge (B), amplified (C), and recorded on a strip chart recorder (D).*

reflected by a proportional decrease in muscle force[1,3-5]. Upper motor neuron damage results in positive signs, such as hyperreflexia and positive Babinski signs, as well as negative signs, such as difficulty in initiating and ceasing movement, decreased speed of movement, decreased ability to isolate movement, and decreased maximal force production.[30] Therefore, quantitation of MVIC measures only one aspect of voluntary motor deficit due to upper motor neuron damage.

Clinically, an upper motor neuron deficit is often screened by asking the patient to perform rapid alternating movements, such as opposing the thumb and index finger repeatedly. Slowed movement and a decrease in movement excursion suggests a deficit. To quantitate this deficit, an event counter/timer is used with a low-resistance finger- and foot-tapper. The validity of this test is under investigation. Measurements of MVIC and finger- and foot-tapping in patients with pure upper motor neuron lesions are being compared to those in patients with pure lower motor neuron disease. Comprehensive measurement of upper motor neuron deficit remains a major challenge.

THE TUFTS QUANTITATIVE NEUROMUSCULAR EXAMINATION

An important principle in designing any test battery is to construct a protocol that addresses specific research questions. The Tufts Quantitative Neuromuscular Examination (TQNE) was developed to quantitate neuromuscular deficit and measure the rate of disease in ALS.[31] It was designed to quantitate accurately the amount of change during a given period and to use items measured in standard units to permit adequate statistical analysis.

The TQNE is a standardized test battery consisting of 32 items that measure

Table 7.1   TQNE Composition

	Number of Items
Pulmonary function[a]	
FVC	1
MVV	1
Bulbar function	
Diadochokinetic rates: "pa"	1
"pata"	1
Timed activities	
Dialing a 7-digit phone number	2
Purdue pegboard	2
15-foot walk	1
Arm strength	
Isometric arm strength, measured with an electronic strain gauge	8
Grip strength, measured with a Jamar dynamometer	2
Leg strength	
Isometric leg strength, measured with an electronic strain gauge	10
Functional rating scale	
Speech, arm, and leg function, measured with a graded scale	3
Total	32

[a]FVC denotes forced vital capacity; MVV, maximal voluntary ventilation.

pulmonary function (forced vital capacity and maximal voluntary ventilation), bulbar function (speech rates), timed hand activities (phone-dialing and the Purdue pegboard test), strength (isometric force), and rated functional capacity (Table 7.1). The major components of the TQNE is MVIC testing with an electronic strain gauge that measures 18 muscle groups in the arms and legs. A Jamar dynamometer is used to measure grip strength.

We now have computer-stored TQNE data for more than 2,300 patient visits. The TQNE has been used to determine the natural history of ALS[32] and to assess the efficacy of therapy.[33-35] Reliability was determined by testing 10 patients with ALS and 35 normal subjects twice within a 3- to 5-hour period. Data were analyzed using both correlation coefficients and percent change (Tables 7.2 and 7.3).[31]

Test-retest variation is a function not only of testing or measurement error but also of human performance variation.[26] Positioning, instructions to the patient, verbal encouragement, muscle contraction and relaxation time, and stabilization can influence the results.[26,27] Such variables can be minimized if strict standardized procedures are followed, but it may be impossible to reduce human performance variation to less than 5%.

Since MVIC testing, in our view, has been shown to be a valid and sensitive indicator of disease progression, it can be used to assess the validity and sensitivity of other testing instruments. To evaluate the relative sensitivity of MMT versus MVIC

Table 7.2 Analysis of 3- to 5-Hour Test-Retest Reliability (Intra-Rater Testing)

Item	Normal Controls (n = 35)		ALS Patients (n = 10)	
	r	Percent Change	r	Percent Change
Isometric Force				
Shoulder flexion R	0.97	5.5	0.99	8.2
Shoulder flexion L	0.97	6.3	0.99	6.0
Shoulder extension R	0.98	7.0	0.97	7.3
Shoulder extension L	0.98	6.0	0.99	5.6
Elbow flexion R	0.97	5.3	0.99	5.5
Elbow flexion L	0.96	4.3	0.99	8.9
Elbow extension R	0.96	6.8	0.99	8.7
Elbow extension L	0.98	5.2	0.97	10.9
Grip R	0.95	7.4	0.99	6.5
Grip L	0.96	5.1	0.99	17.2
Hip extension R	0.95	10.3	0.98	12.4
Hip extension L	0.98	8.1	0.97	12.4
Hip flexion R	0.97	7.7	0.99	10.8
Hip flexion L	0.98	7.0	0.99	7.1
Knee extension R	0.97	7.2	0.99	6.0
Knee extension L	0.98	7.1	0.99	7.6
Knee flexion R	0.96	6.5	0.98	9.6
Knee flexion L	0.92	8.7	0.99	8.9
Dorsiflexion R	0.94	6.7	0.99	9.0
Dorsiflexion L	0.93	7.2	0.98	8.7

R denotes right; L, left. Reprinted with permission of *Neurology*.

testing, 7 patients were tested monthly for a mean of 6 months with both MMT and MVIC testing techniques. Preliminary results indicate that MMT is far less sensitive than MVIC testing in tracking disease progression (Figures 7.7 and 7.8).

Table 7.3 Analysis of 3- to 5-Hour Test-Retest Reliability for Isometric Force (Inter-Rater Testing)

Item	Normal Controls (n = 10)		ALS Patients (n = 10)	
	r	Percent Change	r	Percent Change
Isometric Force				
Shoulder flexion R	0.99	3.9	0.99	6.5
Shoulder flexion L	0.95	7.5	0.99	6.2
Shoulder extension R	0.96	9.3	0.98	8.5
Shoulder extension L	0.97	8.2	0.99	6.0
Elbow flexion R	0.99	3.7	0.99	9.1
Elbow flexion L	0.97	5.4	0.99	8.3

Table 7.3 *(continued)*

Item	Normal Controls (n = 10)		ALS Patients (n = 10)	
	r	*Percent Change*	*r*	*Percent Change*
Elbow extension R	0.96	7.5	0.99	6.7
Elbow extension L	0.99	5.7	0.99	8.2
Grip R	0.98	5.8	0.99	5.1
Grip L	0.94	6.8	0.99	7.5
Hip extension R	0.98	8.2	0.94	11.3
Hip extension L	0.99	8.9	0.92	13.8
Hip flexion R	0.96	6.7	0.95	9.1
Hip flexion L	0.94	10.0	0.96	11.0
Knee extension R	0.99	4.2	0.99	6.8
Knee extension L	0.97	8.0	0.98	5.5
Knee flexion R	0.91	7.9	0.98	9.8
Knee flexion L	0.94	5.6	0.97	8.1
Dorsiflexion R	0.82	15.1	0.97	8.5
Dorsiflexion L	0.85	13.1	0.97	7.5

R denotes right; L, left. Reprinted with permission of *Neurology*.

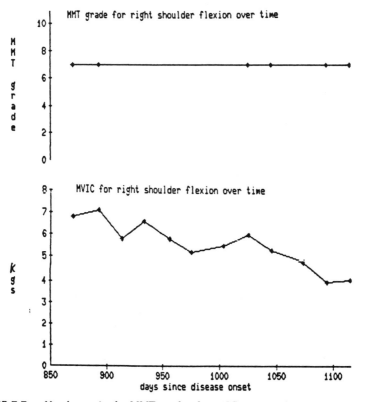

FIGURE 7.7   *No change in the MMT grade of an ALS patient whose MVIC measurement of right shoulder flexion demonstrates a 40% decline over 10 months.*

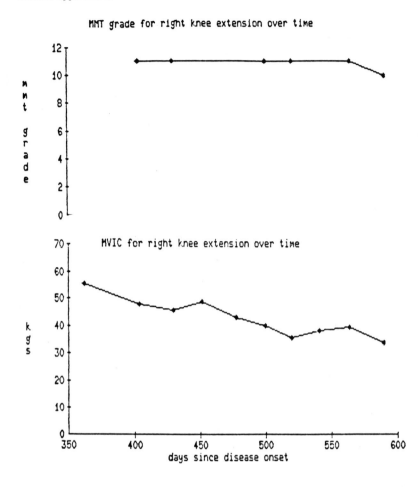

FIGURE 7.8   *Strength of right knee extension in an ALS patient. The strength is graded normal 11 by MMT until day 600, when it drops to Good + (10).* During this time, MVIC measurement shows a linear decline.

FUTURE PLANS

Further development of our testing protocol will include expanding our normal data bank. This will allow us to predict normal values for each muscle group on the basis of sex, age, and size. Such data may be used to determine functional predictors based on sex, age, and size, as well as the amount of strength needed for such activities as ambulation, transfers, writing, and feeding.

In addition, we plan a formal comparison of MVIC testing, MMT, and graded scales (ALS score) in a longitudinal study of patients with ALS. We will also focus on the development of items to measure upper motor neuron deficit for inclusion in the TQNE protocol.

REFERENCES

1. Edwards RHT, Hyde S. Methods of measuring muscle strength fatigue. Physiotherapy 1977; 63:51–5.
2. Smidt GL. Rogers WM. Factors contributing to the regulation and clinical assessment of muscular strength. Phys Ther 1982; 1283–90.
3. Sobue G, Sahashi K, Takahashi A, et al. Degenerating compartment and functioning compartment of motor neurons in ALS: possible process of motor neuron loss. Neurology 1983; 33:654–7.
4. McComas AL. Neuromuscular function and disorders. London: Butterworths, 1977.
5. Grinrod, S, Tofts P, Edwards RHT. Investigation of human skeleton muscle structure and composition by x-ray computerized tomography. European J Clin Invest 1983; 13:465–8.
6. Edwards RHT. Physiological analysis of skeletal muscle weakness and fatigue. Clin Sci 1978; 54:463–70.
7. Shenton DW Jr, Heppenstall RB, Chance B, et al. Electrical stimulation of human muscle studied using 31P-nuclear magnetic resonance spectroscopy. J Orthop Res 1986; 4:204–11.
8. Edwards RHT, Wiles CM, Mills KR. Quantitation of muscle contraction and strength. In: Dyck PJ, Thomas PK, Lambert EH, et al., eds. Peripheral Neuropathy. Philadelphia: W.B. Saunders, 1984:1093.
9. Wright W. Muscle training in the treatment of infantile paralysis. Boston Med Surg J 1912; 167:567.
10. Medical Research Council. Aids to the investigation of peripheral nerve injuries. In: War Memorandum. London: HMSO, 1943; 2:11–46.
11. Kendall H, Kendall F, Wadsworth G. Muscle testing and function. Baltimore: Williams and Wilkins, 1971.
12. Daniels L. Worthingham C. Muscle Testing: technique of manual examination. Philadelphia: W.B. Saunders, 1980.
13. Florence JM, Pandya S, King WM, et al. Clinical trials in Duchenne dystrophy. Standardization and reliability of evaluation procedures. Phys Ther 1984; 64:41–5.
14. Lilienfeld AM, Jacobs M, Willis M. A study of reproducibility of muscle testing and certain other aspects of muscle scoring. Phys Ther Rev 1954; 34:279.
15. Beasley WC. Quantitative muscle testing. Arch Phys Med Rehabil 1961; 42:398–425.
16. van der Ploeg RJO, Oosterhuis HJGH, Reuvekamp J. Measuring muscle strength. J Neurol 1984; 231:200–3.
17. Rothstein J. Measurement in physical therapy. New York: Churchill Livingstone, 1985.
18. Brooke MH, Fenichel GL, Griggs RC, et al. Clinical investigation in Duchenne dystrophy. II. Determination of the "power" of therapeutic trials based on the natural history. Muscle Nerve 1983; 6:91–103.
19. Bohannon RW. Manual muscle test scores and dynamometer test scores of knee extension strength. Arch Phys Med Rehabil 1986; 67:390–2.
20. Norris FH, Callachini PR, Fallat RJ, et al. Administration of guanidine in amyotrophic lateral sclerosis. Neurology 1974; 24:721–8.

21. Vignos PJ, Watkins M. The effect of exercise in muscular dystrophy. JAMA 1966; 197:843-8.
22. Ziter FA, Allsop KG, Tyler FH. Assessment of the muscle strength in Duchenne muscular dystrophy. Neurology 1977; 27:981-4.
23. Hislop HJ, Perrini JJ. The isokinetic concept of exercise. Phys Ther 1967; 47:114.
24. Molnar GE, Alexander J, Gutfeld N. Reliability of quantitative strength measurements in children. Arch Phys Med Rehabil 1979; 60:218.
25. Mayhew TP, Rothstein JM. Measurement of muscle performance with instruments. In: Rothstein JM, ed. Measurement in Physical Therapy. New York: Churchill Livingstone, 1985.
26. deBoer A, Boukes RJ, Sterk JC. Reliability of dynamometry in patients with neuromuscular disorders. Eng Med 1982; 11:169-74.
27. Potvin AR, Tourtelotte WW, Syndulko K, et al. Quantitative methods in assessment of neurologic function. CRC Crit Rev Biomed Eng 1981; 6:177-224.
28. Wiles CM, Karni Y. The measurement of strength in patients with peripheral neuromuscular disorders. J Neurol Neurosurg Psychiatry 1983; 46:1006-13.
29. Hyde SA, Scott OM, Goddard CM. The myometer: the development of a clinical tool. Physiotherapy 1983; 69:424-27.
30. Landau WM. Spasticity: what is it? what is it not? In: Feldman RG, Young RR, Koella WP, eds. Spasticity: disordered motor control. Chicago: Year Book Medical Publishers, 1980:17-24.
31. Andres PL, Hedlund W, Finison L, et al. Quantitative motor assessment in amyotrophic lateral sclerosis. Neurology 1986; 36:937-41.
32. Munsal TL, Andres PL, Burnside S, et al. The natural history of ALS. Ann Neurol 1985; 18:157.
33. Munsat TL, Easterday CS, Levy S, et al. Amantadine and quanidine are ineffective in ALS. Neurology 1981; 31:1054-5.
34. Bradley WG, Hedlund W, Cooper C, et al. A double-blind controlled trial of bovine brain gangliosides (cronassial) in amyotrophic lateral sclerosis. Neurology 1984; 34:1079-82.
35. Keleman J, Hedlund W, Murray-Douglas P, et al. Lecithin is not effective in amyotrophic lateral sclerosis. Neurology 1982; 32:315-6.

Chapter 8

Clinical Measurements of Fatigue and Exercise in Neuromuscular Disease

Michael H. Brooke

In any clinical arena, the topic of quantitation is almost guaranteed to provoke controversy. So varied are the methods of measurement and so vehement the supporters of the various systems that it is sometimes difficult to concede the usefulness of quantitation at any price. Perhaps the initial premise that might be examined is that we do not need quantitation.

The populist view might be that if a clinical effect is so small as to need some complicated instrument for its detection, then it probably does not have any clinical relevance. Related to this is the statement sometimes heard with regard to therapeutic trials: if a medication works, its effect will be apparent without the aid of any measurements. The benefit of pyridostigmine (Mestinon) in myasthenia gravis, for example, was demonstrated without resorting to intraesophageal pressure measurement.

If one examines the premise, it will be noted that quantitation is yet lurking within it. Assume that a boy with Duchenne dystrophy is treated with an experimental drug, and after two months of treatment he is no longer confined to a wheelchair but is walking and climbing stairs with normal strength. Obviously, the drug cures the illness; neither manual muscle strength testing nor myometry is required to determine this. In fact, a very accurate system of quantitation is involved, but it is internalized. Experience has taught the observer that the change in the quantity of strength in the natural history of the illness varies in proportion to the age of the child. Experience, moreover, has taught the observer that there is a quantitative difference in strength between a boy who is confined to a wheelchair and one who is walking normally—and that the difference between these two states is far greater than could be accounted for by chance.

We are thus not debating whether quantitation is worthwhile, but whether it should be sharpened in order to detect the smaller changes. Common sense would seem to say

Supported by a grant from the Muscular Dystrophy Association and a Public Health Service Research Grant (RR-36) from the General Clinical Research Center Branch, Division of Research Facilities and Resources, Bethesda, MD.

yes. The real answer, however, is that it depends. In the case of the boy with Duchenne dystrophy and the magic pill, it would be ludicrous to set up a complicated (and expensive) system of measurements when a very simple evaluation would suffice. On the other hand, there are many clinical situations in which more precise measurements are mandatory. Therefore, the first statement about quantitation that should be made is that the system of quantitation should be tailored to the clinical situation to which it is applied. A particular system of measurement is only "good" or "bad" when considered in the light of what it is required to do in a given clinical situation. Just how good or bad it is must be judged by the evaluation of its reliability, variability, and reproducibility—not in the abstract but in a particular situation.

Just as the appropriateness of a measurement cannot be cited without knowledge of the clinical situation in which it is to be used, the "meaning" of a measurement is difficult to interpret in isolation. One might say, for example, that an individual's height is 100 cm. This can be interpreted only when one knows some additional facts—for example, that his weight is 80 kg, or that her age is 8 years. This is self-evident with respect to everyday measurements but not to laboratory measurements. A creatine kinase level of 500 IU, for example, cannot be interpreted without knowing the patient's sex, state of training, and prior exercise activity.

An additional aspect of quantitation could be termed the "usefulness" of the method. Obviously, a test that is invasive and causes a lot of discomfort is less useful than one that is non-invasive. Similarly, the necessity for complex and expensive laboratory equipment operated by highly trained personnel may render a good system of measurement useless in the clinical arena.

A final problem with many of our measurements is that they require the patient's cooperation. This is not always freely given, especially if the patient has a vested interest in the outcome of the test.

Thus, the ideal measurement should be obtained by methods that are noninvasive, simple to perform, and independent of patient cooperation whenever possible. It should also offer high sensitivity and reproducibility and low variability. Unfortunately, such measurements are few and far between.

The need for standardized normative data and inter- and intraobserver reliability is beyond discussion and must be met before any measurement takes its place as a useful test.

FATIGUE AND EXERCISE

Fatigue and exercise are not two independent aspects of muscle function. They are related as closely as opposite sides of the same coin. It is impossible to experience one without the other. There are semantic problems with the word *fatigue,* which is used to refer to many different states. It is often used by people with multiple sclerosis to indicate how they feel. It is experienced by the neurasthenic, and even by neurologists on their way home late at night. In this discussion we will use the word only as it is used by exercise physiologists, who define it as the failure to maintain the required expected power output.[1]

It is important to recognize that there are at least two types of exercise. The first is exemplified by jogging, swimming, bicycling, and walking. Such exercise can be sustained for half an hour or longer, is often repetitive in nature, and is best thought of as endurance exercise. It is traditionally associated with type 1 muscle fibers with high oxidative capacity, and the biochemical mechanisms supporting it are aerobic. The second type of exercise is exemplified by weight-lifting and occurs when the subject exerts maximum muscular power for brief periods of time. It is carried out mainly by type 2 glycolytic fibers, and the biochemical pathways behind it are relatively anaerobic. The delineation between the two types of exercise is not absolute; for example, it is difficult to decide whether the pathways supporting an olympic marathon runner at the end of a close race are aerobic or anaerobic.

Muscular fatigue may be due to one of four mechanisms: failure of oxygen delivery, failure of adenosine triphosphate (ATP) supplies, failure of the contractile mechanism, and failure of the central mechanisms of muscle excitation. All may be tested, although it may be difficult to isolate a single factor. Bicycle ergometry is used to obtain information on cardiovascular and respiratory function (it also requires normal muscle biochemistry). To some extent, forearm exercise tests bypass the demands on the cardiovascular system and give more information on the ATP support systems of muscle. Failure of contractile mechanisms can be adduced from some interesting studies on evoked contractions that have received little attention from clinicians. The studies outlined in this chapter are all related to fatigue in the muscles rather than fatigue due to central or neural influences. This important type of fatigue is beyond the scope of this chapter, but is well covered in the work of Edwards[1] and others.

INCREMENTAL BICYCLE ERGOMETRY

An adequate supply of oxygen to muscles working at maximum capacity can be provided only if pulmonary function, cardiac output, oxygen-carrying capacity of the blood, and vascular supply to the limbs are normal. Pulmonary function can be assessed by measuring forced vital capacity (FVC), maximum voluntary ventilation (MVV), and maximum expiratory pressure (MEP). In addition, the amount of air exhaled in the first second of a forced expiration (FEV_1) can be useful in evaluating obstructive pulmonary disease. Normally, 85 to 95% of the total FVC should be expired during the first second of a forceful expiration. The MVV is an important measurement because during heavy exercise the demand for pulmonary ventilation may be greater than 180 L/min in young people[2] (Table 8.1).

There is also a change in cardiac output, which may increase sixfold or more to values of 20 to 30 L/min in the trained individual.[3] Cardiac output is difficult to measure (although noninvasive metholds are available), but in the normal individual it is reliably reflected by the heart rate.

The oxygen-carrying capacity of the blood is often forgotten as a possible cause of exercise failure. Any degree of anemia will impair the individual's ability to exercise. The symptoms may not be noticed at rest, but such an individual will not be able to exercise up to the normal maximum levels for his or her age.

Table 8.1   Formulas for Forced Vital Capacity (FVC) and Maximum Voluntary Ventilation (MVV) in Adults

FVC (L)
  Men: $0.052 \times$ height (cm) $- 0.022 \times$ age (years) $- 3.60 \pm 0.58$
  Women: $0.0508 \times$ height (cm) $- 0.032 \times$ age (years) $- 3.02 \pm 0.52$
MVV (L/minute)
  Men: $(86.5 - 0.522 \times$ age$) \times$ body surface area (m^2)
  Women: $(71.3 - 0.474 \times$ age$) \times$ body surface area (m^2)

The increase in blood supply to an exercising muscle is quite large and is, of course, responsible for the increased cardiac output. Any diminution in the capacity of the vascular system to provide the additional blood will be associated with fatigue. Intermittent claudication is the hallmark of a limb compromised in this fashion.

It is common in exercise physiology laboratories to use the incremental bicycle exercise test to evaluate many of these factors. The requirements for the test are a properly calibrated bicycle ergometer and a means of evaluating oxygen and carbon dioxide concentrations in the inspired and expired air. In addition, the patient's electrocardiogram (ECG) should be monitored. This test is not entirely benign and should be done in a well-controlled environment. Strenuous exercise in elderly patients or in patients who may be susceptible to myoglobinuria can have serious consequences. At the beginning of the test, the subject is seated on the bicycle ergometer, either resting or pedaling against a very low load. The subject then pedals against a known load while the oxygen consumption and carbon dioxide production are measured for that level of work. At regular intervals, usually every minute, the work is increased until the subject is physically exhausted and cannot continue at the demanded load. The measurements obtained are the maximum work output (Wmax), the oxygen consumption for each level of work (VO$_2$), the maximum oxygen consumption (VO$_2$max), the maximum heart rate, and the amount of carbon dioxide exhaled at each level. Values derived from these measurements include the hyperventilation or anaerobic threshold, the respiratory exchange ratio (RER), and the "efficiency" of the muscle, which may be expressed by the ratio of oxygen consumed to work performed.

Before relying on such an analysis, one has to decide whether the test was successful or not. In the normally fit individual, there is a steady increase in heart rate and oxygen consumption as the test proceeds. Because an individual can draw on energy reserves in muscle that utilizes anaerobic pathways, he or she can exercise beyond the work load at which maximum oxygen consumption occurs. If the oxygen consumption is plotted against the work load, this phenomenon is evident as a steady increase that reaches a definite plateau (Figure 8.1). It is important to see this plateau to be sure that the test was successful and that the VO$_2$ was indeed maximum. If the VO$_2$max is not evident in this fashion, the patient either has insufficient motivation or an abnormality in the metabolic supply to the muscle. If the test is satisfactory, the values obtained may be compared against those in normal subjects as follows.

Maximum heart rate varies considerably according to the age of the patient. In a 20-year-old, maximum heart rate may be expected to be around 200 beats per minute.

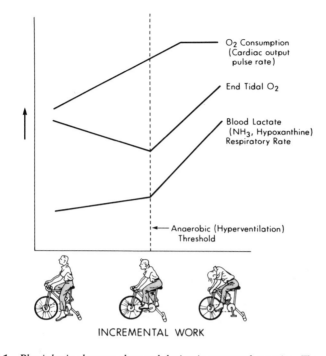

INCREMENTAL WORK

FIGURE 8.1 *Physiologic changes observed during incremental exercise. The vertical axis represents increasing values for each of the factors. The horizontal axis represents increasing levels of work. Oxygen consumption reaches a maximum plateau; this is the VO_2max. Blood lactate and respiratory rate show a discontinuous relationship with a threshold (indicated by the broken line) that occurs at about 60% of the maximum level of work in an untrained individual. This hyperventilation threshold is also detected by measuring the end-tidal oxygen level, which initially decreases but then increases as exercise-induced hyperventilation occurs. (If each breath is not held in the lung long enough to permit maximum oxygen extraction, the percentage of oxygen in the exhaled air is increased.)*

A rule of thumb is that it decreases by 1 beat per minute every year after this age. There is, however, a disproportionately large decrease in heart rate in the decade after 40, making it about 165 beats per minute at 50 years of age.[4,5]

The VO_2max is more variable. It is higher in men than in women and is affected by an individual's level of training. Normal values in the healthy individual are upwards of 3 L/min in men and 2 L/min in women, with both being higher in youth.[6] The VO_2max is markedly influenced by body weight, and for this reason the oxygen uptake is often expressed as milliliters per kilogram of body weight per minute. Values of 35 ml/kg/min and above may be considered normal. However, it should be noted that the normal values found in the literature are rather high when related to patients in a neuromuscular clinic (Table 8.2). The reason is simply that normative data requires the participation of normal volunteers. Most exercise physiology laboratories attract people who are particularly interested in athletics and exercise. Therefore, the population from which they draw their ''normal'' volunteers tends to be on the

Table 8.2   Maximum Oxygen Consumption (VO_2max) (ml/kg/min)

	Students	Controls	Paranormals
Men	49.9 ± 7 (N = 15)	38.3 ± 2.7 (N = 6)	30.8 ± 9 (N = 8)
Women	—	37.1 ± 5.8 (N = 8)	—

muscular side and is perhaps not truly representative of the average person, who is more likely to spend time watching television than jogging. It is more accurate to calculate the oxygen uptake relative to lean body mass rather than total body weight, but accurate assessment of lean body mass is technically difficult. For the ordinarily proportioned person, the percentage of body weight that represents fat is 20% in women and 10% in men.[7] Unfortunately, patients in the neuromuscular clinic are often not of a typical habitus, so it may not be very safe to use these numbers.

Respiratory effort also increases during the performance of an incremental exercise test. This increase is not linear. The curve is discontinuous, with a sharp acceleration in ventilation occurring about two thirds of the way to maximal performance (Figure 8.1). Traditionally, this threshold is believed to be associated with the greater participation of anaerobic mechanisms of energy supply and the appearance of lactate in the blood. It is sometimes called the onset of blood lactate accumulation (OBLA) and has also been called the anaerobic or hyperventilation threshold.[8,9] It does not seem to be specifically related to lactate, however, since a definite anaerobic threshold was noted in a patient with McArdle's disease.[10] Perhaps the threshold is associated with the activation of nonoxidative mechanisms of energy supply in general. Lactate accumulation is only one result. The importance of the anaerobic threshold lies in its correlation with the individual's state of training. There is a definite association between the anaerobic threshold expressed as the percentage of the VO_2max and the individual's performance.[11] For example, the higher the anaerobic threshold of marathon runners, the faster they can complete a race.

The last measurement that can be obtained from the incremental test is the respiratory exchange ratio (RER), which can be of great importance in neuromuscular disease. The RER is the ratio of the amount of carbon dioxide produced to the amount of oxygen used. When fat is the predominant source of energy, as it is at rest, the ratio is approximately 0.7. When carbohydrate is utilized as the predominant fuel, the ratio is 1; for protein, the number is 0.82. During the incremental test, the RER starts out at around 0.8 and climbs as exercise becomes progressively more strenuous. At very high levels of exercise, it usually exceeds 1, because with the exercise-induced hyperventilation, the amount of CO_2 that is eliminated exceeds the amount produced by the actual combustion of fuels in muscle.

Another useful derived statistic is the relationship between the oxygen uptake and the work load. This relationship is a linear one until the point of VO_2max (Figure 8.2). The ratio represents the oxygen cost of performing a given amount of work. In a control population, the average figure is 1.65 ± 0.14 ml of oxygen kpm/min.[12]

In the normal population, many of these measurements are interrelated. Forced vital capacity and VO_2max show a linear correlation, as might be expected (Figure 8.3). Heart rate and oxygen uptake, as well as Wmax and VO_2max, are also related to each other in linear fashion.

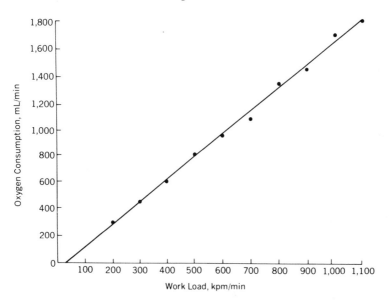

FIGURE 8.2   *The relationship between oxygen consumption and work load is linear until levels equivalent to the VO₂max are reached. The slope of this line is a measure of the body's efficiency in converting chemical energy to work.*[12]

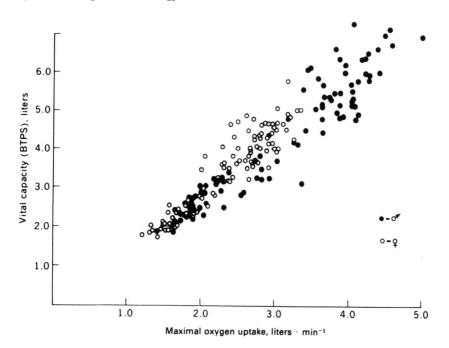

FIGURE 8.3   *Individual data on vital capacity (measured in the standing position) in relation to maximal oxygen uptake during running or cycling in 190 subjects from 7 to 30 years of age. BTPS denotes at body temperature and ambient pressure. (Reprinted by permission from Astrand PO and Rodahl K.* Textbook of work physiology, *3rd Edition, McGraw Hill, 1986.)*

Use of Incremental Bicycle Ergometry in Neuromuscular Disease

A 14-year-old boy complained that for three years he had experienced muscle soreness after vigorous exercise. The pain would often begin about 10 minutes after the start of prolonged heavy exercise. If he then rested, the pain gradually subsided and disappeared within an hour or so. His symptoms were neither exacerbated nor relieved by manipulation of his diet. He had not noticed that fasting made them worse. Although he had no real weakness, he was not able to keep up with his peers in competitive sports. Muscle biopsy revealed no definite structural abnormality. An incremental exercise test was carried out. The Wmax was 1050 kpm, maximum heart rate was 196 beats per minute and VO_2max was 35.6 ml/kg/min. The respiratory exchange ratio was 0.98 at the beginning of the test and 1.22 at the end of the test (values indicated in Table 8.2).

The fact that his heart rate was close to 200 beats per minute, which is the normal maximum heart rate for his age, indicates that the effort he put into this test was indeed maximal. This is reassuring, since both the final work rate and the oxygen consumption were rather low for his age group. Without the evidence of the maximum heart rate, one might suspect that poor motivation was the limiting factor. Evidence to the contrary was reinforced by the fact that the VO_2 reached a definite plateau at the higher levels of work, indicating that the patient's effort had not ceased before the work demanded was greater than the level that could be supplied by increased oxygen consumption (i.e., when mainly anaerobic mechanisms were being used). The RER, even at rest, never dropped far below 1. This implies that fatty acids were not being used as a source of energy. After the incremental exercise test, it was concluded that the boy had a defect in fatty acid utilization, which was lowering both his power output and oxygen utilization. Biochemical studies of the muscle showed an absence of carnitine palmityl transferase (CPT), confirming the diagnosis. Table 8.3 also includes the results on a second patient with CPT deficiency, for comparison.

In patients with myophosphorylase deficiency, incremental bicycle ergometry has suggested a defect in muscle oxidative metabolism.[13-15] In these cases, both Wmax and VO_2 were abnormally low. The respiratory exchange ratio was lower than normal and reached a maximum of 0.96, rather than the more usual maximum of 1.1 or more. This was presumably due to an inability to utilize carbohydrate and a dependence on fatty acid energy sources. An attempt to correct this abnormality by infusing glucose (which in theory should bypass the block caused by phosphorylase deficiency) increased VO_2max but did not return the value to normal; neither did it return the RER to normal. In addition, cardiac output and ventilatory response to the stress of exercise were greater than normal. The authors postulated that these were compensatory mechanisms to attempt to increase the blood-borne metabolites to the muscle. The excessive ventilatory response was returned to normal by glucose infusion and fasting. Few studies have been done in other glycolytic disorders. In phosphoglycerate mutase deficiency, no abnormality was noted.[16]

Patients with disorders of mitochondrial function have not been extensively tested. Uncoupling oxidative phosphorylation leads to fatigue, excessive lactate production,

Table 8.3 Results of Incremental Bicycle Ergometry in Two Patients with Carnitine Palmityl Transferase Deficiency

	Patient 1[a]	Patient 2
Age (yr)	17	21
VO$_2$max (ml/kg/min)	35.6	37.9
Maximum heart rate	196	200
RER at rest	0.98	0.96
RER at end of test	1.22	1.18
Wmax (kpm/min)	1050	1300

[a] Patient 1 is discussed in the text.

and hyperkinetic cardiac and ventilatory responses. In patients with complex I or complex III deficiency, a markedly abnormal increase in heart rate and lactate production occurred at very low levels of exercise.[17-19] This type of response is predictable, since the patient's inefficient utilization of oxygen would be expected to produce the same physiologic effects as strenuous exercise in the normal subject. A useful screening measure in patients suspected of having a mitochondrial disorder is the oxygen cost of the work performed. The change from resting oxygen consumption to maximal oxygen consumption is fairly linear, proportional to the change in work load. The appropriate regression analysis gives a measure of the oxygen cost per increase in load. In the normal population, this is about 1.7 ± 0.14 in men and 1.6 ± 0.12 in women. One aspect of this test that diminishes its usefulness in practice is that for this coefficient to be calculated reliably, it is necessary to measure enough points to permit the performance of a regression analysis for the appropriate correlation coefficient. Many patients in the neuromuscular clinic are not strong enough, or cannot exercise long enough, to provide sufficient data. Nevertheless, if the basal VO$_2$ is abnormally high or if the VO$_2$max is out of proportion to the maximum work load, a defect in mitochondrial function may be suspected. In one 16-year-old boy, the Wmax was 750 kpm, which is too low for his age, but the corresponding VO$_2$max, at 40 ml/kg/min, was disproportionately high and indicated inefficient oxygen utilization.

Endurance or aerobic training can produce a marked change in the measurements discussed above.[20] For effective training to occur, the exercise must be taken regularly for a given length of time, and the level of work must be set in relationship to the subject's maximum potential. In practical terms, exercise that is carried out four days a week, lasts 30 to 40 minutes, and is at a level sufficient to increase the heart rate to 60 to 70% of maximum is adequate to produce a training effect. Such training increases the VO$_2$max, reduces the heart rate at any given absolute level of work (but does not decrease the maximum heart rate), and reduces the amount of lactate produced by the working muscle. It also affects the release of CK from the muscle. In the untrained muscle, moderate exercise ordinarily causes a release of CK, which usually peaks 10 to 18 hours after the exercise. In the trained muscle, there is either no release of CK or a decreased release of CK.[21,22]

FOREARM EXERCISE

Incremental bicycle exercise employs large groups of muscles and tests the body's response to exercise rather than evaluating individual muscles. Forearm exercise is a popular method of evaluating the response of a small group of muscles.[23] A strong repetitive hand grip over a brief period of time does not tax the cardiovascular system. This, coupled with the availability of venous blood draining the muscles of the forearm, makes it easy to study the biochemical response to muscle stress. It was McArdle's early observation that ischemic exercise in a young man with exercise-induced symptoms did not result in lactate production that prompted his speculation about the presence of a glycolytic defect.[24] The ischemic exercise test has since been used almost routinely in the diagnosis of McArdle's disease (though Munsat has noted that it is unlikely to be successful unless proper attention is given to quantitation[23]). The subject grips with the hand at a frequency of 60 Hz against a spring, allowing measurement of the work performed. A cuff is inflated around the upper arm at a pressure sufficient to prevent the circulation of blood through the forearm, and the correlation between work done and lactate is noted. The correlation is most accurate for short period of work (about a minute or so). The use of the ischemic forearm test has been limited to screening for lactate production, perhaps because in McArdle's time the known metabolic disorders were those involving glycolytic enzymes.

In 1978 an interesting enzyme deficiency was noted in the muscle of several patients.[25] Although these patients produced lactate quite normally with forearm exercise, the normal rise in ammonia did not occur. Ammonia is normally produced by deamination of adenosine monophosphate (AMP), which was absent in these patients. The association of ammonia production with myoadenylate deaminase gave an interesting insight into the adenosine/triphosphate (ATP) support systems. The well-known adenylate kinase reaction converts two molecules of adenosine diphosphate (ADP) to ATP and AMP. The deaminase then eliminates the AMP, promoting the reaction in favor of ATP production. The more ATP supplies are depleted, the more they will be replenished by this reaction, and the more ammonia will be produced. Rumpf et al. noted abnormally brisk production of ammonia in a patient with McArdle's disease and postulated that this was a compensatory mechanism to correct for the abnormal biochemical stress.[26]

Since the deamination of ammonia results in the formation of inosine 5'-monophosphate (IMP), which is converted to hypoxanthine, one would expect hypoxanthine and ammonia levels in the blood to behave similarly. Forearm exercise studies have shown that the presence of hypoxanthine in the venous blood is entirely due to the deamination of AMP after exercise and that in a number of metabolic disorders, the presence of biochemical stress on the muscle may be deduced from the presence of an exaggerated hypoxanthine response (Figure 8.4).[27,28]

The majority of laboratories and clinics use an ischemic forearm test (as outlined in Table 8.4)) or some modification of it.[29] This test has certain limitations. Unless the degree of fatigue is extreme, it is difficult to detect subtle differences in such a short time period. Similarly, since all of the biochemical mechanisms are heavily stressed by this form of exercise, it is suitable for detecting an absence of metabolites but is

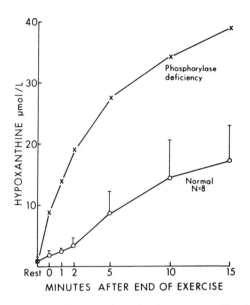

FIGURE 8.4 *Measurements of hypoxanthine levels in venous blood (μmol/L) after forearm exercise show exaggerated hypoxanthine response in a patient with McArdle's disease, compared with eight normal controls. The standard deviations of the measurements are indicated by the vertical bars.*

relatively insensitive in detecting an overproduction of metabolites at low work levels. For example, in some of the mitochondrial myopathies, even small amounts of work produce abnormally high amounts of lactate. The ischemic exercise test does not give this a chance to happen. Even without the occlusion of the blood supply, maximum repetitive grip sustained for a minute calls for an amount of work from the forearm muscles that cannot be supported by the resting blood flow. Even low to moderate work loads will necessitate a more than fivefold increase in the resting blood flow to reach a steady state,[30] and this increase does not take place for some minutes. We found no difference in lactate production when the occluding cuff was omitted. We have designed an incremental forearm test that gives information on maximum grip strength and fatigue and also allows lower levels of work to be structured into the test.

The literature offers few good statistics on hand-grip strength in normal individuals. The reason is fairly simple. Grip strength is dependent on muscle bulk, and an individual's maximum grip may vary from 50 newtons in an elderly lady to over 450 newtons in a husky young man.

Prior to the performance of the incremental forearm test, the patient's maximum grip is measured. The arm is then rested, and after 20 minutes the patient repetitively grips a device at 30 Hz (1.5 seconds grip, 0.5 seconds rest). The device is a force transducer coupled to an oscilloscope so that the patient, by gripping with more or less force, can match two lines on the oscilloscope screen. By programming the "target" line, the patient can be made to grip with a given force. The program is set up in such

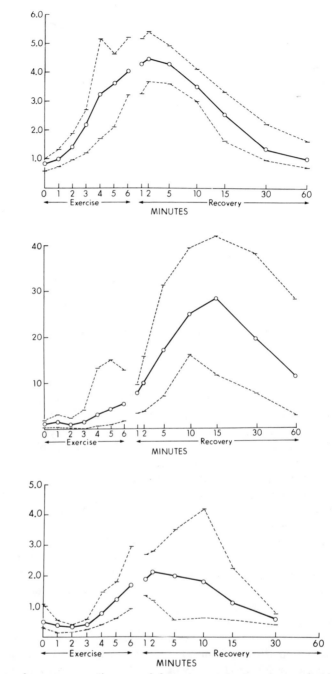

FIGURE 8.5 *Normal responses to incremental forearm exercise in ten normal volunteers. (A) venous lactate (μmol/ml), (B) venous hypoxanthine (μmol/ml), and (C) venous ammonia (μg/ml). The solid line represents the mean. The broken lines represent the highest and lowest values.*

Table 8.4 Peak Forearm Test Values Attained in Normal Subjects (μmol/L)

Method	Ischemic	Lactate	Ammonia	Hypoxanthine
80% MVC @ 30 Hz until exhausted[23]	Yes	5.7 ± 1.8	1.75 ± 0.47	
4–7 kpm @ 60 Hz for 1 min[29]	Yes	3 – 5 × resting level (2.5 – 5)		
Incremental forearm until exhausted	No	4.8 (range, 4.4–5.4)	2.5 mg/L (range, 1.4–4.2)	30.0 (range, 19.8–42.0)

a way that during the first minute of the test the subject grips at 10% of the predetermined maximum load, during the second minute at 20%, during the third at 30%, and so on, until the subject cannot attain half of the demanded load. This usually occurs after 5 or 6 minutes. The results of this test are illustrated graphically in Figures 8.5 and 8.6. In summary, there is an early rise in lactate, with the greatest change usually occurring in the second minute. The ratio of lactate to pyruvate changes accordingly. Ammonia appears somewhat later (the early slight drop in ammonia levels may be due to an increase in blood flow). The relative change in hypoxanthine is greater than that in any of the other metabolites, but the peak levels in the blood are reached about 15 minutes after the end of exercise.

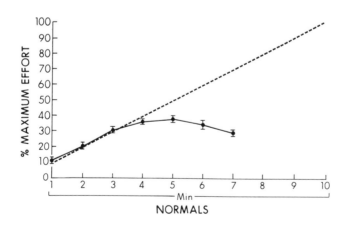

FIGURE 8.6 *Mechanical fatigue in incremental forearm exercise. The straight diagonal line (broken) represents the effort demanded of the patient, which can be contrasted with the force actually exerted. The vertical bars represent the standard errors of the means.*

31P NUCLEAR MAGNETIC RESONANCE SPECTROSCOPY

New techniques using nuclear magnetic resonance (NMR) have added another dimension to forearm exercise. To obtain direct information about ATP levels in the working muscle has always been difficult and is now possible for the first time.

The technique of NMR spectroscopy, which is concisely reviewed by Meyer et al.,[31] is based on the fact that phosphorous nuclei behave like magnetic dipoles. When placed in a strong magnetic field and exposed to bursts of radio frequency, their rotations change in such a way as to induce a signal in the spectrometer. Because the characteristics of the dipole are very sensitive to changes in the environment, the signal from each phosphorus group differs. Those of ATP will differ from each other and from the signals of phosphorous in other compounds. Similarly, changes in the pH in the cell will change the appearance of the resulting spectra.

There are both advantages and disadvantages to NMR spectroscopy. The less "mobile" the phosphorous, the less likely it is to be detected. Thus, phosphorous firmly bound to large molecules (such as the ADP associated with actin) is not detected. This may be an advantage, since this ADP is inactive in intermediary energy metabolism and confuses the more standard biochemical assays. On the other hand, NMR is not a very sensitive technique, and large amounts of tissue are therefore needed to provide a signal for interpretation. The lack of sensitivity requires that repetitive signals be averaged over a certain time period. This means that NMR spectroscopy is less useful in evaluating rapidly changing states than in evaluating those that are relatively stable. Nevertheless, it is the first noninvasive test that gives fundamental information about the behavior of muscle in vivo (Figure 8.7). Because of the size of magnets currently available, the forearm represents about the largest group of muscles that can be consistently investigated. In several laboratories, repetitive forearm exercise has been studied in both normal controls and patients with exercise-related ill-

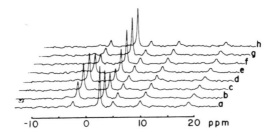

FIGURE 8.7 *Stimulation-recovery cycle, showing 31P NMR spectra of cat soleus muscle. Five-minute scans recorded before (a), during (b thorugh d), and after (e through h) 15 minutes of isometric stimulation at 60 twitches per minute. PPM denotes peaks per minute. The tracings are aligned so that individual peaks can be compared. The three small peaks at the right of each tracing represent the phosphorus groups in ATP. The peak at the left, which is initially low but becomes progressively higher until tracing d, represents inorganic phosphate. The largest peak (second from the left) represents creatine phosphate. As can be seen, this decreases during exercise and then returns to normal during the recovery phase. (Reprinted with permission of Meyer et al.[31])*

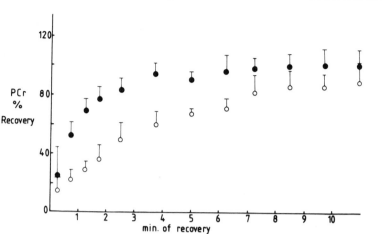

FIGURE 8.8 *Phosphocreatine levels after forearm exercise in a patient with a mitochondrial disorder and in normal subjects. The means and standard deviations in 13 normal subjects (open circles) are shown with those of four examinations of the patient (closed circles). Levels of phosphocreatine fall lower in the patient and recover more slowly toward normal. (Reproduced with permission of Arnold et al.[32])*

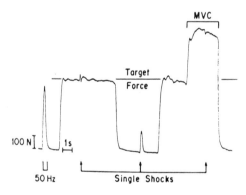

FIGURE 8.9 *Force records of the soleus muscle. Shown are electrical stimulation of the muscle by 8 pulses at 50 Hz (far left); the twitch produced by a single electrical shock superimposed on the target-force voluntary contraction (left arrow); the twitch produced by a single electrical shock from the relaxed muscle (middle arrow); and the maximum voluntary contraction (MVC) (right arrow). In the middle of the MVC, a single electrical shock evoked no additional tension from the contracting muscle. (Reproduced with permission from Bigland-Ritchie et al.[35])*

nesses.[32,33] Most exercise protocols have used repetitive voluntary grip as the exercise stimulus. Electrical stimulation of the muscle has also been used and shown to be roughly equivalent.[34] The major change is a decrease in the peak representing creatine phosphate and an increase in the inorganic phosphate peak (Figure 8.7). The signals from the phosphates in ATP do not change. NMR also provides new information about the recovery of these exercise-provoked changes (Figure 8.8). Studies in patients with various mitochondrial disorders have shown an abnormally low ratio of phosphocreatine to inorganic phosphate at rest, suggesting that the energy supplies were depleted.[32] A long period of many minutes was often needed for the restoration of phosphocreatine to its resting levels, which would also suggest energy depletion.

WHEN IS A VOLUNTARY CONTRACTION NOT A MAXIMAL CONTRACTION?

As noted above, there is an important difference between normal volunteers undertaking exercise studies and patients with a variety of neuromuscular symptoms. One can be fairly certain that the normal volunteers are motivated to produce their best efforts. This is not so for the patients. Sometimes it is difficult to tell whether patients are not trying or whether their illness is limiting their ability to exert. A technique is available to shed some light on this, and it has been little used in human neuromuscular disease.[35] If a muscle is required to sustain a voluntary contraction, and if in the middle of the contraction an electrical stimulus is delivered to the muscle, a superimposed twitch may be noted, unless the contraction is a maximal voluntary one (Figure 8.9). The amplitude of this evoked superimposed twitch is proportional to the difference between the voluntary contraction and the maximum voluntary contraction. The twitch will be large in a muscle that is minimally contracted, and small in a muscle that is contracted almost to the maximum. This technique has been used to investigate the fatigue associated with sustained or repetitive contractions. A sustained contraction of any muscle can be maintained for a limited period of time. As the force of the contraction approaches maximum, this time is shortened to as little as a few seconds. The force of the quadriceps muscle was recorded during repetitive contractions lasting 6 seconds, interspersed with rest periods of 4 seconds. The target force was 50% of the maximum voluntary contraction. After approximately 4½ minutes, subjects were unable to sustain this degree of contraction. The amplitude of the evoked twitch had also declined during the same interval, indicating a progressive failure of the maximum contractile force that could be exerted by this muscle. During the period of fatigue, the integrated electromyographic data did not change, even though the maximum voluntary contraction dropped by 50%. This implies that the fatigue is due to a failure of contractile apparatus rather than any fatigue in the neural apparatus. It would be of great interest to apply this type of technique to patients with neuromuscular fatigue.

REFERENCES

1. Edwards RHT. Human muscle function and fatigue. In Edwards RHT, ed. Human muscle fatigue: physiological mechanisms. CIBA Foundation Symposium #82. London: Pittman Medical, 1981; 1–18.
2. Ruppel G. Manual of pulmonary function testing. St. Louis: C.V. Mosby, 1982; 3.
3. Astrand PO, Rodahl K. Textbook of work physiology. New York: McGraw Hill, 1986; 3.
4. Astrand I. Aerobic work capacity in men and women with special reference to age. Acta Physiol Scand 1960; 49 (suppl 169).

5. Astrand I, Astrand PO, Rodahl K. Maximal heart rate during work in older men. J Appl Physiol 1959; 14:562.
6. McArdle WD. Comparison of continuous and discontinuous treadmill and bicycle tests for max VO_2. Med Sci Sports Exerc 1973; 5:156.
7. Von Dobeln W. Human standard and maximum metabolic weight in relation to fat free body mass. Acta Physiol Scand 1956; 37(suppl 126):287.
8. Wasserman K, Whipp BJ, Koyal SN, et al. Anaerobic threshold and respiratory gas exchange during exercise. J Appl Physiol 1973; 35:236.
9. Karlsson J, Jacobs I. Onset of blood lactate accumulation during muscular exercise as a threshold concept. Int J Sports Med 1982; 3:190.
10. Hagberg JM, Coyle EF, Carroll JE, et al. Exercise hyperventilation in patients with McArdle's disease. J Appl Physiol 1982; 52:991–4.
11. Karlsson J, Sjodin B, Jacobs I, et al. Relevance of muscle fiber type to fatigue in short, intense, and prolonged exercise in men. In: Edwards RHT, ed. Human muscle fatigue: physiological mechanisms. London: Pittman Medical, 1981; 59–74.
12. Carroll JE, Hagberg JM, Brooke MH, et al. Bicycle ergometry and gas exchange measurements in neuromuscular diseases. Arch Neurol 1979; 36:457–61.
13. Haller RG, Lewis SF. Abnormal ventilation during exercise in McArdle's syndrome: modulation by substrate availability. Neurology 1986; 36:716–9.
14. Lewis SF, Haller RG. The pathophysiology of McArdle's disease: clues to regulation in exercise and fatigue. J Appl Physiol 1986; 61:391–401.
15. Haller RG, Lewis SF, Cook JD, et al. Myophosphorylase deficiency impairs muscle oxidative metabolism. Ann Neurol 1985; 17:196–9.
16. Kissel JT, Beam W, Bresolin N, et al. Physiologic assessment of phosphoglycerate mutase deficiency: incremental exercise tests. Neurology 1985; 35:828–33.
17. Land JM, Morgan-Hughes JA, Clark JB. Mitochondrial myopathy. Biochemical studies revealing a deficiency of NADH-cytochrome B reductase activity. J Neurol Sci 1980; 50:1–13.
18. Morgan-Hughes JA, Darvenica P, Kahn SM, et al. A mitochondrial myopathy characterized by a deficiency in reducible cytochrome B. Brain 1977; 11:617–40.
19. Kennaway NG, Buist NRM, Darley-Usmar VM, et al. Lactic acidosis and mitochondrial myopathy associated with deficiency of several components of complex 3 of the respiratory chain. Pediatr Res 1984; 18:991–9.
20. McArdle WD, Katch FI, Katch VL. Exercise physiology. Philadelphia: Lea & Febiger, 1986; 2.
21. Brooke MH, Carroll JE, Davis JE, et al. The prolonged exercise test. Neurology 1979; 29:636–43.
22. Brooke MH. A Clinician's View of Neuromuscular Diseases. Baltimore: Williams & Wilkins, 1986.
23. Munsat TL. A standardized forearm ischemic exercise test. Neurology 1970; 20:1171–8.
24. McArdle B. Myopathy due to a defect in muscle glycogen breakdown. Clin Sci 1951; 10:13–33.
25. Fischbein WN, Armbrustmacher VW, Griffin JL. Myoadenylate deaminase deficiency: a new disease of muscle. Science 1978; 200:545–8.
26. Rumpf KW, Wagner H, Kaiser M, et al. Increased ammonia production during forearm ischemic work test in McArdle's disease. Klin Wochenschr 1981; 59:1319–20.
27. Patterson VH, Kaiser KK, Brooke MH. Exercising muscle does not produce hypoxanthine in adenylate deaminase deficiency. Neurology 1983; 33:784–6.
28. Brooke MH, Patterson VH, Kaiser KK. Hypoxanthine and McArdle disease: a clue to metabolic stress in the working forearm. Muscle Nerve 1983; 6:204–6.
29. Sinkeler SP, Wevers RA, Joosten EM, et al. Improvement of screening in exertional myalgia with a standardized ischemic forearm test. Muscle Nerve 1986; 9:731–7.
30. Wahren J, Hagenfeldt L. Human forearm muscle metabolism during exercise. I. Circulatory adaptation to prolonged forearm exercise. Scand J Clin Lab Invest 1968; 21:257.

31. Meyer RA, Kushmerick MJ, Brown TR. Application of 31P NMR spectroscopy to the study of striated muscle metabolism. Am J Physiol 1982; 242:C1-11.
32. Arnold DL, Taylor DJ, Radda GK. Investigation of human mitochondrial myopathies by phosphorous magnetic resonance spectroscopy. Ann Neurol 1985; 18:189-96.
33. Eleff S, Kennaway NG, Buist NRM, et al. 31P NMR study of improvement in oxidative phosphorylation by vitamins K3 and C in a patient with a defect in electron transport at complex 3 in skeletal muscle. Proc Natl Acad Sci 1984; 81:3529-33.
34. Shenton DW, Heppenstall RB, Chance B, et al. Electrical stimulation of human muscle studied using 31P nuclear magnetic resonance spectroscopy. J Orthoped Res 1986; 4:204-11.
35. Bigland-Ritchie B, Furbush F, Woods JJ. Fatigue of intermittent and submaximal voluntary contractions: central and peripheral factors. J Appl Physiol 1986; 61:421-9.

Chapter 9

A Methodologic Approach to Studying the Effects of Age and Disease on the Spatiotemporal Properties of Ambulation

A.M. Ferrandez, Jean Pailhous, and Georges Serratrice

The behavioral aspects of ambulation have received little attention in the neurology literature. Published work is primarily devoted to the neurobiologic basis of locomotion and more commonly focuses on normal rather than differential aspects, such as pathological or ontogenetic features. Very few works have compared ambulation in the young adult to that in older adults or children.[1-4] Studies of locomotor development usually use as their upper limit the earliest age at which children are able to walk, and use as their lower limit the first few weeks after birth.[5,6] Although these studies investigate the structural aspects of locomotion, they neglect adaptive capabilities. For the purposes of this chapter, we have examined the studies on ambulation and will propose a methodologic approach to studying the effects of age and disease on spatiotemporal aspects of walking.

The lack of studies on disturbances of ambulation in adults and on the evolution (and degeneration) of locomotor adaptation may reflect the perception of locomotion as a stereotyped movement. Generally, automatic aspects have been emphasized in studies of the rhythmic structure and morphology of locomotion.[7-9] Winter[10] found that joint angle patterns and electromyographic profiles are invariable, and Bernstein[11] used the force pattern to analyze the structural elements involved in muscular activity. Other unchanging elements, such as kinesthetic constants, have been observed in the stride, and invariable ratios have been found to exist in the duration of the stance versus swing phase in both walking and running.[12,13]

Studies on the structure of locomotion have been reviewed by two of us (A.M.F. and J.P.).[14] Most such studies focus on characteristics of the stride, which is generally defined as the distance covered or time elapsed between heel strikes of the same foot.

By emphasizing the stereotypic aspects of walking, these studies consider the apparatus more than the function. Thus, the first biologic function of locomotion—displacement—has been ignored. The effects of displacement on vision (especially on optical flow[15]) and the voluntary aspects of displacement (particularly movement-triggering and modulation) have also been neglected.

In short, the adaptive capabilities of ambulation have often been overlooked—yet because of its repetitive nature, locomotion is capable of significant correction. For example, when we cross the street, we step onto the opposite curb with our preferred foot. This is true for well-lateralized adults but not for small children, even those who have already learned to walk. In the adult, gait is adjusted in the course of several steps; thus, when one is walking, the step just reaching the curb is neither very long nor very short and the correction is performed unconsciously. The implications of this activity are twofold: the first is that locomotion parameters are kept constant unconsciously; the second is that these parameters are modified in a subtle and repetitive way.

Study of the adaptive capabilities of locomotion would naturally differ from the study of locomotor structure. Adaptations may be elicited centrally (e.g., through voluntary acceleration) or environmentally (e.g., through one's adaptation to irregular ground). Study of the structure involves determining the gait-patterning mechanisms, whereas study of the adaptive capabilities examines the laws governing the variations on gait patterns. Discovering these laws involves determining the correlations between stride length and velocity values and calculating the percentage of variation from one step to the next. Both efforts require quantification.

DATA COLLECTION METHODS

The study of adaptive capabilities in locomotion is a dual process. First, phasic and tonic ability must be measured while the subject's walking behavior is observed. Second, spatiotemporal parameters (stride length, cadence, and velocity) must be measured. Given the sequential nature of locomotion, data must be collected over several consecutive strides. The data concern four areas.

The first area to observe is gait stability from one stride to the next, which can be determined by calculating the percentage of variation between two consecutive strides and repeating this calculation for all the strides. Usually the value obtained is about 2 or 3% in a given experimental condition and can be reduced to 1% if the subject is asked to "always walk the same way."

The second area to observe is the links between parameters, which are calculated as correlations (e.g., cadence/velocity, stride length/velocity, stride length/cadence). These correlations obey well-defined laws. In adults and 6- to 8-year-old children with no locomotor deficits, we found strong links when analyzing velocity (i.e., correlations between cadence and velocity and between stride length and velocity) and weak links between cadence and stride length. A subject's velocity could be inferred from the stride length, but his or her cadence could not (Figure 9.1)[16]

The third area of concentration is modulations of locomotion. The word *modulation* is used when the values of parameters are modified but the correlations remain the

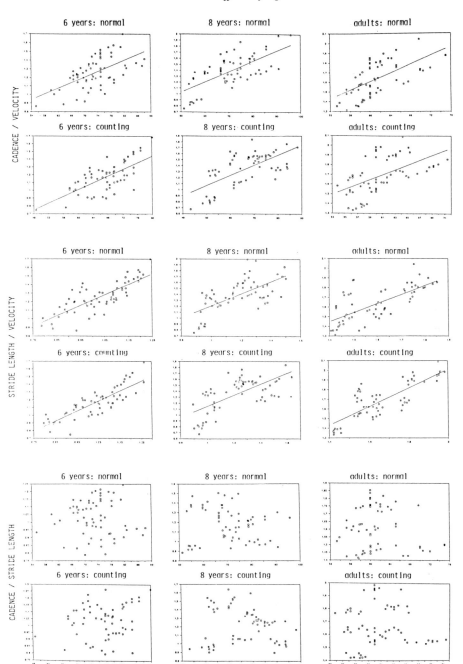

FIGURE 9.1 *Spatiotemporal structuring of locomotion. Correlations were calculated for each pair of parameters. Strong links were found between cadence and velocity and between stride length and velocity; weak links were found between cadence and stride length.*

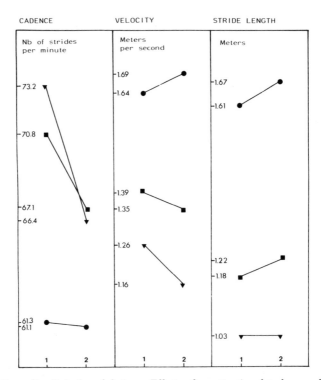

FIGURE 9.2 *Centrally elicited modulations. Effects of an attentional task on walking parameters in 6- and 8- year-old children and in adults. The subjects' attention was focused on cadence (they had to count their steps). Cadence decreased in children but not in adults.*

same. Modulations are obtained by varying the experimental conditions (Figures 9.2 and 9.3).[16] There are several ways to calculate the significance of modulations, although we generally use statistical tests (analysis of variance [ANOVA] being the most popular) to judge whether the difference between two values was a random event or caused by experimental factors.

The final area of testing involves determining the relative role of stride length and cadence in an observed increase or decrease in velocity. Usually, an increase in velocity involves increases in both cadence and stride length; this participation is termed cooperative. But in some cases, stride length and cadence are rival (e.g., when the increase in velocity is produced by a significant increase in cadence despite a decrease in stride length). It is important to determine what type of participation is involved in the accelerative or decelerative processes. When the participation is cooperative, it is useful to calculate precisely what percentage of the velocity variation is due to stride length and what percentage is due to cadence (Figures 9.4 and 9.5).[16,17] Whether the velocity variation is significant can be determined by ANOVA.

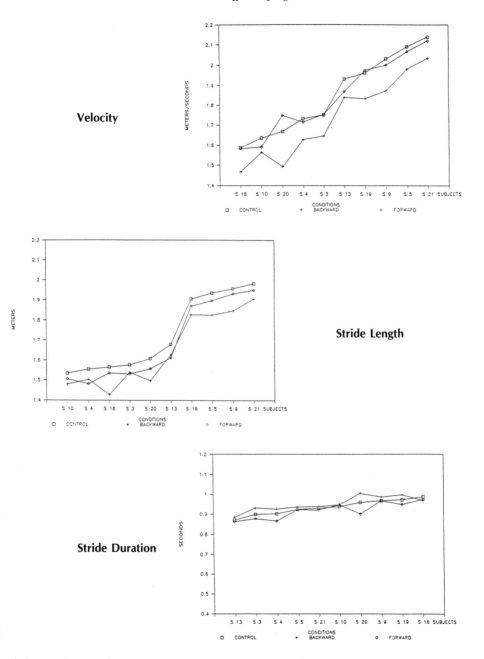

Velocity

Stride Length

Stride Duration

FIGURE 9.3 *Environmentally elicited modulations. Effects of different optical flows on walking parameters. The subjects were required to always walk in the same way. All parameters decreased when the optical flow was directed against the subject's direction of locomotion (backward condition).*

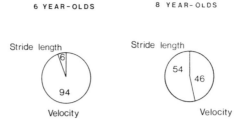

FIGURE 9.4   *Relative participation of stride length and velocity in the variation of cadence. The observed decrease in cadence between the free-walking situation and the counting-steps situation was due to decreases in stride length and velocity. The decrease in velocity was most important in 6-year-old children, whereas decreases in velocity and stride length were almost equally important in 8-year-old children.*

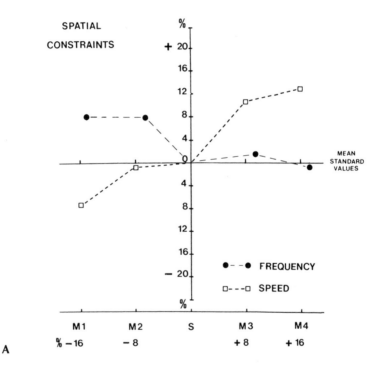

A

FIGURE 9.5   *Constraints on cadence and stride length. (A) Variations in stride frequency and walking speed when stride length was imposed. The figure shows the mean percentage variation in speed and stride frequency relative to free gait(s). Under conditions M1 and M2, the subject walked with shorter strides than when moving freely (16 and 8% shorter than the reference stride length, respectively). Under conditions M3 and M4, the subject had to lengthen his or her stride (8 and 16% more than the reference stride length, respectively).*

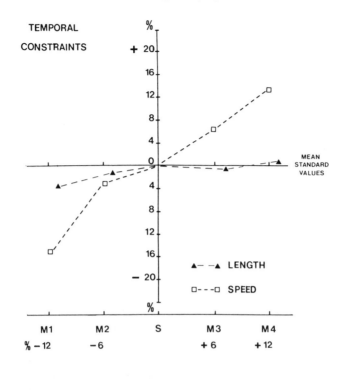

FIGURE 9.5 (Continued) *(B) Variations in stride length and walking speed when stride frequency was imposed. The figure shows the mean percentage variation in speed and stride length relative to free gait(s). Under conditions M1 and M2, the subject walked at a slower stride frequency than when moving freely (12 and 6% less than the reference stride frequency, respectively). Under conditions M3 and M4, the subject walked with a greater stride frequency than when moving freely (6 and 12% greater than the reference stride frequency, respectively).*

EXPERIMENTAL CONDITIONS

One experimental condition for studying locomotion deficits involves having subjects walk at a lively pace (i.e., that spontaneously used in walking toward an object to pick it up) without giving them any specific instructions regarding pace. Locomotor characteristics, particularly the patterns of links between parameters, are more apparent at a higher velocity.[17] The "lively pace" study is the only one that permits fine evaluation of locomotor problems due to aging or disease. By comparing the data from that study with data from a control group (nondisabled), one is able to determine what kind of locomotor problem is involved. The affectation of small steps or general slowing of all motor activity can be quantified. Thus, a comparison of stride length or duration data in experimental and control subjects allows for a rapid and precise evaluation of locomotive disorders. Alterations less easily discerned, such as deterioration of links between parameters, can also be demonstrated through comparative studies of experimental and control subjects.

Acceleration and deceleration are useful experimental conditions. They should be combined in a two-part process by first using the $N, N - 1$ computations to predict changes in velocity between strides and then calculating the percentage change in velocity due to the increased stride length and cadence.

CENTRAL VERSUS ENVIRONMENTAL FACTORS

Central factors to be considered in the control of locomotion include such things as the effect on locomotion when a subject is instructed to count his or her steps. When children count their steps while walking, their cadence decreases; this alteration is not seen in adults (Figure 9.2).[16] Synchronization between the rhythms of walking and counting requires attentional processes that are not fully developed in children. In adults, problems with this mechanism are generally seen in either elderly subjects or subjects with attentional disorders.

Environmental factors, such as the effect of loads on walking gait, can also alter locomotion.[18] One can investigate the effects of different load-carrying conditions on posture and locomotion (e.g., have the subject carry a backpack, or a double pack that distributes the load equally between the subject's front and back).

Finally, the perceptual conflict paradigm (e.g., the conflict between proprioceptive and visual information) and the resulting deviation in directional displacement can be studied by having the subject wear prismatic glasses to create the illusion of walking up or down a slope. How a subject adapts to the altered visual perspective can provide important information on locomotor disorders. Analysis of posture and gait in such situations can also provide important clues to the general motor-adaptive capabilities of elderly patients and may increase our understanding of the variations in locomotion that occur in advanced age.

CONCLUSION

The proposed methods of observing locomotor patterns and modulations thereof permit a fine degree of quantification of disorders related to aging or disease. In particular, they enable the investigator to distinguish between problems that lead to abnormalities in individual parameters and problems that affect the correlations between parameters. For example, the effective stride length can be diminished in older adults. Thus, one may postulate that older adults could walk slowly with smaller steps at a slower cadence without altering the pattern of links between parameters (for example, correlations between velocity and cadence and velocity and stride length would be maintained). Disorders affecting locomotor structure, such as a waddling or shuffling gait, can exist without affecting adaptive capabilities. Likewise, these disorders may not affect the stability of the gait (i.e., they may cause only a slight percentage of variation from one stride to the next) or the relative participation of cadence and stride length involved in acceleration.

By using this program in conducting research, investigators will be able to dissociate disorders affecting the structure of ambulation from those affecting modulation capabilities. They will also be able to investigate various pathological disorders efficiently. In doing so, they will contribute to a better understanding of locomotor problems caused by disease and of the motor problems that arise in aging populations.

REFERENCES

1. Crowninshield RD, Brand RA, Johnston RG. The effects of walking velocity and age on hip kinematics and kinetics. Clin Orthop 1966; 132:140–4.
2. Grieve DW. Gear RJ. The relationships between length of stride, step frequency, time of swing and speed of walking for children and adults. Ergonomics 1966; 5:379–9.
3. Murray MP, Drought AB, Kory RC. Walking patterns of normal men. J Bone Joint Surg 1964; 46:335–60.
4. Murray MP, Kory RC, Clarksson BH, et al. Comparison of free and fast speed walking patterns of normal men. Am J Phys Med 1966; 45:8–24.
5. Forssberg H. Ontogeny of human locomotor control: 1. Infant stepping, supported locomotion and transition to independent locomotion. Exp Brain Res 1985; 57:480–92.
6. Thelen E, Bradshaw G, Ward JA. Spontaneous kicking in month-old infants: manifestations of human central locomotor program. Behav Neural Biol 1981; 32:45–53.
7. Delcomyn F. Neural basis of rhythmic behavior in animals. Science 1980; 210:492–8.
8. Grillner S. Control of locomotion in bipeds, tetrapods and fish. In: Brooks VB, ed. Handbook of physiology. Section 1: The nervous system. Washington, DC: American Physiological Society. 1981; 2.
9. Shik ML, Orlovski GN. Neurophysiology of locomotor automatism. Physiol Rev 1976; 56:465–501.
10. Winter D. Biomechanical motor patterns in normal walking. J Motor Behav 1983; 15: 302–30.
11. Bernstein N. The co-ordination and regulation of movements. Oxford: Pergamon, 1967.
12. Grillner S, Halbertsma J, Nilsson J, et al. The adaptation to speed in human locomotion. Brain Res 1979; 165:177–82.
13. Shapiro DC, Zernicke RF, Gregor RJ, et al. Evidence for generalized motor programs using gait pattern analysis. J Motor Behav 1981; 13:33–47.
14. Ferrandez AM, Pailhous J. From stepping to adaptive walking: modulations of an automatism. In: Whiting HTA, Wade MG, eds. Themes in motor development. Dordrecht, Netherlands: Martinus Nijhoff, 1986; 265–78.
15. Gibson JJ. Visually controlled locomotion and visual orientation in animals. Br J Psychol 1958; 49:182–94.
16. Ferrandez AM, Pailhous J. A note on modulations and structuring of locomotion in children and adults. J Motor Behav 1986; 18:475–85.
17. Laurent M, Pailhous J. A note on modulation of gait in man: effects of constraining stride length and frequency. Hum Movement Sci 1986; 5:333–43.
18. Kinoshita H. Effects of different loads and carrying systems on selected biomechanical parameters describing walking gait. Ergonomics 1985; 28:1347–62.

Chapter 10

The Use of Quantitative Techniques to Define Amyotrophic Lateral Sclerosis

Theodore L. Munsat, Patricia L. Andres, and Linda M. Skerry

Over the past decade, the Neuromuscular Research Unit at Tufts–New England Medical Center has had a primary interest in the clinical therapeutics of neuromuscular disease, particularly amyotrophic lateral sclerosis (ALS).[1-5] We have assumed that if an effective drug were found, it would most likely provide modest or temporary amelioration of the disease rather than total cure. We have therefore sought to devise a measurement process capable of detecting change that is less than clinically obvious.

A review of existing measurement techniques suggested that a new approach was essential; in our judgment, even the most commonly used testing procedure, the ALS score,[6] has major methodologic deficiencies. The ALS score consists of 34 items rated on a scale of 0 to 3, with a normal score of 100. The items include an admixture of functional assessments, symptoms, reflexes, and signs, all of which are weighted equally and summated to achieve a single value. Items such as bowel and bladder function (rarely involved in ALS) and plantar reflexes (rarely abnormal) are given significance equal to that of items such as speech, respiratory function, and the ability to stand. Reliability and validity data for the ALS score are not available. The data generated are ordinal.

We were interested in designing a test battery that was sensitive to minor change, clinically meaningful, reliable (i.e., reproducible), inexpensive, time-efficient, and valid (i.e., as direct as possible in its measurement of the voluntary motor system). This thinking led us to select maximum voluntary isometric contraction (MVIC) as the essential element in our test battery, which we call the Tufts Quantitative Neuromuscular Exam (TQNE). MVIC measurements were supplemented by a limited number of timed repetitive functional tests in attempt to assess the upper motor neuron

(UMN) component of ALS (measurement of UMN deficit continues to be a very difficult problem). In its early forms, the TQNE was used in several negative clinical drug trials.[2-5] We have now published the current version, a 28-item examination that takes about 40 minutes to administer.[1]

DATA TRANSPOSITION

One of the several major problems with existing rating and grading scales is that values of individual performance items do not reflect the relative clinical and pathological significance of a given neurologic deficit. This considerably reduces the sensitivity of the test battery. For example, the ALS score[6] values equally a positive Babinski sign and whether or not the patient is able to stand unaided. Similarly, using the mean absolute strength loss of a small muscle and a large muscle gives a distorted picture of the actual clinical change and the contribution of the individual muscles to the composite score. Also, many items in existing scales are measured disparately (e.g., in kilograms, in seconds, and "present or absent"), which precludes effective statistical analysis.

It became clear to us in the early development of the TQNE that a data transformation step was essential. This would simultaneously compensate for improper item-weighting and the use of different measurement units. Although several such transformations are available (e.g., in the Blom score[7]), we elected to use a z-score transformation, which relates derived raw data to the mean performance of a large representative group of ALS patients as follows:

$$\text{z-score} = \frac{\text{raw score} - \text{ALS population mean}}{\text{ALS population standard deviation}}$$

To represent the "world" of ALS patients against which each raw value is judged, ALS population means and standard deviations were calculated by randomly selecting a single value for each test item from each of 176 carefully defined ALS patients in our data bank. Alternatively, we could have related raw data to a normal population, but we considered this less desirable, given our interest in studying therapeutic intervention as well as natural history. We concluded that the comparison to other similarly affected individuals was more appropriate. We assumed that our patient population was indeed representative of all ALS patients, as there was nothing in our referral patterns to suggest otherwise. There was nothing unique about the way ALS patients entered our clinical facilities, as compared with ALS patients elsewhere. The z-score values are thus expressed in standard deviation units, so that a value of +1 means that a patient's score is 1 SD above the mean of "all" ALS patients, whereas a score of −1 indicates that it is 1 SD below that mean. The transformed data can be displayed as a regression line against time to reflect the disease's natural history or analyze a therapeutic intervention (Figure 10.1).

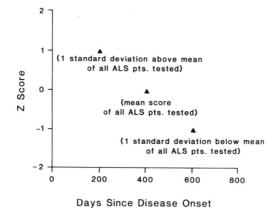

FIGURE 10.1 *Technique of plotting z-scores against time. This technique can be used for individual TQNE items or for megascores. Score values are thus expressed as standard deviation units.*

DATA REDUCTION: THE USE OF COMPOSITE SCORES (MEGASCORES)

The next stage of development was a data reduction step. A meaningful data reduction process was considered necessary for a number of reasons. The most obvious one—an enlarging data base that becomes increasingly cumbersome to manage—is only a relative issue in these days of advanced computer capability. A more important consideration was the statistical probability of a "positive" therapeutic effect resulting from the large number of evaluations carried out. With a probability level of 0.05, there is one chance in every 20 evaluations of observing "benefit" fortuitously. Studies using large numbers of outcome variables, including the analysis of multiple subgroups, are in danger of a Type I error—i.e., finding a therapeutic intervention to have limited benefit when in fact it does not. It is more statistically sensitive to work with a smaller number of measurement outcomes, preferably five to eight.

In ALS, data reduction has clinical relevance. Our early observations led us to believe that muscles innervated by adjacent spinal cord segments behave similarly. This observation was strongly supported by our factor-loading analyses (Figure 10.2), which clearly demonstrated the regional character of the disease. For example, muscles of the arm behaved more like other muscles of the arm than like muscles of the leg or bulbar muscles. The aggregation of muscle functions into anatomically relevant groupings thus had biologic as well as statistical significance. In addition, using the mean of a number of related z-scores would further enhance the sensitivity of the measurement by balancing out positive and negative measurement errors.

As part of our factor-loading analyses, we carefully pulled out test items found

		FACTOR 1	FACTOR 2	FACTOR 3	FACTOR 4	FACTOR 5	FACTOR 6
FVC	3	0.215	0.763	0.003	0.199	-0.008	-.0.039
MVV	4	0.105	0.728	-0.114	0.339	0.020	0.138
PA	8	0.114	-0.056	0.141	-0.904	-0.016	0.083
PATA	12	0.043	0.013	0.182	-0.907	-0.072	0.089
BLOW	18	-0.013	0.238	-0.233	0.804	-0.144	0.116
SPEECH	19	-0.151	0.056	-0.066	0.930	0.101	-0.058
swallow	20	-0.212	0.189	-0.051	0.810	-0.080	0.127
distance	24	0.769	0.106	0.185	-0.125	0.047	0.425
gait	25	0.859	-0.024	0.086	-0.225	0.156	0.299
stairs	26	0.862	0.060	0.188	-0.173	0.123	0.272
curbs	27	0.874	0.060	0.184	-0.141	0.142	0.282
floor	28	0.595	0.245	0.289	-0.224	0.218	0.359
toilet	29	0.803	0.085	0.227	-0.111	0.360	0.095
bed	30	0.729	0.055	0.136	-0.129	0.373	0.172
chair	31	0.790	0.155	0.203	-0.073	0.297	0.188
tlegstan	33	0.311	0.107	0.039	0.074	-0.170	0.645
comb	39	0.108	0.179	0.825	-0.155	0.108	0.271
teeth	40	0.052	0.176	0.869	-0.162	-0.108	0.156
faucet	42	0.108	-0.026	0.806	-0.143	-0.012	0.124
wash	43	0.149	0.281	0.712	-0.235	0.346	0.162
feed	44	0.003	0.118	0.910	-0.205	-0.054	-0.054
cut	45	0.038	0.185	0.695	-0.124	0.498	-0.018
dressUE	46	0.156	0.172	0.773	-0.250	0.290	-0.022
dressLE	47	0.314	0.020	0.387	-0.289	0.555	0.198
write	48	-0.034	0.088	0.720	-0.023	0.269	-0.061
phoneR	51	-0.045	-0.056	-0.637	-0.265	-0.454	0.158
phoneL	52	-0.210	-0.137	-0.136	-0.187	-0.709	0.070
pegbdR	57	0.119	0.044	0.710	-0.007	0.486	-0.253
pegbdL	58	0.135	0.023	0.296	-0.025	0.812	-0.087
shdflexR	61	0.142	0.804	0.464	0.070	-0.009	0.086
shdflexL	62	0.130	0.882	0.219	-0.056	0.171	0.131
shdextR	63	0.234	0.829	0.361	0.140	-0.019	0.010
elbflexR	65	0.165	0.698	0.612	0.108	-0.003	0.038
elflexL	66	0.114	0.795	0.241	-0.015	0.282	0.137
elbextR	67	0.121	0.745	0.512	0.131	-0.012	0.049
elbextL	68	0.259	0.791	0.223	0.004	0.195	-0.004
gripR	70	0.150	0.510	0.707	0.056	0.133	-0.129
gripL	71	0.140	0.479	0.250	-0.107	0.496	-0.010
hipextR	74	0.650	0.570	-0.124	0.086	0.09	-0.177
hipextL	75	0.572	0.679	-0.095	0.027	0.045	-0.099
hipflexR	76	0.640	0.643	-0.043	0.106	-0.170	-0.220
kneextR	78	0.709	0.539	0.069	0.078	-0.113	-0.181
kneextL	79	0.717	0.498	-0.018	-0.076	-0.001	-0.174
kneflexR	80	0.773	0.378	-0.100	0.099	-0.035	-0.189
kneflexL	81	0.812	0.362	-0.154	0.064	0.047	-0.112
dorsiR	82	0.841	0.162	0.132	-0.035	-0.078	-0.114
dorsiL	83	0.807	0.063	0.064	-0.101	0.030	0.004

FIGURE 10.2   *Rotated factor loadings (pattern).*

to be both clinically and statistically redundant (i.e., providing no additional information). Prior to data reduction, the TQNE contained 48 items (Figure 10.2). Subsequently, 28 items remained, which conveniently and appropriately sorted into 5 composite scores, termed *megascores* (Table 10.1). We most commonly excluded items of functional performance that were adequately covered by MVIC measurements. This allowed us to omit items that were both statistically redundant and clinically less desirable because of the less direct nature of the measurement. For example, we deleted timed one-leg stands from Mega 5; cough rating, forehead movement, and timed

Table 10.1. TQNE Composition

Megascores	*Number of Items*
Mega 1 (pulmonary function)	
FVC	1
MVV	1
Mega 2 (bulbar function)	
Diadochokinetic rates	
"pa"	1
"pata"	1
Mega 3 (timed activities)	
Dialing a 7-digit phone number	2
Purdue pegboard	2
Mega 4 (arm strength)	
Isometric arm strength, measured with an electronic	
strain gauge	8
Grip strength, measured with a Jamar dynamometer	2
Mega 5 (leg strength)	
Isometric leg strength, measured with an electronic	
strain gauge	10
Total	28

drinking from Mega 2; and fastening a safety pin and tapping a pencil from Mega 3.

At the end of this analytic process, we were left with five megascores that had both statistical and biologic relevance to the disease and that could be used to analyze its natural history as well as therapeutic interventions.

NATURAL HISTORY OF ALS

Studies purporting to define the natural history of ALS almost exclusively examine the clinical aspects of age of onset, region of onset, and time of death.[8-12] There are no studies available that document the rate of motor neuron loss—which, in our view, should be the main focus of a natural history study. Thus, our present knowledge of the rate and pattern of motor loss remains descriptive, anecdotal, and subjective. This lack of knowledge of the true natural history of ALS is unfortunate, as valid data on true disease progression are essential for appropriate patient management, interpretation of therapeutic intervention, proper design of clinical trials, and generation of new theories of pathogenesis and etiology.

In an attempt to provide more meaningful data, we used the TQNE in sequential measurement for up to 67 months (mean $\pm$SD, 21 $\pm$13.5; range, 8 to 67) in 50 representative patients. Our goal was to define more accurately the pattern of motor neuron loss that characterizes this disease. The 50 patients selected for this study all had carefully defined ALS.[13] Patients with atypical features were excluded. All patients had eight or more complete TQNEs over a period of eight or more months. Patients with incomplete data points were excluded. Data were stored in a VAX 750 computer in formats of the CLINFO system (National Institutes of Health). Statistical packages resident in CLINFO and BMDP were utilized for analyses. The basic determinants analyzed were the regression plots of individual and composite (megascore) items, plotted against time. The date of disease onset was established by patient interview. Megascore regression lines are referred to as *Megaslopes*. A megaslope of -1 indicates that the megascore declined by 1 SD per year. Figures 10.3 through 10.7 illustrate representative megaslopes. Repeated measures of ANOVA were used for calculation of statistical significance between several subgroups, and two-tailed t tests were used for two group comparisons.

Details of the results of this analysis have been submitted for publication and can be summarized as follows:

1. Analysis of the five regional megaslopes for all 50 patients (Table 10.2) revealed that bulbar function deteriorated more slowly than respiratory function, hand dexterity, and arm strength. Leg strength deteriorated slightly less rapidly than arm strength.

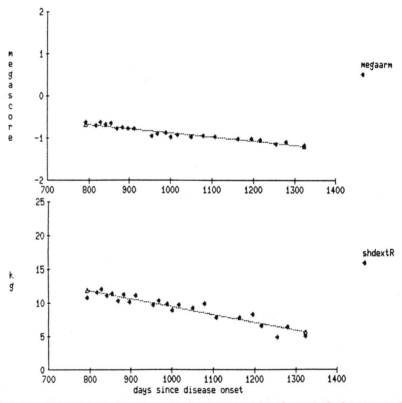

FIGURE 10.3   *ALS Patient 1 demonstrating deterioriation plots for a single function (right shoulder extension [shdextR]) and a composite function for arms (mega-arm).*

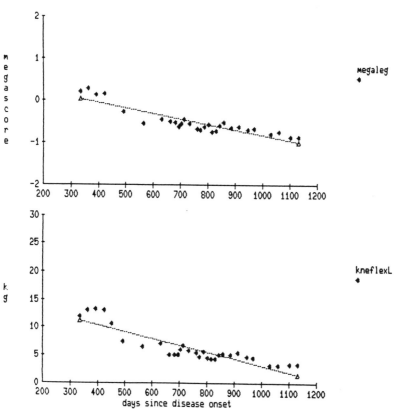

FIGURE 10.4   *ALS Patient 2 demonstrating deterioration plots for a single function (left knee flexion [kneflexL]) and a composite function for leg (mega-leg).*

2.   Subgroup analyses suggested that sex, age of onset, and region of onset did not significantly influence deterioration rates, with the exception that arm strength showed somewhat more rapid decline in men.

3.   Deterioration rates indicative of motor neuron loss were remarkably linear in form (Figures 10.3 through 10.7). Detectable plateaus or significant alterations in the rate of deterioration were not seen. Once linear deterioration had begun, we did not observe significant flattening of the slope, with the exception that several patients "bottomed out" at a low level of function. That is, just prior to complete loss of function, when only a small number of motor units remained, there seemed to be an arrest of further loss.

4.   Although ALS may begin asymmetrically, deterioration rates were found to be similar between the two sides of the body and between proximal and distal muscles.

Most papers on the natural history of ALS have focused on patient longevity as the major course determinant. This may give a false impression of the true character of motor neuron loss. In our experience, time of death is often more closely related

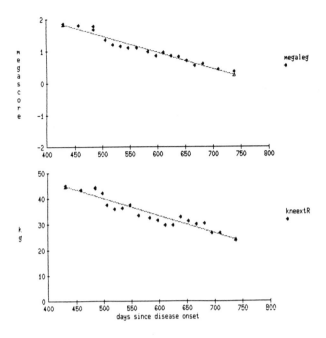

FIGURE 10.5   *ALS Patient 3 demonstrating deterioration plots for a single function (right knee extension [kneextR]) and a composite function for leg (mega-leg).*

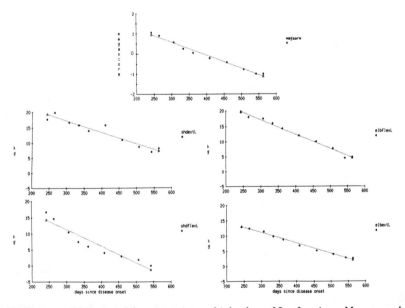

FIGURE 10.6   *ALS Patient 4 demonstrating multiple plots of five functions. Mega-arm denotes megaslope for arms; shdextL, left shoulder extension; elbflexL, left elbow flexion; shdflexL, left shoulder flexion; elbextL, left elbow extension.*

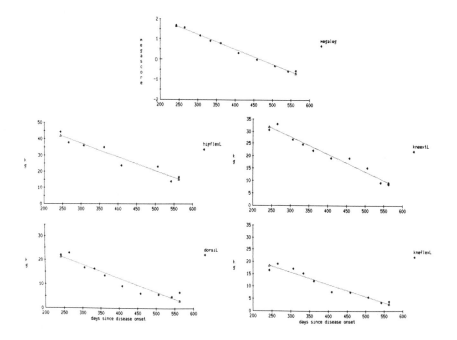

FIGURE 10.7   *ALS Patient 5 demonstrating multiple deterioration plots. Megaleg denotes leg megascore; hipflexL, left hip flexion; kneextL, left knee extension; dorsiL, left foot dorsiflexion; kneflexL, left knee flexion.*

to the adequacy of pulmonary function. Thus, factors such as chronic obstructive pulmonary disease and smoking history are powerful outcome determinants.

We believe the above data represent a more accurate characterization of the disease, which should prove useful in the design of future clinical trials. For example, if patients who are deteriorating rapidly are selectively randomized in a controlled drug trial, it will be possible, knowing the linearity of the disease and the measurement error, to make a preliminary judgment of the drug's efficacy in as few as four patients within a period as short as 4 months. This would allow the time-efficient screening of a large number of different drugs or drug analogues with therapeutic potential.

APPLICATIONS TO CLINICAL PRACTICE

Do these results and observations have relevance to the daily practice of neurology? We believe they do. We would like to suggest that the traditional neurologic examination is inadequate for documenting motor performance impairment with reliability. In fact, the motor examination is grossly deficient in this respect, as it does not allow the objective documentation of change in performance. Performance change with time is usually assessed on the basis of the patient's history. That is, if the patient and his

Table 10.2   Deterioration Rates among 50 Patients, Expressed as Decline in Standard Deviation Units per Year

Megaslope	Mean (±SD)	Range	P Values				
			1	2	3	4	5
1	−1.001 ±0.82	−0.080 to −4.033					
2	−0.776 ±0.58	−0.009 to −2.143	0.002				
3	−1.073 ±0.89	−0.020 to −4.176	0.649	0.0001			
4	−0.978 ±0.66	−0.031 to −3.139	0.964	0.004	0.591		
5	−0.828 ±0.62	−0.230 to −3.770	0.173	0.648	0.135	0.043	

family say things are better, then the neurologist usually records that information. Major changes, of course, are apparent to both patient and neurologist, but more subtle and often meaningful modifications are difficult, if not impossible, to determine with accuracy. Thus, we suggest that the need for quantitation, so clear in clinical research, is increasingly apparent in clinical practice as well. This need cannot be met by the manual muscle test, and certainly not by the traditional neurologic examination. The reproducible measurement of MVIC is not difficult or expensive; it should become an integral part of the study of any patient with weakness. For the individual practitioner, we suggest two alternatives. MVIC could be measured at the bedside with one of the several hand-held myometers available. In a hospital, a physical therapist could be trained to use a strain-gauge tensiometer. For the neurologist practicing as part of a group, we suggest a dedicated measurement table in the group practice area or adjacent physical therapy department. Data can be reported in a clinically useful manner, becoming an integral part of the patient's chart (Figures 10.8 and 10.9).

A dedicated motor measurement laboratory could gradually expand into a broader neurofunction measurement facility with capabilities for measuring extrapyramidal, sensory, autonomic, and cognitive function as well. Such a laboratory would serve as an extension of the bedside neurologic examination, providing meaningful data for important management and therapeutic decisions. The information so gained would clearly lead to more cost-effective management, with ineffective therapies quickly identified.

ISOMETRIC TESTING

New England Medical Center
Neuromuscular Unit
Quantitative Isometric Strength Test

Date	Female Norms mean(s.d.)				
Weight					
FVC					
MVV					
Shd Flex R	15.9(2.7)				
Shd Flex L	15.1(2.5)				
Shd Ext R	19.4(3.7)				
Shd Ext L	17.9(3.8)				
Elb Flex R	18.9(3.2)				
Elb Flex L	17.8(2.6)				
Elb Ext R	12.4(2.2)				
Elb Ext L	11.7(2.4)				
Grip R	25 (6)				
Grip L	22.0(4)				
Hip Ext R	24.8(6.6)				
Hip Ext L	24.5(6.8)				
Hip Flex R	34.7(8.4)				
Hip Flex L	34.1(7.9)				
Knee Ext R	35.9(8.6)				
Knee Ext L	34.8(9.1)				
Knee Flex R	17.7(4.5)				
Knee Flex L	17.9(4.8)				
DorsiFlex R	21.1(4.6)				
Dorsiflex L	20.2(4)				

Scores indicate maximal isometric strength in kgs measured by strain gauge
tensiometer with pt. in specified position. Testing variability is about
9% from mean of serial scores.

Examiner:_____   DOB_____HEIGHT_____
Meds.:_____
Comments:_____
_____
_____

FIGURE 10.8   *Form for isometric testing.*

LONGITUDINAL STRENGTH TESTING

New England Medical Center
Neuromuscular Unit
Quantitative Isometric Strength Test

Patient J.K.

Date	Female Norms mean (s.d.)	7-14-82	2-24-84	8-2-85	8-14-86
Weight		93	91	93	90
Shd Flex R	16.0(3.7)	11.0	10.0	9.3	10.6
Shd Flex L	15.5(3.6)	2.7	4.0	3.7	4.3
Shd Ext R	20.0(5.1)	13.5	13.0	12.2	13.0
Shd Ext L	17.5(4.5)	13.0	12.0	12.7	11.3
Elb Flex R	18.5(3.4)	14.3	15.0	14.2	14.6
Elb Flex L	18.0(3.3)	14.3	14.2	15.3	13.8
Elb Ext R	12.5(2.7)	11.5	10.0	10.7	10.9
Elb Ext L	11.5(2.4)	10.3	9.3	10.3	9.7
Grip R	24.5(6.3)	10.0	10.0	9.0	6.0
Grip L	22.0(4.7)	20.0	19.0	20.0	20.0
Hip Ext R	24.0(8.0)	18.2	15.0	17.0	16.1
Hip Ext L	24.0(7.9)	9.3	6.5	4.7	6.2
Hip Flex R	33.5(9.5)	25.0	24.0	20.3	20.1
Hip Flex L	33.5(8.5)	23.0	20.7	16.0	17.2
Knee Ext R	36.0(8.9)	5.0	4.3	4.5	4.7
Knee Ext L	34.5(9.8)	6.7	6.2	3.3	3.8
Knee FlexR	18.5(5.7)	5.5	5.7	4.7	5.1
Knee FlexL	18.0(5.4)	5.5	5.5	4.5	4.2
DorsiflexR	21.0(3.8)	13.2	10.0	11.2	12.2
DorsiflexL	20.0(3.1)	14.7	13.0	11.2	12.6

Scores indicate maximal iosmetric strength in kgs measured by strain gauge
tensiometer with pt. in specified position. Testing variability is about 9%.

Examiner: _____P.A._____ DOB__8-14-62____ HEIGHT___5' 0"____
Meds.: _____none_____
Comments:_____

FIGURE 10.9   *Results of longitudinal testing in a representative patient.*

REFERENCES

1. Andres PL, Hedlund W, Finison L, et al. Quantitative motor assessment in amyotrophic lateral sclerosis. Neurology 1986; 36:937–41.
2. Keleman J, Hedlund W, Murray–Douglas P, et al. Lecithin is not effective in amyotrophic lateral sclerosis. Neurology 1982; 32:315.
3. Keleman JK, Hedlund W, Orlin JB, et al. Plasmapheresis with immunosuppression in amyotrophic lateral sclerosis. Neurology 1983; 40:752.
4. Munsat TL, Easterday CS, Levy S, et al. Amantadine and guanidine are ineffective in ALS. Neurology 1981; 31:1054.
5. Mora JS, Munsat TL, Kao KP, et al. Intrathecal administration of natural human alpha interferon in amyotrophic lateral sclerosis. Neurology 1986; 36:1137–40.
6. Norris FH, Calanchini PR, Fallat RJ, et al. The administration of guanidine in amyotrophic lateral sclerosis. Neurology 1974; 24:721–8.
7. Miller JP. A parsimonious approach to data transformations. Proceedings of the 1977 Statistical Computer Section of the American Statistical Association. 1977; 327–31.
8. Garruto RM. Bibliography of amyotrophic lateral sclerosis and parkinsonism-dementia of Guam. Bethesda, MD.: National Institutes of Health, 1983.
9. Juergens SM, Kurland LT, Okazaki H, et al. ALS in Rochester, Minnesota, 1925–1977. Neurology 1980; 30:463–70.
10. Mortar P, Chio A, Leone M, et al. Motor neuron disease in the province of Turin, Italy, 1966–1980. J Neurol Sci 1984; 66:165–73.
11. Mulder DW. The diagnosis and treatment of amyotrophic lateral sclerosis. Boston: Houghton Mifflin, 1980.
12. Reed DM, Brody JA, Holden EM. Predicting the duration of Guam amyotrophic lateral sclerosis. Neurology 1975; 25:277–80.
13. Munsat TL, Bradley WG. Amyotrophic lateral sclerosis. In: Tyler HR, Dawson DM, eds. Current Neurology. Boston: Houghton Mifflin, 1979.

Chapter 11

Isokinetic and Functional Evaluation of Muscle Strength Over Time in Amyotrophic Lateral Sclerosis

Benjamin Rix Brooks, Robert L. Sufit, Jo Ann Clough, Jill Conrad, Mohammed Sanjak, Martha Schram, and Lynelle M. Erickson

As described by Cook and Glass[1] and Andres et al.,[2] there are different ways to assess motor function; depending on the task, each has its advantages and disadvantages. Studies of patients with amyotrophic lateral sclerosis (ALS) must be performed longitudinally in order to follow the natural history of the disease and assess treatment trials. These needs require a robust methodology that will encompass the assessment of patients with various degrees of strength and capability, the evaluation of changes in these parameters in a given patient, and the involvement of different examiners.

At present, the clinical tool most widely used to evaluate patients with ALS is the manual muscle test (MMT) in its various forms. Although widespread use has made it a familiar technique, clinicians may not be sufficiently aware that the MMT is an ordinal scale,[1] and that its limited number of ranks (e.g., 5 in the Medical Research Council [MRC] scale, 10 in the Daniels and Worthingham scale) restricts its sensitivity to change. Increasing the number of ranks, however, introduces inter-rater subjectivity and a decrease in reliability.

Isometric dynamometry circumvents the ordinal difficulties found in the MMT and introduces equipment that is new but quite stable. Unfortunately, isometric dynamometry requires scrupulous attention to joint position and muscle substitution, which are difficult to keep consistent with each patient and from examiner to examiner across time and patients. Instruments that measure strength in proximal (and therefore stronger) muscles are not as readily available as those that measure strength in smaller, more distal muscles.

Griffin et al.[3] have looked at isometric testing in the ordinal MMT and compared it to isokinetic muscles strength testing. They studied patients with all forms of neuromuscular disease, including two with ALS. They found that isokinetic testing was a more sensitive barometer of improvement than the MMT. For that matter, improvement would not be documented by MMT. However, when weakness and a deteriorating condition were present, isokinetics did not yield clinically significant information.

ISOKINETIC TESTING IN ALS

Isokinetic assessment overcomes many of the deficiencies of MMT and isometrics. For example, proximal muscles are easily assessed with isokinetics. Accuracy over time and from patient to patient is easily maintained because torque and joint angle can be measured simultaneously, and peak torques can be chosen regardless of the angle used for testing. The accommodating resistance produced by isokinetics allows measurements to be made over a wide range of strengths. Furthermore, muscle substitution is almost impossible because the patient is restrained by the apparatus. The only disadvantages are the cost of the equipment and the occasional inability of some patients to perform parts of the test because of respiratory insufficiency.

Isokinetic dynamometers are useful for measuring muscle strength in terms of torque at various velocities, typically from 0 to between 300 and 400°/sec. Muscle torque changes at a varying angle throughout the range of motion because the muscle torque produced is dependent on the length/tension relationship of the muscle. The greatest tension occurs at midrange of the arc of movement. Thus, velocities of 180°/sec or higher are useful for predicting some functional deficiencies. Functional deficits in upper motor neuron (UMN) disease are largely the result of delayed activation and reversal of the order of activation, as demonstrated by Shumway and Cook,[4] and isokinetics is limited in its ability to study these deficits. Nevertheless, isokinetic assessment remains a valuable tool for the quantification of muscle torque.

Even with the advantages of isokinetics, no one test should be used exclusively. A combination of zero-based linear scales of strength (such as isokinetics) and more functionally based measures (such as walking velocity) gives one the ability to follow patients with greater sensitivity to change and to functionally relevant tasks. The combination also allows correlations to be drawn that may be more powerful measures than any single test. For the purpose of this study, we also included isometrics and MMT to test the validity of isokinetic assessments and as a source of possible correlations.

We used bilateral isokinetic measurements of the knee and elbow flexors and extensors to assess longitudinal change, as well as treatment effects on muscle strength, in ALS patients. Isokinetic testing uses a fixed speed with an accommodating resistance throughout the range of motion. The advantage of this form of assessment is that one can maximally load the force applied at every point throughout the range of motion without risking injury to the patient, since the resistance is equal to the force applied.

In order to ensure that patients were physically able to participate in our study and that they constituted a homogeneous group, we selected only those who had the Charcot variety of ALS with both upper and lower motor neuron involvement. Additionally, at least three extremities had to be involved, as judged by electromyographic criteria. All patients were ambulatory at the beginning of the study period, and their respiratory competence was assured by a normal arterial carbon dioxide tension and forced vital capacity (FVC) greater than 50% of the predicted value. We excluded patients who had significant cardiovascular, pulmonary, or endocrine disease. Patients whose motor neuron disorder could be associated with a paraneoplastic or other cause were also excluded.

METHODS OF ASSESSMENT

Isokinetic Assessments

The patients were placed in the short-sitting position (i.e., sitting with the chest and lower extremity stabilized by adjustable straps) for evaluation of the knee torque. They were instructed to grasp handgrips to further stabilize their position; patients who were unable to do so were instructed to place their hands on their laps. The patients' upper extremities were evaluated as they lay supine on a universal body exercise table. Straps were used to stabilize the pelvis and chest and to minimize substitution. If a patient was unable to generate sufficient force to maintain contact, the hands were strapped to the handgrip.

Patients were carefully monitored for signs of cardiovascular or respiratory compromise arising from the very strenuous nature of the muscle assessment and the difficulty (in patients with bulbar or respiratory involvement) of maintaining the supine position. If necessary, a wedge was placed under the patient's head and chest to facilitate adequate ventilation. We allowed the patients brief rest periods if they became dyspneic, developed muscle cramps that interfered with testing, or experienced significant muscle fatigue. Rest periods varied in length and were dependent on the patient's ability to regain respiratory stability and comfort.

Data were generated and recorded on a single- or dual-channel recorder. The patients' maximum torque output was assessed throughout the velocity spectrum. Velocities of 0, 30, 60, 180, 240, and 300°/sec were selected to obtain data on how patients with neuromuscular disease would perform at slow and fast contractile rates, as well as to construct functional correlates (unpublished data). Because of the learning effect and the variability of torque output in UNM disease, six repetitions were tested at 0, 30, and 60°/sec, and 10 repetitions were assessed at 180, 240, and 300°/sec. The subjects were assessed every 6 to 8 months to document changes in torque production over time (the assessments were performed at these intervals to eliminate the possibility of a training effect).

Functional Assessment

To increase the utility of our findings, we included functional measures (a subset of those originally proposed by Brooke[5]). We timed the patients walking 30 ft (8.5 m) as fast as they could safely go. Eight repetitions were measured, and the mean was calculated. We then timed the patients' ability to step onto a low footstool with both their strong and weak leg. Finally, we timed the patients' ability to rise from sitting to a standing position. We permitted upper-extremity assistance and noted its use. Again, multiple measures were made, and the mean was used for longitudinal regression analysis.

Manual Muscle Testing

A subset of the ALS patients was also evalutated by two investigators using the MMT technique, as described by Kendall.[6] Eighty-nine measures of peak torque (performed with the isokinetic dynamometer at 0°/sec, and with 90° of elbow flexion for biceps and triceps for the upper extremities, and 45° of knee flexion for the quadriceps and hamstrings) were compared to MMT grades to determine the most sensitive tool and the torque variability in each muscle grade.

Data Analysis

Data were collected from a single-channel system on a strip chart. Peak torque was determined for every contraction at each velocity. Means and standard deviations were calculated for every velocity tested in the spectrum. We tracked patients over a 16-month period in order to assess changes in maximum torque production as related to the natural progression of the disease and to the effect of thyrotropin releasing hormone (TRH) on muscle strength. Comparisons were made between torque production and functional activities (e.g., standing, stepping, and walking velocities) to determine if isokinetic evaluation could be used as a predictor of function in this population. Force/velocity curves were constructed from the means to determine if there was an inverse linear relationship between torque production and velocity (Hill equation[7]). Graphs were constructed to determine which muscle groups experienced the greatest change in peak torque over the 16-month period. Finally, comparisons were made between peak torque and MMT grades to assess the variability of torque production within each muscle grade.

ISOKINETIC DYNAMOMETRY IN ALS

The typical force/velocity relationship in patients with ALS is different from that in controls (Figure 11.1). The patients generated less torque at 0°/sec with 90° of elbow flexion and 45° of knee flexion than at 60°/sec, as shown by the line labeled "saline." Torque demonstrated a linear decline from 60°/sec to 300°/sec. The dashed line shows the utility of isokinetic testing in the evaluation of treatment protocols, such as trial of TRH.

Reduction in torque output of leg muscles during a 16-month study is evident at

0, 60, and 180°/sec (Figure 11.2). At all three velocities, the reduction in strength was greater in the stronger muscle groups in the lower extremities than in the weaker groups. The reduction in torque was linear at 0°/sec for the stronger muscles and nonlinear at 60 and 180°/sec. In fact, if one assumes that the strong leg will follow the time curve of the weak leg, the break in the curve becomes much clearer and reflects an asymptotic relationship.

The percent change in muscle torque for strong and weak muscle groups over study periods of 0 to 8 months and 8 to 16 months shows a statistically significant ($P < 0.05$) decrease over time in the strength change of the stronger extremity at 180°/sec (Figure 11.3); isometric measures (presumably including MMT) have failed to demonstrate this greater loss of torque at higher velocities in stronger muscles. The mechanism of the loss is unclear and may involve both the upper and lower motor neurons.

FUNCTIONAL TESTING IN ALS

The change in velocities for functional tests was linear during the 16-month study period (Figure 11.4). The subjects demonstrated group means of 90, 50, and 70% reduction over time in their velocities for standing, stepping onto a stool, and walking, respectively.

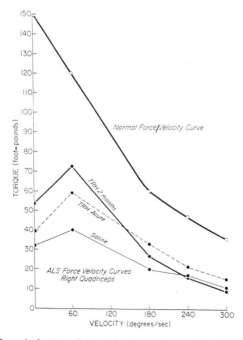

FIGURE 11.1 *Force/velocity relationships in patients with ALS. TRH denotes thyotropin releasing hormone. Reproduced with permission from Sufit et al.*[8]

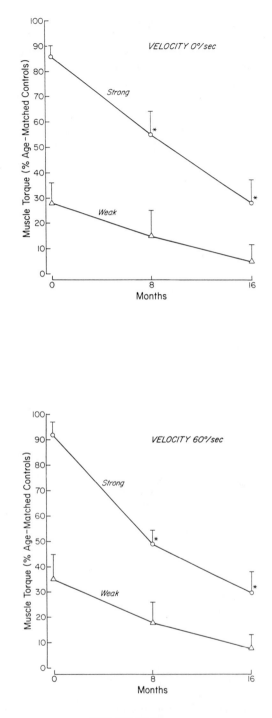

FIGURE 11.2

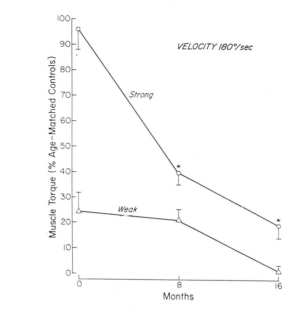

FIGURE 11.2   *Reduction in torque output of strong and weak muscle groups. Reduction at (A) 0°/sec, (B) 60°/sec, and (C) 180°/sec. Asterisks indicate statistical significance. Reproduced with permission from Sufit et al.*[8]

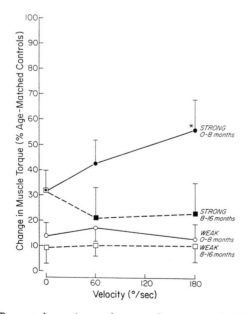

FIGURE 11.3   *Percent change in muscle torque for strong and weak muscle groups. Asterisk indicates a statistically significant difference at P < 0.05. Reproduced with permission from Sufit et al.*[8]

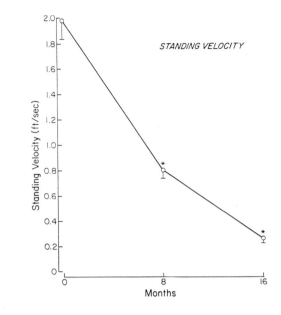

A

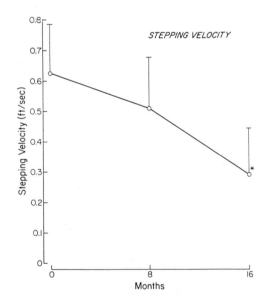

B

FIGURE 11.4

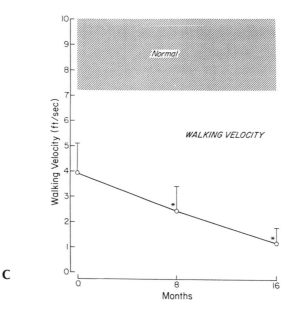

C

FIGURE 11.4   *Changes in velocity over time. Changes in (A) standing velocity, (B) stepping velocity, and (C) walking velocity. Asterisks indicate statistical significance. Reproduced with permission of Sufit et al.[8]*

At each time point studied, walking velocity correlated significantly with knee flexor torque at 180°/sec (Table 11.1). Stepping onto a stool also correlated with knee

Table 11.1.   Correlation of Functional Tests over Time, with Knee Flexor Torque at 180°/Sec

	Torque Measurement Interval		
Function	0 Months	8 Months	16 Months
Walking 30 feet			
0 months	0.9327[a]	0.9515[b]	0.2449
8 months	0.9754[b]	0.9598[b]	0.0625
16 months	0.8580	0.6743	0.6666
Stepping onto stool			
0 months	0.9040[a]	0.7782	0.6060
8 months	0.9697[b]	0.8818[a]	0.5361
16 months	0.6060	0.3900	0.7578
Standing from chair			
0 months	0.8836[a]	0.9293[a]	0.6054
8 months	0.8281	0.9406[b]	0.5075
16 months	0.9461[b]	0.8989[a]	0.8913[a]

[a]$P < 0.05$.

[b]$P < 0.01$.

flexor torque at 180°/sec. Standing up from a chair did not. Walking velocity and stepping velocity, as well as the velocity of standing up from a chair, correlated strongly with each other (Table 11.2).

CORRELATION OF ISOKINETIC TESTING AT 0°/SEC WITH MMT

The relationship of MMT grades and isokinetic torque measures in the lower extremity comparisons shows a broad and overlapping range of torque production at each MMT grade (Figure 11.5). A grade of 5 reflected torques of 32 to 80 foot-pounds, whereas a grade of 4 showed a range of 12 to 57 foot-pounds. Even a grade of 3, which by definition should show a torque of zero or slightly more (if one includes the plusses in the grade), showed torques of up to 57 foot-pounds, although all the values above 30 were graded 3 by one examiner and 4 by the other. Although the overlap from grade 5 is less in the upper extremities than in the lower, there is still a broad range of torque values, from 26 to 70 foot-pounds (Figure 11.5). Grades 4 and 3 were virtually indistinguishable on the basis of torque output (with grade 4, ranging from 8 to 21 foot-pounds, with grade 3, from 0 to 21).

CONCLUSION

The use of isokinetics and functional evaluations to test the progressive course of ALS proved to have significant benefits. As stated earlier, by combining the sensitivity and range of isokinetics with the functionality of the MMT, clinicians are able to follow ALS patients more closely than is possible with either alone. In our study, we found an asymptotic relationship in the decline of muscle strength between stronger and weaker muscle groups, which the MMT alone had been unable to document at higher velocities. We also noted correlations between walking and stepping functions and knee flexor torque, but not standing. These results may lead to further analyses of the correlations (or lack thereof) between functional activities and isokinetic parameters. None of the tests by themselves would have produced these data. Although the pathogenetic mechanisms of ALS are still ambiguous, the use of combined testing strategies will better document the deficits that result and may aid in our understanding of the disease.

Table 11.2   Correlation between Functional Tests Over Time

Function	0–8 Months	0–16 Months	8–16 Months
Walk	0.9159[a]	0.7367	0.7494
Chair	0.9522[b]	0.2432	0.0208
Step	0.9675[b]	0.8024	0.6866

[a]$P < 0.05$.
[b]$P < 0.01$.

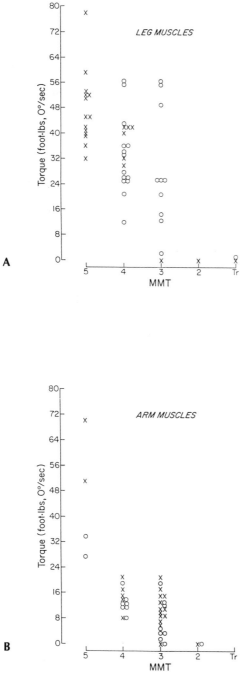

FIGURE 11.5 *The relationship of MMT grades and isokinetic measures in torque production. (A) The lower extremities, and (B) the upper extremities, as graded by two examiners (X and O). Reproduced with permission from Sufit et al.[8]*

REFERENCES

1. Cook JD, Glass DS. Strength evaluation in neuromuscular disease. Neurol Clin 1987; 5(2):101–24.
2. Andres PL, Thibodeau LM, Finison L, et al. Quantitative assessment of neuromuscular deficit in ALS. Neurol Clin 1987; 5(2):125–42.
3. Griffin JW, McClure MH, Bertorini TE. Sequential isokinetic and muscle testing in patients with neuromuscular disease. Phys Ther 1986; 66:32–5.
4. Nashner LM, Shumway-Cook A, Marin O. Stance posture control in select groups of children with cerebral palsy: deficits in sensory organization and muscular coordination. Exp Brain Res 1983; 49:393–409.
5. Brooke MH. A clinician's view of neuromuscular diseases. Baltimore: Williams and Wilkins, 1977; 30–3.
6. Kendall HO, Kendall FP, Wadsworth GE. Muscles: testing and function, Second edition. Baltimore: Williams and Wilkins, 1971; 1–15.
7. Gilliam TB, Sady SP, Freedson PS, et al. Isokinetic torque levels for high school football players. Arch Phys Med Rehabil 1979; 60:110–14.
8. Sufit RL, Clough JA, Schram PT, et al. Isokinetic assessment in ALS. Neurol Clin 1987; 5(2):197–212.

ACKNOWLEDGMENTS

This study was supported in part by a Muscular Dystrophy Association (MDA) Midwest Regional Amyotrophic Lateral Sclerosis (ALS) Research and Treatment Center Grant (BRB, RLS), an MDA Task Force on Drug Development Grant (BRB, RLS), and a Veterans Administration (VA) Merit Review Grant (BRB). The excellent administrative and secretarial skills of Kim Kallembach and Laurie Weigt are gratefully appreciated.

Chapter 12

Quantitative Techniques in the Assessment of Multiple Sclerosis: The Problems and Current Solutions

Labe C. Scheinberg and Chris Anne Raymond

No other branch of medicine lends itself so well to the correlation of signs and symptoms with diseased structure as neurology, but it is only by means of a systematic examination and an accurate appraisal that one can properly elicit one's findings . . . Quantitative evaluation of neurologic abnormalities may be used for the accurate determination of a patient's clinical status, the study of the natural history of the disease and the measurement of response to either medical or surgical treatment.

Thus said DeJong,[1] an authority on clinical neurology. In our opinion, few other neurologic diseases lend themselves so poorly to correlation of signs and symptoms with disease structure, accurate determination of clinical status, prediction of natural history, and measurement of response to treatment as does multiple sclerosis (MS).

MS is a protean disease of the central myelin; its cause is unknown. Onset typically occurs early in adult life and runs a chronic, variable course. The patient usually experiences gait problems, urinary dysfunction, and fatigue, although any finding may occur. Although major advances have been made in diagnosing the illness and relieving its symptoms, arresting its progress remains elusive.[2-4]

A neurologic wag, long frustrated in managing patients with MS and disillusioned by annual announcements of cures, once stated: "He whom the gods would destroy, they first set out to do clinical trials in multiple sclerosis."[5] Clinicians face three problems in assessing MS: variability, variability, and variability. The disease varies,

The authors wish to thank Drs. Aaron Miller and Ute Traugott for their review and criticism of this manuscript. Supported by National Institute on Disability and Rehabilitation Research grant (G008300040) from the Medical Rehabilitation Research and Training Center for Multiple Sclerosis.

155

the patient varies, and the doctor varies. Before discussing these three factors in more detail, some definitions are in order.

DEFINITIONS

Symptoms are subjective sensations or other observations a patient reports about his or her body or its products. (Yet Lhermitte's sign is called a symptom.)

Signs are entities observed by the clinician during physical examination of the patient. Certain signs may be observed both by the patient and physician and are called *subjective signs* or *objective symptoms.* Jaundice is an example. Others, called *iatric signs,* are detected only with special examination techniques (e.g., ophthalmoscopic examination for disc pallor[6]).

Findings refers to symptoms or signs.[6]

Onset is the first appearance of any symptom(s) that can be attributed to a lesion in the nervous system.[2]

Relapse (attack, bout, exacerbation) is the appearance of a new symptom or the return of a previous symptom. Most neurologists define an attack as symptom(s) of neurologic dysfunction (with or without objective confirmation) lasting more than 24 hours. Certain symptoms (e.g., Lhermitte's sign, tonic seizures, facial myokymia, or episodic dysarthria) may last only seconds. Generally speaking, these do not constitute an attack unless they persist for a period of days or weeks.[2] *Temporary exacerbation* or *pseudoexacerbation* is used to describe phenomena, such as fever, that produce transient worsening. *Pseudoremission,* or improvement, may result from symptomatic treatment, such as that for spasticity, that does not modify the course of the disease. Generally, a remission must last at least one month to be considered significant.

In the context of disordered function in disease, the scheme of Wood[7] has gained widespread acceptance. It defines the illness in terms of *disease (pathology), impairment, disability, and handicap.*

Impairment is any loss or abnormality of psychological, physiologic, or anatomical structure or function. The term is usually interchangeable with *disability,* as originally used by Kurtzke.[8] In the Minimal Record of Disability (MRD) for MS,[9] it is measured with the Disability Status Scale (DSS) or more recently, the Expanded Disability Status Scale (EDSS).[10] Impairment usually is described quantitatively by physicians or other trained health professionals, but recently it has been demonstrated to be valid as a patient self-assessment measure.[11]

Disability is the inability to perform a human activity successfully as the result of an impairment. Disability usually is interchangeable with *incapacity,* as used in the Incapacity Status Scale (ISS) of the MRD[9]; typically, it is assessed by nonphysician health care professionals, such as physical or occupational therapists. It may be recorded by patient or family reporting ("can do") or by more time-consuming testing ("does do"). In the latter case, the activities tested are those covered in the Activities of Daily Living (ADL) scale, frequently employed by rehabilitation professionals.

Handicap is a disadvantage, resulting from an impairment or a disability, that limits or prevents an individual from fulfilling the expected behaviors of a particular social role (e.g., spouse, employee). Handicaps may be measured with the Environmental Status Scale (ESS) of the MRD; in general, they are assessed by nonphysician health care professionals, such as medical social workers or rehabilitation counselors.

Because of the lack of a close correlation between disease pathology and clinical findings, it is quite possible to have pathology without impairment, disability, or handicap. In some cases, if the patient is highly motivated and has extensive social supports, it is possible to have extensive pathology and impairment with minimal disability and no handicap. Conversely, there are cases of minimal pathology with major impairment, disability, and handicap. Although lesions may occur in any part of the CNS, not all have equal effect in producing findings. One small but critically placed plaque may result in quadriplegia, whereas multiple large plaques situated in "silent areas" may be clinically undetectable.

Other terms, although less widely used, should be defined. *Primary findings* are symptoms or signs that can be directly correlated with the presence of lesions (e.g., blurred vision, gait disturbances) or those that are thought to have a morphologic or physiologic basis (e.g., fatigue, dementia). *Secondary findings* are symptoms or signs that result from primary findings and represent complications, avoidable or otherwise (e.g., contractures, decubiti, urinary tract infections). These are not specific to multiple sclerosis (which can, of course, also be the case with primary findings). *Tertiary findings* are features that result from the above and are to a certain extent synonymous with handicap.

VARIABILITY OF DISEASE FACTORS

The course of MS is variable, and the length of illness may be months or many years. Some individuals die from unrelated causes without having neurologic findings during their lives but are found at autopsy to have widespread pathology characteristic of MS.[12] Others have severe impairment with only a few lesions.

In many cases, patients present with a brief period of blurred vision of paraparesis and no previous history of neurologic dysfunction or other findings. Using electrophysiologic techniques or neuroimaging, one can detect paraclinical evidence of other sites of pathology that may have occurred silently sometime in the past but produce no findings. In a recent study, Jacobs et al.[13] noted that 75% of lesions detected by magnetic resonance imaging (MRI) were clinically silent. These usually were located in the centrum semiovale, temporo-occipital, and/or periventricular white matter. Only 5% of the lesions were associated with a diagnosis of clinically definite MS, and 20% with a diagnosis of possible MS. The study can loosely be interpreted as showing that as many as 95% of lesions in the patient with MS may fail to produce clinical findings. We can only state that although clinical examination is valuable for the diagnosis and management of symptoms, it can be misleading in assessing the effects of disease-modifying agents during the usual length of clinical trials.

In many instances, the onset of clinical findings is not synonymous with the onset of disease. In MS, the interval may be many years. For purposes of research, the Poser criteria[14] state that clinical onset occurs between 10 and 59 years of age, though there are autopsy-proven cases with clinical onset as early as the first decade of life and as late as the eighth decade.

Almost any finding may be present at onset, but it is obvious that findings characteristic of central myelin dysfunction (weakness, incoordination, sensory dysfunction, visual disturbances) are predominant, whereas those characteristic of neuronal dysfunction (seizures, dementia, focal atrophy, language dysfunction, fasciculations) are rare. (It is not the purpose of this chapter to tabulate the relative frequencies of findings; these can be obtained in any textbook of neurology.)

The course of MS has been described in a variety of ways, but for the sake of simplicity, we propose that it be described in one of two: (1) mild or benign, with a long period of minimal impairment and disability, or (2) severe or grave, with a rapid downhill course leading to marked impairment and disability. Others have used a different scheme:

1. Benign—sudden onset, few attacks; complete or almost complete remission, no permanent disability (20% of cases).
2. Exacerbating/remitting—sudden onset, repeated attacks; complete or almost complete remission, minimal permanent disability (20 to 30% of cases).
3. Remitting/progressive—sudden onset, repeated attacks; partial or no remission, progressive permanent disability (40% of cases).
4. Progressive—insidious onset with steady progression; no remission; often, permanent disability (10 to 20% of cases).[15]

As implied by this scheme, the rate of disease progression in MS may vary from weeks to years. A patient may have an almost "malignant" form and progress relentlessly and rapidly from good health to complete disability, or have slowly progressive weakness of the legs without remission yet remain ambulatory after many years.

In our opinion, whether the disease is exacerbating/remitting or remitting/progressive depends entirely on the seemingly random occurrence of lesions, coupled with the response of the host's CNS to the plaque-forming process and its physiologic "reserve" in affected neurologic tracts. Cases have been observed in which the clinical symptoms were improving while pathology (detected by neuroimaging) was worsening, and vice versa. Cases that have a "benign" course for several years can become progressive. Patients with MS of apparently benign onset (e.g., those with sensory findings such as paresthesia or optic neuritis that lead to complete remission) may eventually have a lesion in the cervical cord, where it produces severe permanent disability.

There have been many efforts to predict the severity of future impairment and the rate of disease progression on the basis of such factors as the type of onset, age at onset, nature of initial findings, and degree of remission. All such efforts have been controversial and, in the experience of the first author (L.C.S.), of little predictive value at the time of initial patient assessment. Some of these prognostic guidelines seem to do no more than restate the obvious. For example, if a patient initially is not ambulatory, then he or she is given a bad prognosis. But if the patient is currently unable to walk, this is already a bad sign.

In a series of 70 cases, other workers reported[16] that the disease began earlier in women. They reported that cerebellar or oculomotor signs at onset were not considered to be bad prognostic signs. On the other hand, they felt that those with optic neuritis, sensory disturbances, and weakness tended to have a poorer course. This somewhat contradicts the observations of Kraft et al.[15]

In the experience of the first author (L.C.S.), two features have held up well in predicting disability. Early cerebellar signs, especially truncal ataxia, carry a poor prognosis. On the other hand, patients with minimal cerebellar and pyramidal tract signs and low EDSS scores five years after onset have about an 80% chance of showing the same degree of disability at 10 and 15 years after onset.[17] These comments indicate only that cerebellar signs are very disabling and respond poorly to treatment, and that the disease tends to produce its greatest impairment in the first five years after clinical onset.

VARIABILITY OF PATIENT FACTORS

Few investigators have written about the role of patient factors, particularly the decision to consult a physician, in the course of MS. Some patients see a physician shortly after the onset of findings as minimal as paresthesia; others slowly progress to severe paraparesis without seeking medical attention. Many patients overlook, ignore, or fail to report findings later documented by evoked-response testing.

Often during the period between perceiving symptoms and seeing a physician, patients attribute their complaints to such causes as "nerves," fatigue, poor posture, or arthritis and consider them trivial. At some point, whether because of family urging, anxiety, inability to function, or other reasons, they do seek attention.

After the initial physican contact, there is a variable time period until a diagnosis is established. Some physicians may never determine the diagnosis, or some patients may never learn the diagnosis by name. In many instances, both patient and physician may know or suspect the diagnosis, but each keeps it secret from the other.

Other factors that influence whether a patient will report symptom progression include emotional factors such as depression, anxiety, boredom, stress, and fatigue; environmental changes (high temperatures and humidity worsen symptoms); intercurrent infection; other treatable complications, such as decubiti or spasticity; and, *mirabile dictu,* the desire to enter highly touted clinical trials.[5]

Patients often will report new findings and the progression of old ones that cannot be validated. When the patient is carefully examined, and the clinician records impairment, disability status, and handicap with the MRD, these can be refuted. One should be concerned when changes in impairment are not reflected by changes in disability and handicap, and vice versa. A patient may have an EDSS score of 7.0 (on a scale of 9.5), with moderate disability and minimal handicap. This often indicates successful rehabilitative management. On the other hand, a low EDSS score and moderate or severe disability and handicap point to intervening emotional factors or the need for rehabilitative measures.

VARIABILITY IN PHYSICIAN FACTORS

If the role of patient factors in evaluating MS has been overlooked, even more so has the role of physician factors. We all are sensitive to our faults, but one need only read the progress notes in hospital records or office charts to observe how poorly patient status is documented. Brief notes such as "patient reports worsening, paraparesis has increased. ACTH to be given intravenously," are all too common. Some physicians make little effort to describe the examination in quantitative terms. Others are unaware of many available scales, and those who are aware may use them rarely and poorly.

Doctors are influenced by conscious and unconscious motives to report improvement where none exists. This often is the case when an investigator has some type of investment in the trial and is not adequately blinded. Few effective agents have so few side effects as to make complete double-blinding possible, and patients and physicians unconsciously collaborate to report fallacious improvement. When no treatment is being given, the patient may report deterioration while the doctor reports improvement or stabilization. Only quantitative, objective measures of patient status, applied routinely, will resolve these conflicts.

ATTEMPTS AT QUANTITATIVE EVALUATION OF MS

Unlike disorders such as muscular dystrophy, in which impairments are primarily motor, or Alzheimer's disease, in which they are primarily mental and behavioral, MS has protean features. Patients present with pyramidal, cerebellar, sensory, visual, urinary, or mental findings. One or two may worsen while others improve. There is no universally accepted single indicator by which to assess the patient's overall status. If one uses a profile such as PULSES,[6] the resulting data are difficult to handle in monitoring and comparing large series of patients in clinical trials. This is why PULSES has been used only to evaluate rehabilitation needs and outcomes, not clinical trials of therapeutic agents.

In certain studies (cited by Potvin et al.,[1] functions assessed by different parts of a larger scale are scored and presented as a profile of functions, but no one has attempted to reduce these into a meaningful overall score. Most assessment efforts, sparked by Kurtzke's work, have used an unintentionally or intentionally weighted score of a single ability, such as walking, to devise an overall status score.

In 1955 Kurtzke developed the major impairment-recording system;[8] it was subsequently expanded in 1983.[10] Called the Expanded Disability Status Scale (EDSS), it is actually a scale of impairment of neurologic function. The principal functional systems—i.e., pyramidal, cerebellar, brainstem, sensory, bowel and bladder, visual, cerebral (or mental)—are assessed on a scale from 0 (normal) to 5 or 6 (complete or almost complete loss of function). These Functional Systems (FS) are scored on the basis of neurologic history and examination. The patient's gait is then evaluated on the basis of history (when impairment is minimal) or observation (when gait abnormality is greater), and the patient is scored on the EDSS, with scores ranging from 0 to 9.5. Zero indicates a normal examination with full range of activity, and 9.5 signifies a totally helpless, bedridden patient. An EDSS score within the 4.0 to 8.0 range is essentially an ambulation index. The lower-range scores (0 to 3.5) depend on the functional system scores: e.g., 1.0 indicates minimal signs (such as a Babinski) on examination without disability, and 2.0 indicates minimal disability in one functional system (such as mild ataxia).

In the EDSS, impairments are judged on both objective neurologic examination (vision) and self-reporting (bowel and bladder). Severe visual loss in one eye (FS score, 5) may result in an EDSS of 4.0 or 4.5, whereas on other evaluations,[18] this would represent 19% of the impairment of the whole person. However, since the EDSS is an ordinal scale, not an interval or ratio scale, this may not matter. A patient with an EDSS score of 3.0 may certainly not be three times more impaired than one with an EDSS score of 1.0. Suffice it to say that although the system is flawed, it is widely accepted and easy to use. It has become the standard for evaluating the results of clinical trials and is probably the best measure we have.

In an effort to develop a weighted rating scale, Sipe[19,20] has produced a neurologic rating scale (NRS). It is based on the standard neurologic examination, with normal being a cumulative score of 100. The primary emphasis is on motor function, which contributes a maximum score of 52 (gait and station, 10; cerebellar, 10; power, 20; reflexes, 12). Sensory functions, since they result in less disability, contribute 12 points; mental function contributes 10 and vision 5. Other cranial nerves contribute 21 points. Bladder dysfunction is subtracted from the total score. (Hence, a totally disabled patient with incontinence would be scored −10.) Sipe and coworkers consider this scoring system to be complementary to the EDSS.

Mickey et al.[21] developed another single score—the Illness Severity Score (ISS)—because they thought the EDSS lacked sensitivity. They and others have noted that significant clinical changes in the patient are not always reflected by a change in the EDSS. In the ISS, pyramidal and cerebellar findings are given greater weight, sensory and visual findings less. Disease activity and course also play a significant role in determining the final ISS.

CONCLUSION

There is no ideal clinical scoring system for MS clinical trials. Disease progression and remission often do not correlate well with clinical findings. Modifying the EDSS to include some elements of the NRS and ISS would be an improvement, but it appears that use of the EDSS is so entrenched that further change is unlikely. Even if modifications improved the test's sensitivity to changes in function, EDSS scores would probably still not correlate well with disease pathology. Perhaps the reason for this can be found in Freud's famous reply when asked how he knew when patients had benefited from psychiatric treatment: *"Arbeiten und lieben."* If the MS patient could work and love, the treatment would probably show some measure of success.

REFERENCES

1. Potvin AR, Tourtellotte WW. Quantitative examination of neurology functions. Boca Raton, FL: CRC Press, 1985; 1:28.
2. Hallpike JF, Adams DW, Tourtellotte WW, eds. Multiple sclerosis: pathology, diagnosis and management. Baltimore: Williams & Wilkins, 1983.
3. McDonald WI, Silberberg DH, eds. Multiple sclerosis. London: Butterworths, 1986.
4. McAlpine D, Lumsden CE, Acheson ED, eds. Multiple sclerosis: a reappraisal. Edinburgh/London: Churchill Livingstone, 1972.
5. Raymond CA. Can fewer patients studied more intensively solve historic problems of MS clinical trials? JAMA, 1986; 256:691-2.
6. Feinstein AR. Clinical Judgement. Baltimore: Williams & Wilkins, 1976.
7. Wood PHN. Classification of impairments and handicaps. World Health Organization, 1975. (unpublished document WHO/ICD-9/Conf 75.15.)
8. Kurtzke JF. A new scale for evaluating disability in multiple sclerosis. Neurology 1955; 5:580.
9. Haber A, LaRocca N, eds. Minimal record of disability for multiple sclerosis. New York: The National Multiple Sclerosis Society, 1985.
10. Kurtzke JF. Rating neurologic impairment in multiple sclerosis: an expanded disability status scale. Neurology 1983; 33:1444.
11. Scheinberg L, Feldman J, Ratzker P, et al. Self-assessment in multiple sclerosis. Paper presented at the Annual Meeting of the American Academy of Neurology, New Orleans, May 1, 1986.
12. Gilbert JJ, Sadler M. Unsuspected multiple sclerosis. J Neurol Neurosurg Psychiatry 1974; 37:1259-64.
13. Jacobs L, Kinel WR, Polachini I, et al. Correlations of nuclear magnetic resonance imaging, computerized tomography and clinical profiles in multiple sclerosis. Neurology 1986; 36:27-34.
14. Poser CM, Paty DW, McDonald WI, et al., eds. The diagnosis of multiple sclerosis. New York: Thieme-Stratton, 1984.
15. Kraft GH, Freal JE, Coryell JK, et al. Multiple sclerosis: early prognostic guidelines. Arch Phys Med Rehabil 1981; 62:54-8.
16. Izquierdo G, Hauw JJ, Lyon-Caen O, et al. Analyse clinique de 70 cas neuropathologiques de sclerose en plaques. Rev Neurol (Paris) 1985; 141:546-52.
17. Kurtzke JF, Beebe GW, Nagler B, et al. Studies on the natural history of multiple sclerosis and early prognostic features of the later course of the illness. J Chronic Dis 1977; 30:819-30.
18. Guides to the evaluation of permanent impairment. Chicago: American Medical Association, 1984; 2.
19. Knobler RL, Panitch HS, Braheny SL, et al. Systemic alpha interferon in multiple sclerosis: a controlled clinical trial. Neurology 1984; 34:1273-9.
20. Sipe JC, Knobler RL, Braheny SL, et al. A neurologic rating scale for use in multiple sclerosis. Neurology 1984; 34:1368.
21. Mickey MR, Ellison GW, Myers LW. An illness severity score for multiple sclerosis. Neurology 1984; 34:1343-7.

Chapter 13

Disability Rating Scales for the Assessment of Multiple Sclerosis

Sigrid Poser

In the management of multiple sclerosis (MS), there is a long tradition of constructing and using disability rating scales to predict disease progression and assess the results of treatment. Unfortunately, these scales have often been either too complex to be easily used, not detailed enough to be thoroughly sensitive to change, or too narrowly designed for multicenter use. Furthermore, data from studies using these scales have been subjected to inappropriate statistical analyses. The purpose of this chapter is to examine the use of disability rating scales in MS research and, on the basis of past trials and practices, to make recommendations for the future use of scales and the choice of appropriate analyses. (The reader is referred to Chapter 12, by Scheinberg and Raymond, for further description of rating scales for MS.)

HISTORICAL PERSPECTIVE

Alexander[1] was one of the first investigators to develop a documentation system for studies of therapy in patients with MS, but many problems with his weighting scale have yet to be resolved. In his system, described in 1951, score values were assigned to significant functional variables to weight them according to importance. In addition to signs and symptoms, ambulation and other measures of physical performance were weighted up to a maximum score of −200 for total disability. The method proved cumbersome and complex, and has not remained in use.

Disability Status Scale

Kurtzke's method,[2] published only a few years later, has survived—probably because it is less complicated. The method consists of assessing functional systems individually and using the results to assign a disability score. The utility of the Disability Status Scale (DSS) was tested in a cooperative study on the effect of adrenocortico-trophic hormone (ACTH) in acute exacerbations of MS. The final report was encouraging:

> The Disability Status Scale, together with the Functional Systems, comprises an adequate system of evaluating change in a therapeutic trial of MS and, of all the measures used in this study, apparently is the most consistent indicator of change.[3]

However, it should be noted that this study focused on acute bouts, during which dramatic changes are often expected. In spite of the positive judgment from the ACTH trial, many investigators have found the Kurtzke scales insufficiently detailed and therefore not sensitive enough to detect change in therapeutic trials, particularly in evaluating a drug's influence on disease progression rather than its effects in the treatment of exacerbations. Kurtzke tried to overcome this problem by introducing half-steps in order to expand his original 10-point scale to 19 points between 0 and 10, but this Expanded Disability Status Scale (EDSS)[6] had other difficulties, which I will mention later.

In addition to Kurtzke's two-part system, the ACTH study used a standard neurologic examination, a 7-day symptom score, and a battery of quantitative tests (administered by physical therapists) as parameters of impairment. The DSS does not measure disability according to the World Health Organization (WHO) definition,[4] but rather rates it in terms of impairment. The inclusion in therapeutic trials of scales that assess performance in activities of daily living is a more recent development. Kurtzke's incapacity scale is commonly used for this purpose.[6]

Fog and Linnemann Scale

Following the early example of Alexander, Fog and Linnemann[7] developed a scale that scored the items of the neurologic history and examination according to a weighting procedure. Fog never published the detailed instructions for this scale (39 pages), and I am not aware that anyone besides the Copenhagen group has used this system. Fog, however, used it for many years, and his papers on the different types of disease progression are based on the system. In them he observed patients over a period of years and predicted their future courses by constructing computer models to extend the patterns they had exhibited in the past. He found that in most patients, the disease followed a linear progression. He also used his system in clinical trials of drugs such as transfer factor and azathioprine. When Patzold et al.[8] conducted a controlled study of azathioprine versus levamisole, their results confirmed Fog's assumptions on the different patterns of disease progression. Although their weighting procedure was different from Fog's, Patzold's group obtained very similar curves and found, again, that the disease followed a linear progression in most patients.

COMPARISON OF SCALES

The entire range of problems to be found in any rating procedure was summarized by Grynderup in 1969.[9] He compared data in 400 patients classified according to five different rating scales, including the Hyllested scale, the McAlpine and Compston method, the Ry system, the classification of the Committee for Medical Rating of Physical Impairment (CMRPI), and the Kurtzke scale. The Hyllested scale divides patients into six grades according to a combination of walking capacity and the need for help or nursing care. With the method developed by McAlpine and Compston, patients are divided into six grades according to their degree of mobility. The Ry system, as developed by Pedersen, gives a topographical picture of the disease by rating six different systems on a scale of 5 to 0, with maximum impairment scored as 30. The CMRPI classification is designed to evaluate all types of CNS impairment. It separately rates three sections—cranial nerves, brain, and spinal cord—which are ultimately combined to a maximum total of 100. The Kurtzke DSS has already been described.

Grynderup found that patients were ranked mainly in the upper half of the scale when classified by the methods of Kurtzke and of McAlpine and Compston, and mainly in the lower half with the methods of Hyllested and Ry, whereas the CMRPI resulted in a more even distribution. A comparison of these distributions suggests systematic differences in scoring procedures. Although the analysis showed good agreement between the various systems in their capability for ranking patients, each is helpful in rating different types of impairment; they are not equally suitable for specific problems. As Grynderup stated, "Hellested's and McAlpine and Compston's short systems may be used with advantage in large series of patients of whom only second-hand information of varying reliability is available."[9]

Grynderup also concluded, "If a rating system is to be used in the assessment of the effect of a given therapy on the course of the disease, it must be an advantage to use a system with a relatively larger number of grades, because this makes it possible for the examiner to record even minor changes, and thus a better numerical measure of the effect, if any, obtained."[9] That statement is still valid, particularly in studies that monitor the chronic progressive type of course.

The DSS might have been appropriate for the ACTH study, because dramatic improvement occurs when an acute exacerbation remits. However, the more interesting question is whether a therapeutic agent influences the progressive phase of the disease. The DSS is not detailed enough to register the more subtle changes one would expect in this kind of study.

Kurtzke points out another reason that most studies using his scales are not reliable.[10] In an analysis of studies based on his scales, he found that most authors used the wrong statistical tests. According to Kurtzke, the use of means or other numerical values derived from the DSS is inappropriate because the scale is not ordinal, and only nonparametric tests should be used to calculate significance levels. For a recent summary of the available nonparametric tests, the reader should consult Forrest and Andersen.[11]

THE MULTICENTER APPROACH

A multicenter study to evaluate aspects of MS was started in Germany in 1970. Whereas the studies mentioned earlier were restricted to a single researcher or center, our study needed a documentation system that could be used by researchers at numerous sites. Also, the method chosen had to take into account the facilities available at participating institutions. The ideal approach would have been direct entry of information into a data-display terminal, but at the time our project began, there were not enough terminals available for an on-line procedure. From among the off-line possibilities, we chose a documentation system that would permit data retrieval by an optical character reader.

We conducted a pilot study with 812 patients, reported in 1978,[12] to identify the methodologic difficulties the multicenter study would face. A committee then developed a two-page form to be used for collecting data from the patient history and neurologic examination. To ensure diagnostic uniformity and to avoid the need for an instruction manual, the most important definitions were printed on the reverse side of each sheet. A total of 21 hospitals participated in the study. After initial interest waned, the number of participating hospitals decreased; unfortunately, the introduction of a computerized form failed to raise this number. Although fewer hospitals participated, the number of documented patients increased, indicating that a certain number of investigators broadened their use of the system once it could be performed by a computer.

Applications

Many statistical analyses can be carried out with the resulting data bank. One example is our study of symptomatology at the onset of MS, at the time the patient was entered in the study, and over the entire course of the disease.[13] We are now conducting a multicenter epidemiologic study in Europe, using the same reporting forms. In The Netherlands, Minderhoud's group (personal communication, 1986) performed a weighting procedure, using data from the neurologic examination portion of our study and a few additional items. Their overall score correlated fairly well with the Kurtzke scale.

However, the principle of Kurtzke's two-part system[2]—the scoring of functional systems and integration of the scores within an overall scale—differs from our procedures. Kurtzke criticizes scales based on combining scores because they record items cumulatively that are the result of a single lesion (e.g., the spasticity, paresis, and abnormal reflexes of a pyramidal lesion). He also objects that combining scores is analogous to "adding apples and pears." Kurtzke's functional groups (e.g., pyramidal, cerebellar, brainstem) are scored according to severity of impairment, and these single scores form the basis for determining the grade of disability—at least in grades 1 to 3 of the EDSS. Beginning with grade 3.5, the scale is defined mainly by ability to walk.

Although walking disorders are the most common problem for patients with MS, a certain number of patients cannot be categorized satisfactorily by this scale. Kurtzke claims that in his experience, any sample of MS patients exhibits a bell-shaped distribution over the 10 grades of the DSS. However, most other investigators have found a double bell-shaped distribution around DSS 2 and DSS 7. This discrepancy is important to consider when choosing an appropriate statistical test for the research planned.

Progression Index

Although the DSS is not sufficiently detailed for short-term therapeutic studies, it can be valuable for comparing groups of patients over longer periods of time. We were interested in the question of prognosis and devised an index to measure disease progression among our study patients. By dividing the present grade of disability by the duration of the disease in years, a quotient may be calculated that reflects the rate of deterioration.[14] But this quotient is not justifiable in patients with disease duration of less than 2 years, patients examined during an exacerbation, or patients with disability at grade 8 or 9 and disease duration of more than 10 years (since they cannot deteriorate by more than 1 or 2 grades when they are analyzed statistically over many years, they falsely appear to improve).

The index was developed on the assumption that progression is linear, as Fog and Patzold found in the majority of their patients. When appropriately utilized with observation of the aforementioned limitations, the quotient is a reliable prognostic indicator; it has been used by others with little or no modification.[15,16] In a subsequent study, when a logarithmic transformation was performed after the probit analysis, we found that the resulting progression index yielded a very good approximation of the normal distribution curve.[14]

We used this parameter to compare groups of patients and were able to confirm earlier results obtained through a different methodology. In the study of 812 patients, we grouped subjects with the same degree of present disability according to the duration of their disease. With both procedures, we found no difference in prognosis between the sexes. We also demonstrated that a representative sample of patients from an epidemiologic area has a much better prognosis than one would generally infer from statistics based on hospital studies.

SCORING PROCEDURES IN THE PRESENT STUDY

We encountered several difficulties with scoring procedures in a study of cyclosporine A versus azathioprine. We included the following parameters: (1) a standardized neurologic examination, including evaluation of visual acuity and a drawing and writing test (signs and symptoms were weighted and summed to produce an overall score); (2) the functional systems of Kurtzke; (3) the expanded disability scale of Kurtzke; (4) the incapacity scale of Kurtzke; and (5) the ambulation index of Hauser et al.[17]

Certain subjects could not be satisfactorily rated by the EDSS because they had a deficit that carried a high score and their impairment in that particular category remained stable. For example, three subjects with a visual score of 5 (i.e., visual acuity less than 20/200 in the weakest eye) experienced considerable improvement in other systems, but their vision was unaffected. Because the highest score in the functional groups determines the grade, the DSS remained unchanged. In such a situation, when a therapy produces significant positive change in some functions, these results must be considered false negatives. At the same time, patients with walking difficulties whose degree of spastic paresis remains stable may be assigned to a new impairment category, depending on the number of canes they require on the day of examination.

Although the final results of the study on cyclosporine A were not available at this writing, preliminary results after 1 year of treatment showed that the correlation between impairment and disability measured by the incapacity score is so high that we would most likely omit the incapacity scale in future studies. The economical use of time and energy must be considered, and we found the items to be too time-consuming, especially in the version in which patients are observed climbing stairs, dressing, and eating. The same is true for the ambulation index of Hauser et al.[17] I did not have an examination room measuring 8 meters in length, so I had to move to another part of the building in order to do a correct classification.

RECOMMENDATIONS

The use of scales in determining the progression of MS is a time-honored practice. As scales have been developed, tested, modified, and sometimes discarded, certain elements in their usage have remained constant. The choice of scale is dependent on the degree of change to be tested; thus, the sensitivity of the scale is a relevant consideration. If data obtained with use of the scale are to be analyzed, it is always advisable to contact a statistician. He or she can not only calculate sample size and perform the randomization but can also evaluate the parameters to be used so that the correct analyses will be performed with the correct scales.

Finally, in choosing a test, one must consider time constraints and data-storage capabilities. Although I mentioned a situation in which we would rule out the use of a time-consuming test, there are circumstances in which these scales are appropriate. The reader is undoubtedly familiar with the Minimal Record of Disability (MRD),[4] which includes a socioeconomic scale in addition to the EDSS, functional groups, and the incapacity scale of Kurtzke. The prospective epidemiologic study we have recently undertaken includes the items of the socioeconomic scale: working ability, financial status, personal residence, personal assistance required, transportation, community services, and social activities. Again, it is time-consuming to gather all this information accurately, and I doubt that it is necessary for the patient's medical management. The information is vital, however, for forecasting social needs—e.g., the required number of nursing homes, ambulatory services, and other relevant facilities.

Whether worldwide use of the MRD can be achieved will not be known for some time. Unless a specific question is formulated for study, I expect that many investigators who have already examined and recorded their patients regularly will be reluctant to adopt this system because it may be incompatible with their own. Others may not be motivated enough to spend an hour or more in the process of examining and recording.

In conclusion, if I were beginning a new therapeutic trial, I would use a standardized neurologic examination, the Functional Systems and EDSS of Kurtzke, and nothing more.

REFERENCES

1. Alexander L. New concept of critical steps in course of chronic debilitating neurologic disease in evaluation of therapeutic response. Arch Neurol Psychiatry 1951; 66:253–71.
2. Kurtzke JF. A new scale for evaluating disability in multiple sclerosis. Neurology 1955; 5:580–3.
3. Cooperative study in the evaluation of therapy in multiple sclerosis. Neurology 1970; 20(part 2):1–59.
4. Kurtzke JF. Disability rating scales in multiple sclerosis. Ann NY Acad Sci 1984; 436: 347–60.
5. World Health Organization. International classification of impairments, disabilities, and handicaps. Geneva: World Health Organization, 1980.
6. Kurtzke JF. Rating neurologic impairment in multiple sclerosis: an expanded disability status scale (EDSS). Neurology 1983; 33:1444–52.
7. Fog T, Linnemann F. The course of multiple sclerosis in 73 cases with computer designed curves. Acta Neurol Scand 1970; 46:1–15 (suppl 48).
8. Patzold U, Pocklington P. Course of multiple sclerosis. Acta Neurol Scand 1982; 65: 248–66.
9. Grynderup V. A comparison of some rating systems in multiple sclerosis. Acta Neurol Scand 1969; 45:611–22.
10. Kurtzke JF. Clinical trials relating to multiple sclerosis. Paper presented at the XIII World Congress of Neurology, Hamburg, 1985.
11. Forrest M, Andersen B. Ordinal scale and statistics in medical research. Br Med J 1986; 292:537–8.
12. Poser S. Multiple sclerosis. Berlin/Heidelberg/New York: Springer, 1978.
13. Poser S, Wikström J, Bauer HJ. Clinical data and the identification of special forms of multiple sclerosis in 1271 cases studied with a standardized documentation system. J Neurol Sci 1979; 40:159–68.
14. Poser S, Raun NE, Poser W. Age at onset, initial symptomatology and the course of multiple sclerosis. Acta Neurol Scand 1982; 66:355–62.
15. Raun NE, Fog T, Heltberg A, et al. Correlation of the course of MS and histocompatibility antigens. In: Bauer HJ, Poser S, Ritter G, eds. Progress in multiple sclerosis research. Berlin/Heidelberg/New York: Springer, 1980; 456–9.
16. Walker JE, Cook JD, Harrison P, et al. HLA and the response of lymphocytes to viral antigens in patients with multiple sclerosis. Hum Immunol 1982; 4:71–8.
17. Hauser SL, Dawson DM, Lehrich JR, et al. Intensive immunosuppression in progressive multiple sclerosis. N Engl J Med 1983; 308:174–80.

Chapter 14

Quantification of Sensibility in Mononeuropathy, Polyneuropathy, and Central Lesions

Ulf Lindblom and Richard Tegnér

Quantification of sensibility disturbances can serve several purposes. First, it may provide diagnostic evidence in patients with suspected nerve lesions, especially when other tests are inconclusive. Second, if several sensory modalities are tested, the type and extent of an impairment can be defined in relation to physiologically different somatosensory systems. Both hypo- and hyperesthesia, as well as aberrant sensations, can be recorded. Such a comprehensive presentation is a convenient document and may help both the doctor and the patient to understand the neural dysfunction and the symptoms. Third, an assessment of the course of the disease and of spontaneous or induced changes (e.g., therapeutic effects) can be obtained by repeated testing at successive intervals.

Sensory quantification in the individual patient is best applied on the basis of a thorough conventional neurologic examination, with bedside techniques that outline the dysfunction with regard to different modalities and the relative contribution of negative and positive manifestations. Except for specific studies, sensory quantification should always be preceded by a neurologic examination to ensure adequate selection of quantitative techniques and application sites.

Another condition for sensory quantification is the access to clinically applicable methods for graded stimulation, which should be as modality-specific as possible. Such methods are available for touch contact, discriminative touch, vibration, pressure, and temperature. Most often, the perception thresholds or the minimum discriminable difference between two stimuli are determined. In some instances (e.g., in patients with

This study was supported by Vivian L. Smith Foundation for Restorative Neurology.

171

hyperesthesia), suprathreshold stimuli and magnitude estimation of the sensation may be applied.

For each stimulus mode, there is a choice of more or less complex test procedures. The sophisticated methods are usually the most exact, but they are also more time-consuming. In most situations, the amount of available time becomes a limiting factor for both the investigator and the patient, whose compliance is reduced by fatigue. The choice of type and number of tests to be applied must therefore be made with due consideration of both the time factor and the suitability of the tests for the particular patient under study, as well as the cost of the necessary equipment. Existing psychophysical techniques can often be modified to suit clinical conditions. The same basic tests may be used in various somatosensory disorders, but there are some differences in their application in mononeuropathies, polyneuropathies, and central lesions.

MONONEUROPATHIES

The simplest case for sensory quantification is a mononeuropathy in a sensory or mixed nerve with pure loss of sensibility. The neurologic examination is uncomplicated and the quantification shows elevated thresholds for touch, warm, cold, and/or thermal pain. Vibrametry may also be used, but one has to consider that the stimulus spreads easily through the tissues and may excite receptors outside the innervation territory of the nerve under study.

A sustained threshold increase may confirm the presence of a lesion if electrophysiologic and other tests have been inconclusive, which is often the case in our practice. The modality profile of the hypoesthesia will indicate the relative affection of A-beta, A-delta, and unmyelinated nerve fibers.

In mononeuropathies with positive manifestations (paresthesia or dysesthesia, hyperesthesia, and allodynia), the result of the neurologic examination may be difficult to interpret because several modalities are stimulated simultaneously with bedside techniques. For example, pins stimulate both touch and pain receptors, and warm or cold objects stimulate both mechanoreceptors and thermal receptors. With modality-specific and graded techniques, a much better analysis can be performed, as illustrated with thermal stimulation in Figure 14.1. The dysfunction can be analyzed in relation to different somatosensory systems; hyperphenomena can be quantified, and aberrant perceptions can be better defined.

Tactile Thresholds

To measure tactile thresholds with von Frey hairs[1] (nowadays, nylon filaments) is an old but still-useful method. A series of 10 or 12 filaments with logarithmically spaced bending pressures between 0.02 and 10 to 40 g (0.2 to 400 mN) will suffice. The threshold is either expressed as the filament closest to that felt half of, for example, ten successive applications, or it is determined by the "staircase method," also known as the method of limits.[2] With this method, the threshold is the average of the first

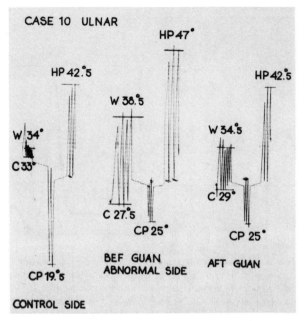

FIGURE 14.1 *Record of thermal sensitivity from patient with ulnar neuropathy and hyperpathia. Note increase of difference limen between warm (W) and cold (C) thresholds, hypoalgesia for heat pain (HP) and cold allodynia (CP) on the abnormal side as compared with the control side. After the administration of guanethidine (GUAN), which blocked the ongoing pain, the cold allodynia persisted, the heat pain threshold was normalized, and the thresholds for warm and cold were improved but still significantly elevated. The greater sensibility loss before guanethidine illustrates superimposed sensibility loss associated with ongoing pain. (From Lindblom, 1985.[14])*

stimulus of an ascending series of strengths to be felt ("yes" value) and the first stimulus of a descending series not to be felt ("no" value). The regular repetition of stimulation may result in the error of rhythmicity and should be avoided.

Through the years, scattered methodologic papers on the von Frey method have been published,[3-6] but there are relatively few original studies in which it has been applied. The advantages of the method are that it is quick, easy, cheap, and applicable everywhere, and that it correlates well with tactile pulses. Its disadvantages are mixed stimulus modes and undefined rate of application.

Tactile pulses from a mechanical stimulator provide precise and adequate stimuli of low-threshold cutaneous mechanoreceptors, all of which are innervated by large myelinated A-beta fibers.[7,8] This method requires equipment costing approximately $15,000. It has been used mostly in psychophysiologic investigations of normal subjects[9] but also in clinical studies[7,10-13] (Figures 14.2 and 14.3). It is probably the best-controlled and most sensitive measure of tactile thresholds, which can be determined by either the method of limits or a forced-choice procedure. The exact timing of the stimulus makes it suitable for studies of reaction time and evoked potential. In combination with magnitude estimation, suprathreshold intensity functions can be produced to quantify hypo- or hyperesthesia[11,12] (Figure 14.3). The method is useful

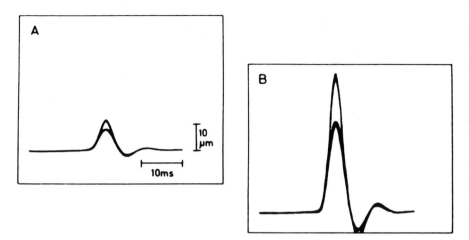

FIGURE 14.2   *Tactile thresholds, determined by short mechanical pulses according to the method of limits, on the index fingers of a patient with a sutured median nerve. Oscillographic records of threshold pulses from normal side (A) and injured side (B). Upper pulse contours indicates the lowest amplitude of the ascending stimulus series that was felt; lower contours indicate the highest pulse of the descending series that was not felt. (Reprinted by permission from Lindblom, 1981.[21])*

for specific investigations but less suitable for the clinical routine, since it is time-consuming and requires substantial laboratory resources. It is noteworthy that measurements with tactile pulses and von Frey hairs correlate surprisingly well.[14]

One advantage of using a mechanical stimulator is that the stimulus provides selective non-noxious activation of large fibers with a choice of defined pulses (single or repetitive pulses, trains, ramps). Also, it is relatively quick and easy to apply to such sensitive areas as face and hands. The method is of limited value for proximal and hypoesthetic areas because of limited amplitude range, and impossible to apply on the chest because of respiratory movements. Considerable intra- and interindividual variance occurs, at least with the method of limits.

Thermal Thresholds

The Marstock method[15] uses a Peltier thermode and provides selective thermal stimulation with graded warmth and cold. Thresholds are determined with a tracking technique. Both hypo- and hyperesthetic phenomena can be quantified as abnormal thresholds for warm, cold, heat pain, and cold pain (Figure 14.1). The method emphasizes the profile of thermal sensitivity and the pattern of abnormalities, while a forced-choice procedure detects the minimum discriminable temperature changes.[16-18] Studies of intensity functions and adaptation are feasible with the Marstock method, whereas recordings of reaction times and evoked potentials require special techniques.[19,20]

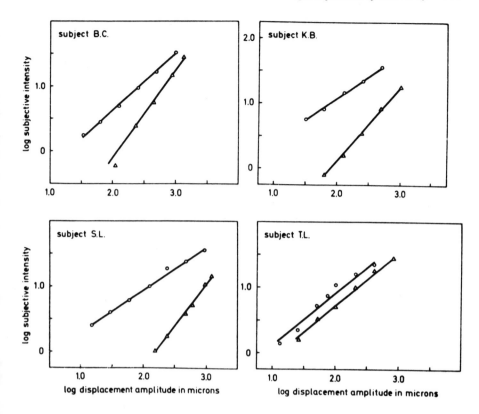

FIGURE 14.3 *Tactile sensation magnitude functions in patients with sutured median nerves after maximum recovery time. Subjective intensity plotted against stimulus strength in log-log coordinates. Test pulses applied to the tip of digit 2 or 3 of sutured side (open triangles) and contralateral normal hand (open circles). Note persisting hypoesthesia with best recovery in subject T.L., who was the youngest. (Reprinted by permission from Franzén and Lindblom, 1976.[11])*

The Marstock method is relatively quick, modality-specific, and applicable to all skin regions that offer a good surface contact with the thermode. Its disadvantages include considerable intra- and interindividual variance, and the method is more dependent on subjective criteria and patient instruction than tactile and vibratory thresholds.

Pain Thresholds for Pinch and Pressure

Thresholds for mechanically evoked pain can be estimated by a strain-gauge receiver mounted in a pair of forceps[21] or in a blunt pressure probe.[22] Since the criteria for pain report vary markedly, the use of an intrapatient reference value from a homologous skin area is recommended. The method is especially useful in acute studies in

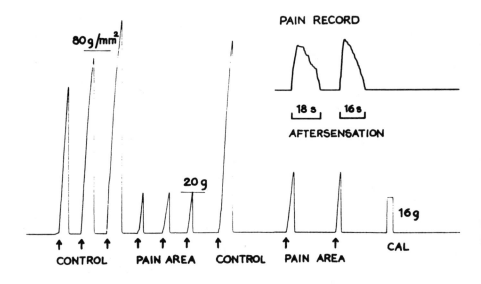

FIGURE 14.4   *Potentiometric recordings of pain thresholds and aftersensations in a 45-year-old woman with sciatic nerve causalgia. A blunt-ended pressure algometer was applied in the pain area (foot sole), where pain was elecited at an abnormally low pressure (20 g/mm²), as compared with 80 g in the normal homologous region contralaterally. About 30 g of pressure in the pain area evoked rather intense pain, with 16 to 18 seconds of aftersensation. (Reprinted by permission from Lindblom 1985.[14])*

which the pain sensitivity is manipulated[10] and also in the documentation of hyperalgesia and tenderness (pressure allodynia) (Figure 14.4).

POLYNEUROPATHIES

There is a growing need for a standardized and easily repeatable diagnostic procedure in polyneuropathy (PNP). First, the prevalence of PNP has increased significantly with the successful long-term management of diseases such as diabetes mellitus and uremia. Severe PNP is now rare, but slight or moderate PNP is a frequent complication of these conditions. The PNP reflects the underlying disease, so that the nerve dysfunction may be used as an index (albeit an indirect one) of the disease state, and repeated assessment of the PNP can help the physician to follow the disease's course and monitor its treatment.

Second, standardized PNP assessment is becoming more pertinent as therapies are developing for the nerve dysfunction itself. Examples of such therapies are plasmapheresis in Guillain-Barré syndrome, corticosteroids in chronic inflammatory polyneuropathy (CIP), and membrane stabilizers for the control of positive PNP symptoms such as paraesthesia and pain. Third, there is a large group of patients with PNP in whom no etiology can be demonstrated. It is important to make a careful assessment of the type and course of nerve dysfunction in these patients for use in further research into its origin. Finally, there is a need for a repeatable screening type of neurologic examination to detect PNP as early as possible in patients undergoing treatment with potentially neurotoxic drugs and in populations at risk for occupational or other environmental neurotoxic exposure.

The following section describes a standardized procedure for the clinical assessment of PNP that has been useful in both cross-sectional and longitudinal studies.[23-26] The selection of diagnostic criteria and the application of instrumental procedures are discussed.

Symptoms and Signs

Most PNP symptoms are of the positive, or irritative, type. They may be graded according to their prevalence, as indicated in Table 14.1. It is important that only bilateral symptoms be scored as significant. Numbness should be both bilateral and sustained to count, and it should preferably be graded according to its distal to proximal distribution. Subjective muscle weakness is usually too indistinct to be graded meaningfully.

Clinical signs can be graded as shown in Table 14.2. Detection of touch with wisps of cotton wool or a camel's hair brush is not a very sensitive test, but it conveniently introduces the idea of sensory testing to the patient. Tests of tactile discrimination with graphesthesia or of two-point discrimination are more sensitive, and these sensibilities are often impaired early, like the tendon reflexes and vibration sense.

The second most common impairment is that of temperature sensibility. Our experience with uremic and diabetic neuropathy indicates that cold and warm sensations are affected in parallel, although they are mediated by different sets of fibers: A-delta and C fibers, respectively.[27] Reduced pin-prick sensation and thermal pain sensitivity are usually noticeable later, but hyperalgesia, which indicates an irritative stage of nerve dysfunction, may occur early. Paresis of the dorsiflexors of the toes and feet, accompanied by atrophy of the short toe extensors, may be early signs and must be looked for during examination; the patient is unaware of them.

Table 14.1   Quantification of Symptoms of Polyneuropathy

Symptom		Grading
Numbness	0	If intermittent or unilateral
	1–3	If sustained and bilateral
	1	If restricted to the feet
	2	If extending above the malleoli
	3	If also in the upper extremities
Paresthesias, dysesthesias	0	If occasional or unilateral
Neuropathic pain	1	If a few times a week and bilateral
Muscle cramps	2	If most days of the week and bilateral
	3	If every day or night and bilateral
Muscle weakness	—	(No grading suggested)

Table 14.2   Quantification of Signs of Polyneuropathy

Type of Function or Sign	Grade of Impairment	
Touch	0	If unilateral
Touch, discriminative	1	If restricted to the feet
Vibration, tuning fork	2	If extending to the lower legs
Joint kinesthesia	3	If also in the upper extremities
Pin prick		
Cold		
Warmth		
Paresis		
Muscle atrophy		
Muscle reflexes (ankle, knee and	0	For unilateral loss
biceps brachii)	1	For loss of one on each side
	2	For loss of 3–4 reflexes
	3	For loss of 5–6 reflexes

For notation of the symptoms and signs, we recommend a form such as the one reproduced in Figure 14.5—with space for some general data on top and for short verbal notes on each line—as a basis for grading. Signs are graded for the right and left sides separately and averaged in the right-hand column (0 for unilateral impairment). For cutaneous sensory modalities, clear-cut bilateral hyperesthesia or paresthetic sensation without apparent loss should be scored in addition to loss of sensibility.

Diagnostic Criteria and Grading

It appears important that the diagnostic criteria are clearly stated by various investigators. Most neurologists put more weight on signs than symptoms and require the presence of at least one bilateral sign in addition to symptoms. In the absence of symptoms, two or more signs may be required, such as a stocking pattern of hypoesthesia or decreased vibratory sensation in the feet, together with loss of ankle reflexes or weakness of toe dorsiflexors. Dyck et al.[28] have recently concluded, on the basis of comparison with a neuropathologic index, that abnormal findings in two of three different evaluations (scored symptoms, neurologic deficits, and abnormalities of nerve conduction) constitute sensitive and reliable minimal criteria for the diagnosis of neuropathy.

Since the diagnostic significance increases with the number and extent of abnormalities, it is reasonable to interpret the number of abnormal tests and the degree of impairment of each function as an overall measure of nerve dysfunction. This is the main rationale for applying an array of several separately graded tests and adding the grades together. Table 14.2 lists ten items for scoring on a scale of 0 to 3; theoretically these constitute a 30-point scale. If the four scored symptomatic items in Table 14.1 are added, the maximum PNP score is 42. In practice, only lower scores are obtained, since all items never score maximally in the same patient. It should be pointed

NEUROPATHY ASSESSMENT   PATIENT   *J.P. male*
                                   age 34
DATE *Oct 19,-83*   BY *B.L.*

DIAGNOSIS *Diabetes*   TREATMENT   *diet + insulin*

SYMPTOMS			GRADE
NUMBNESS *constantly in both feet*			*1*
PAR- or DYSESTHESIA *pins and needles in hands and feet 2-3 times/month*			*0*
NEURALGIC PAIN *0*			*0*
MUSCLE CRAMPS *every night, sometimes even daytime*			*3*
MUSCLE WEAKNESS *0*			
MISCELLANEOUS *general fatigue*			

SIGNS	RIGHT SIDE		LEFT SIDE	
TOUCH CONTACT	*0-1*		*0-1*	*0*
TOUCH DISCRIMI- NATIVE	*1*		*1*	*1*
VIBRATION TUNING FORK	*1*		*1*	*1*
JOINT KINESTHESIA	*0*		*0*	*0*
PIN PRICK	*2*		*1*	*1.5*
COLD	*2*	*28°*	*28.5°*	*2*	*2*
WARMTH	*2*		*2*	*2*
PARESIS	*1 cannot walk on heels on either foot.*		*1*	*1*
ATROPHY	*1 short ext bilat*		*1*	*1*
REFLEX BICEPS	—		—	
REFLEX QUADRICEPS	—		—	*3*
REFLEX GASTROC-SOL	—		—	

Sens.lab. Neurol.Dept. Karol.Hosp.   SUM of GRADES: *16.5*

COMMENTS: *Mixed, moderate polyneuropathy.*

.........*U.L.*.........
Signature

FIGURE 14.5   *Neuropathy assessment form.*

out that the scoring system was developed for slight or moderate PNP, the commonest types seen in neurologic practice. For patients with severe PNP (e.g., those with Guillain-Barré syndrome), the grading must be adapted to the span of clinical severity.

Selection of Tests

The most important reason for using several tests is that they represent different functions and, to some extent, different types of nerve fibers that may be differentially affected, especially in early stages of PNP. Early detection is therefore best achieved with use of several tests.

Once the suggested standardized procedure has been established as a routine, all items of Tables 14.1 and 14.2 can be evaluated within half an hour. However, a reduced number of items may be wanted. The history of symptoms can be limited to the positive ones, which can be noted as present or absent without grading.[29] To simplify the examination, touch contact plus joint kinesthesia, vibration, or reflexes— or even two of these three—may be left out. If so, it is probably best to retain vibration and to use vibrametry instead of the tuning fork. It is important to retain the pin-prick and temperature tests, as these are the only tests of small-fiber function. Warmth and pain are the only available tests for somatic unmyelinated fibers, whereas there are abundant tests for large myelinated fibers.

Instrumental Procedures

The commonest laboratory procedure is electrophysiologic investigation with electroneurography and electromyography. Signs of denervation on electromyography, reduced nerve conduction velocity, and reduced action potential amplitude are well established objective electrophysiologic indicators of peripheral nerve dysfunction. If abnormalities are recorded in at least two nerves, preferably one in each lower leg, a suspected diagnosis of PNP is confirmed. By means of electroneurography, quantitative measures are obtained, as well as indications of the type of nerve lesion and its distal to proximal extension.

Some investigators use only electrophysiologic criteria in the assessment of neuropathy. In most clinical contexts, however, the complementary use of clinical and electrophysiologic tests appears to be more appropriate. One reason is that to some extent they reflect different pathogenetic mechanisms. A reduced conduction velocity, for example, can be the only sign of PNP and may remain subclinical without functional consequences. Normal electrophysiologic data, on the other hand, can coexist with a clinically significant and sometimes severe neuropathy. It is also of interest that therapeutic intervention may act differentially on clinical and electrophysiologic parameters.[25,30]

The second most common instrumental procedure is to measure vibratory perception thresholds with electromagnetic devices. These allow the delineation of abnormal thresholds[31,32] and can also be used for longitudinal studies.[25,33,34] The exactness of the chosen technique is crucial. The tuning fork becomes unreliable in patients with neuropathy and also in screening subjects over 60 years old because of the exponential regression of vibrational sensitivity with age. Generally, changes in vibration threshold appear to reflect short-term deterioration or improvement of nerve function earlier than do electrophysiologic parameters. Vibration thresholds are recordable at later stages of neuropathy than evoked action potentials.

Testing for vibration thresholds is quick in most patients, applicable in most bodily regions, and relatively inexpensive. Disadvantages are stimulus spread and considerable variance, at least with the method of limits.

During recent years there has been a rapidly growing interest in the quantitation of thermal sensibility, and various techniques have been introduced. Their special merit is the early detection of small-fiber impairment in somatic neuropathy. Two methods have been introduced, both based on the Peltier principle of producing temperature changes by applying an electric current to a metal junction. The Marstock method has already been described. The second method uses a forced-choice procedure to measure the least detectable temperature difference.[16,18] This method measures the threshold of discrimination more exactly but takes more time. Both methods have been applied in PNP assessment.[16,17,27,35-38]

CENTRAL LESIONS

Lesions of the spinal cord, brainstem, and thalamus can usually be examined by the same techniques that have been described for the peripheral nerves. This section will therefore deal with sensory quantification in lesions of the parietal cortex, which require a quite different approach. The reasons for this are that (1) thresholds for primary sensory qualities such as touch and temperature are often undefinable, (2) mainly complex sensory functions are involved, and (3) dissociated sensory loss is common. No single test is pathognomonic; it is the profile of sensibility impairment that has diagnostic significance.

A subject's ability to discriminate size, shape, roughness, and weight has been described by Head and Holmes[39] as an important test of somatosensory cortex function. Important technical contributions have recently been made by Roland.[40] He used a computer technique to manufacture micro- and macrogeometric structures (rough surfaces, spheres, ellipsoids, parallelepipeda) that could be carefully defined in terms of energy content, bandwidth, etc. By examining a large group of patients with well-defined cortical lesions, he showed that identification of shape was the most sensitive function, being impaired after partial lesions of the SI hand area, whereas identification of size and microgeometric discrimination were impaired only after destruction of the whole SI hand area.

Weight discrimination is similarly a sensitive and easily administered quantitative test of cortical sensory function.[39] The deficit in weight discrimination may be severe despite normal or only slightly impaired joint kinesthesia and/or tactile sensibility. To our knowledge, no modern studies are available.

The above tests are useful to quantitate sensibility only in the hands. Two other tests, topagnosis and graphesthesia, can be used to study other body parts.

Graphesthesia is the ability to identify figures drawn on the skin. A simpler, more basic test is directional cutaneous kinesthesia, in which the patient is asked to state the direction of a line drawn on the skin by a dull point. Normal subjects can always recognize the direction of lines drawn on the fingertips if the lines are longer than 1 cm, and on other body parts if they are longer than 6 cm. In a study of 12 patients with parietal lesions, it was found that graphesthesia was more often defective than directional cutaneous kinesthesia.[41] Loss of the latter nearly always occurred with loss of directional joint kinesthesia, whereas there was frequently a dissociation between these tests and two-point discrimination and topagnosis. Inability to identify objects (astereognosis) was related either to loss of directional skin and joint kinesthesia or to loss of two-point discrimination, indicating that the nervous system can use different strategies for this task.

Measurement of vibration thresholds are important in cortical lesions only in the sense that they are normal in pure cortical lesions; impaired vibratory sensitivity therefore indicates that lesion extends deeper.[42]

Topagnosis, the ability to localize tactile stimuli on the body surface, has been extensively studied since the nineteenth century (for recent review, see Hamburger[43]). A clinically useful technique, introduced by Noordenbos,[44] is the "goggle method." The test subject is provided with a pair of deep-red goggles with an occluding flap on the front. Standard points are marked on the test area in red ink, which the subject is unable to see. With the flap occluded, the examiner touches one of the points and marks with black ink the spot he believes has been touched. The distance and direction of the error can then be calculated. Topagnosis has been shown to depend on the quality and force of the stimulus, and there is also a distinct effect of practice.[43] For these reasons, normative values are less useful, and it is preferable to compare results from homologous areas. Although topagnosis is often impaired in parietal lobe lesions, topagnosis may occur with lesions anywhere along the neuraxis.

CONCLUSION

Many tests are available and no single laboratory can be expected to use them all. The choice of a set of tests should take into account (1) what part of the neuraxis will be examined, (2) the intended use of the tests—whether they will be used for a specific investigation or if they are intended for routine clinical purposes, and (3) the amount of time that can be spent on each patient. It is sometimes a difficult decision whether to examine many patients with a "quick and dirty" method or only a few patients with a more precise technique.

REFERENCES

1. von Frey M. Untersuchungen über die Sinnesfunctionen der menschlichen Haut: Druchempfindung und Schmerz. Abhandl Sachs Gesell Wiss Math Phys 1886; 23: 175–266.
2. Gescheider GA. Psychophysics. Method and Theory. New York: John Wiley, 1976; 20–38.
3. Weinstein S. Tactile sensitivity of the phalanges. Percept Mot Skills 1962; 14:351–4.
4. Sekuler R, Nash D, Armstrong R. Sensitive, objective procedure for evaluating response to light touch. Neurology 1973; 23:1282–91.
5. Levine Scott BS, Pearsall G, Ruderman RJ, et al. Von Frey's method of measuring pressure sensibility in the hand: an engineering analysis of the Weinstein-Semmes pressure aesthesiometer. J Hand Surg 1978; 3:211–16.
6. Johansson RS, Vallbo ÅB, Westling G. Thresholds of mechanosensitive afferents in the human hand as measured with von Frey hairs. Brain Res 1980; 184:343–51.
7. Lindblom U. Touch perception threshold in human glabrous skin in terms of displacement amplitude on stimulation with single mechanical pulses. Brain Res 1974; 82:205–10.
8. Westling G, Johansson RS, Vallbo ÅB. A method for mechanical stimulation of skin receptors. In: Zotterman Y, ed. Sensory functions of the skin in primates. Oxford: Pergamon, 1976:151–8.
9. Vallbo ÅB, Johansson RS. The tactile sensory innervation of the glabrous skin of the human hand. In: Gordon G, ed. Active touch. The mechanism of recognition of objects by manipulation. Oxford: Pergamon, 1978:29–51.
10. Lindblom U, Meyerson B. Influence on touch vibration and cutaneous pain of dorsal column stimulation in man. Pain 1975; 1:257–70.
11. Franzén O, Lindblom U. Tactile intensity functions in patients with sutured peripheral nerve. In: Zotterman Y, ed. Sensory functions of the skin. Wenner-Gren Center international symposium series, vol. 27. Oxford: Pergamon, 1976:113–18.
12. Lindblom U, Verrillo RT. Sensory functions in chronic neuralgia. J Neurol Neurosurg Psychiatry 1979; 42:422–35.
13. Borg K, Lindblom U. Diagnostic value of quantitative sensory testing (QST) in carpal tunnel syndrome. Acta Neurol Scand 1988; 78:537–41.
14. Lindblom U. Assessment of abnormal evoked pain in neurological pain patients and its relation to spontaneous pain: a descriptive and conceptual model with some analytical results. In: Fields HL, Dubner R, Cervero F, eds. Advances in pain research and therapy. New York: Raven, 1985; 9:409–23.
15. Fruhstorfer H, Lindblom U, Schmidt WG. Method for quantitative estimation of thermal thresholds in patients. J Neurol Neurosurg Psychiatry 1976; 39:1071–5.
16. Dyck PJ, Karnes J, O'Brien PC, et al. Detection threshold of cutaneous sensation in humans. In: Dyck PJ, Thomas PK, Lambert EH, et al., eds. Peripheral neuropathy. Philadelphia, PA: Saunders, 1984; 1:1103–38.
17. Bertelsmann FW, Heimans JJ, Weber EMJ, et al. Thermal discrimination thresholds in normal subjects and in patients with diabetic neuropathy. J Neurol Neurosurg Psychiatry 1985; 48:686–90.
18. Jamal GA, Hansen S, Weir AI, et al. An improved automated method for the measurement of thermal thresholds. 1. Normal subjects. J Neurol Neurosurg Psychiatry 1985a; 48:354–60.
19. Fruhstorfer H, Detering I. A simple thermode for rapid temperature changes. Pflugers Arch 1974; 349:83–5.
20. Fruhstorfer H, Lindblom U. Sensibility abnormalities in neuralgic patients studied by thermal and tactile pulse stimulation. In: von Euler C, Franzén O, Lindblom U, et al., eds.

Somatosensory mechanisms. Wenner-Green Center international symposium series, vol 41. London: Macmillan, 1984:354–61.

21. Lindblom U. Quantitative testing of sensibility including pain. In: Stålberg E, Young RR, eds. Clinical neurophysiology. Butterworths international medical reviews, vol 1. London: Butterworths, 1981:168–90.

22. Jensen K, Andersen HØ, Olesen J, et al. Pressure-pain threshold in human temporal region. Evaluation of a new pressure algometer. Pain 1986; 25:313–23.

23. Bergström J, Lindblom U, Norén LO. Preservation of peripheral nerve function in severe uremia during treatment with low protein high caloric diet and surplus of essential amino acids. Acta Neurol Scand 1975; 51:99–109.

24. Knave B, Persson HE, Goldberg JM, et al. Long-term exposure to jet fuel. An investigation on occupationally exposed workers with special reference to the nervous system. Scand J Work Environ Health 1976; 3:152–64.

25. Tegnér R, Lindholm B. Uremic polyneuropathy: different effects of hemodialysis and continuous ambulatory peritoneal dialysis. Acta Med Scand 1985; 218:409–16.

26. Tegnér R, Lindholm B. Vibratory perception threshold compared with nerve conduction velocity in the evaluation of uremic neuropathy. Acta Neurol Scand 1985; 71:284–9.

27. Lindblom U, Tegnér R. Thermal sensitivity in uremic neuropathy. Acta Neurol Scand 1985; 71:290–4.

28. Dyck PJ, Karnes JL, Daube J, et al. Clinical and neuropathological criteria for the diagnosis and staging of diabetic polyneuropathy. Brain 1985; 108:861–80.

29. Dyck PJ, Sherman WR, Hallcher LM, et al. Human diabetic endoneurial sorbitol, fructose and myo-inositol related to sural nerve morphometry. Ann Neurol 1980; 8:590–6.

30. Greene DA, Winegrad AI. Effects of acute experimental diabetes on composite energy metabolism in peripheral nerve axons and Schwann cells. Diabetes 1981; 30:967–74.

31. Goldberg JM, Lindblom U. Standardized method of determining vibratory perception thresholds for diagnosis and screening in neurological investigation. J Neurol Neurosurg Psychiatry 1979; 42:793–803.

32. Halonen P. Quantitative vibration perception thresholds in healthy subjects of working age. Eur J Appl Physiol 1986; 54:647–55.

33. Nielsen VK. The peripheral nerve function in chronic renal failure. VII. Longitudinal course during terminal renal failure and regular hemodialysis. Acta Med Scand 1974; 195:155–62.

34. Fagius J, Jameson S. Effects of aldose reductase inhibitor treatment in diabetic neuropathy—a clinical and neurophysiological study. J Neurol Neurosurg Psychiatry 1981; 44:991–1001.

35. Fruhstorfer H, Goldberg JM, Lindblom U, et al. Temperature sensitivity and pain thresholds in patients with peripheral neuropathy. In: Zotterman Y, ed. Sensory functions of the skin in primates. Wenner-Gren Center international symposium series, vol 27. Oxford: Pergamon, 1976b:507–19.

36. Guy RJC, Clark CA, Malcolm PN, et al. Evaluation of thermal vibration sensation in diabetic neuropathy. Diabetologia 1985; 28:131–7.

37. Jamal GA, Weir AI, Hansen S, et al. An improved automated method for the measurement of thermal thresholds. 2. Patients with peripheral neuropathy. J Neurol Neurosurg Psychiatry 1985; 48:361–6.

38. Lehmann WP, Haslbeck M, Müller J, et al. Frühdiagnose der autonomen Diabetes-Neuropathie mit Hilfe der Temperatursensibilität. Deutsch Med Wochenschr 1985; 110:639–42.

39. Head H, Holmes G. Sensory disturbances from cerebral lesions. Brain 1911; 34:102–254.

40. Roland PE. Cortical areas in man participating in somatosensory discrimination of microgeometric surface deviations and macrogeometric object differences. In: von Euler C, Franzén O, Lindblom U, et al., eds. Somatosensory mechanisms. Wenner-Gren Center international symposium series, vol 41. London: Macmillan, 1984:125–38.

41. Bender MB, Stacy C, Cohen J. Agraphesthesia. J Neurol Sci 1982; 53:531–55.

42. Roland PE, Nielsen VK. Vibratory thresholds in the hands. Comparison of patients with suprathalamic lesions with normal subjects. Arch Neurol 1980; 37:775-9.
43. Hamburger HL. Locognosia. Rotterdam, Holland: 1980. (Thesis.)
44. Noordenbos W. The sensory stimulus and the verbalization of the response: the pain problem. In: Somjen GG, ed. Neurophysiology studied man. International Congress series, no. 253. Amsterdam: Excerpta Medica, 1972:207-14.

Chapter 15

Approaches to Quantitative Cutaneous Sensory Assessment

Peter James Dyck and Peter C. O'Brien

Disordered function and structure of peripheral and central sensory neurons (axons) are recognized by symptoms, neurologic deficits, abnormality of evoked electrical responses, and morphologic study. The assessment of neurologic symptoms and deficits relating to disease of sensory nerve fibers and tracts is difficult because several modalities of sensation are involved, symptoms do not necessarily relate to severity of deficit, very sophisticated approaches are required to evaluate sensation, and detection thresholds vary markedly with site and age and to a minimal degree with sex and height. Evaluation is nonetheless becoming increasingly important as new treatments are being tested and used. Quantitative cutaneous sensory assessment will be of value in assessing therapy in compression and entrapment neuropathy and repair of severed nerves, in metabolic neuropathies (especially diabetic polyneuropathy), in toxic neuropathies, in immune neuropathies (inflammatory demyelinating neuropathy, monoclonal-protein-associated neuropathy, and necrotizing vasculitis), and in such central nervous system disorders as multiple sclerosis. There is a particularly strong need for commercially available microprocessor-controlled sensory systems that can reliably test sensory threshold and print out the results, expressed as percentiles for site and age.

WHAT IS QUANTITATIVE CUTANEOUS SENSORY ASSESSMENT?

These procedures estimate the slightest cutaneous stimuli that can be perceived—the detection threshold. Slow mechanical deformation or the skin is used to evaluate touch-pressure sensation, and rapid mechanical deformation serves to evaluate vibratory sensation. The sensations experienced usually are named for the stimuli producing them—touch-pressure, vibratory, cooling, and warming. Tissue-damaging stimuli are used to assess nociception. Evaluations of detection thresholds should be distinguished from evaluations of sensation in the above-threshold range. In the latter, the amount of a sensory experience may be ranked or compared with another measurable attribute.

In practice, quantitative assessment of cutaneous sensation ranges from the use of hand-held devices that deliver stimuli whose waveforms and amplitudes are inadequately known or quantitated, to preprogrammed automated systems in which the stimulus is precisely specified and quantified, forced-choice testing is employed, preprogrammed steps (on algorithm) are followed, threshold is estimated by validated approaches, and results are printed out as percentiles specific to site, age, and sex.[1,2] As discussed later, whether the results are sensitive, specific, and reliable depends at least in part on the characteristics of the stimulus, nature of the instrumentation, rules employed in testing and finding the threshold, and adequacy of the controls. It depends further on variables in normal subjects and patients. For example, drowsiness, distraction, or anxiety may affect results. Variable noise in sensory systems themselves may also account for variations.[2] Forced-choice testing is used to exclude the contribution of system noise to estimates of threshold and to reduce patient and observer bias.[3]

WHY ESTIMATE CUTANEOUS DETECTION THRESHOLDS OF SENSATION?

This question needs to be asked because clinical testing appears to be sufficient for some purposes and is more rapid than estimating detection thresholds. Moreover, other surrogate measures of nerve or sensory tract dysfunction are available and provide objective, sensitive, graded, and repeatable measures.[4,5]

For some purposes (e.g., recognizing a region of skin analgesia, as in leprosy, or a sensory lack, such as that resulting from compression of the spinal cord, or hemianesthesia due to stroke), a neurologist's rapid assessment of sensation using cotton wool, stick pins, a tuning fork, and manual positioning of the toe may provide satisfactory results.

Various surrogate measures of nerve or sensory tract function provide objective, sensitive, graded, and repeatable measures.[4,5] Concerning peripheral nerve, possibly the best of these surrogate measures are parameters of nerve conduction. Useful inferences about sensory function can be drawn from data on the amplitude, waveform, latency, and conduction velocity of afferent nerve fibers. Abnormal attributes of nerve conduction are statistically associated with severity of symptoms and deficits (e.g., in diabetic polyneuropathy). However, the statistical associations are not close enough to predict symptoms or sensory deficits from nerve conduction abnormalities.[4,5]

Sometimes attributes of nerve conduction have no predictive value for symptoms and deficits. For example, in certain forms of painful, hereditary sensory and autonomic neuropathy, nerve conduction measurements are normal, but thermal, nociceptive, and autonomic functions are abnormal.

Thus, the reasons for evaluating cutaneous detection thresholds are that one cannot accurately infer threshold from surrogate measurements, and clinical methods are inadequate for some purposes. Clinical methods are not sufficiently standardized, quantitated, reproducible, or accurate to estimate detection threshold with anatomical site, development, age, sex, handedness, and aging. In medical research and practice, evaluation of detection thresholds is needed to detect and characterize the type of sensory loss and the alterations of this loss with time, risk factors, or treatment intervention. Inferences about the anatomical site(s) of pathologic abnormality, class of affected neurons (fibers or tracts), and pathologic alteration can be made on the basis of the type and distribution of sensory loss.[6-8] Selective sensory deficits, by modality of sensation, have been found to relate to selective decrease or absence of classes of sensory fibers revealed by assessment of the compound action potential of the excised sural nerve *in vitro* and study of diameter histograms of myelinated and unmyelinated fibers of the same nerve. The quantitative assessment of cutaneous sensation may also help in quality control of the clinical evaluation.

We are using vibratory and cooling detection thresholds (VDT and CDT) as evaluated by Computer Assisted Sensory Examination (CASE) in a population-based cross-sectional and longitudinal study (the Rochester Diabetic Neuropathy Study) to assess the frequency and severity of neuropathy and its risk factors. We have also used VDT and CDT in a sham-controlled trial of plasma exchange in chronic inflammatory demyelinating polyneuropathy[9] and in two levels of glycemic control in diabetic neuropathy.[10] Others have used quantitative sensory approaches in similar and other studies (see Chapters 14 and 17 and references 11 to 24).

TEST REQUIREMENTS

The thinking on how to quantitate sensory evaluation falls into two categories, which might be called the "doctor's bag" and "laboratory" approaches. In the doctor's bag approach, simple, inexpensive instruments are hand-carried to the bedside, home, or factory, or on field trials. Quality is compromised to a degree in order to make the instruments small, simple, portable, and inexpensive. They are used in any situation in which a doctor or nurse examines patients. In the laboratory approach, the patients or normal subjects come to a laboratory in which the environment and testing approaches are optimized. Irrespective of the approach used, it is important to recognize that results of sensory evaluation may be influenced by the test environment, bias on the part of subject or patient and observer, the medical condition, the stimulus, the instrumentation, the format and steps of testing, the method of finding threshold, and the appropriateness and size of the control population.

To minimize variability, the test should be given in a quiet environment free of visual or auditory distraction. This probably precludes open wards, work places or home settings, in which other people are present. Time should be set aside to administer the test. The subject should be well rested and prepared to concentrate. As mental anguish, distraction, and drowsiness will undoubtedly raise threshold spuriously (even when a two-alternative, forced-choice algorithm is employed), the technician must attempt to recognize these adverse conditions and continue testing only when conditions are appropriate.

It is difficult to give the test in precisely the same way each time because whoever administers it must determine the order of testing, note and record results, and set the conditions for the next testing event. Using a microprocessor and sensory system ensures that all steps of testing, measurement of threshold, and comparison with normal results will be done in the same way. Threshold may be measured more quickly and accurately by a system than by a trained observer, and the result should be more valid. From our experience in the Sensation Laboratory at the Mayo Clinic (presented in more detail in Chapter 16), the cost of hardware and software is readily offset by the lower cost of professional time. A trained technician can administer the test.

As for stimulus, the waveform should be suitable for the sensation tested and should not vary in intensity or shape; it should also be quantifiable and graded over a wide range. Only one stimulus should be presented, and it should be available in any magnitude. The range of intensities should vary from small values (i.e., below the threshold of children at their most sensitive regions) to large values (i.e., above the threshold of old people at their least sensitive sites).

Because receptors are anatomically distributed over the surface of the skin, detection of abnormality may be enhanced by testing a grid pattern of skin. It has been possible to do this with touch pressure and vibration, but we have not found a way to do this with cooling or warming.

Especially in forced-choice testing of mechanoreceptor function, the stimulator should rest on the skin with a constant load before superimposing a waveform. In this way, impact that is variable and that provides a second stimulus with different waveform from the one tested is avoided. Ideally, portable instruments should be applied with a constant load to avoid providing extraneous stimuli from the observer's hand movement or the damping of the stimulus inherent in some instruments.

The algorithm of testing may be a considerable source of variation in results. In developing CASE, we evaluated some of these variables, asking: Should the magnitude of stimulus increase continuously or in steps? Should the increase be linear, or should it be exponential and based on estimates of just-noticeable difference? How many trials are needed to assure that a result is unlikely to have occurred simply by chance? When the limits (supersensitive or insensitive) are reached, should supersensitivity or insensitivity be declared, or should the result be repeated once more or several times more?

COMPUTER-ASSISTED SENSORY EXAMINATION (CASE)

The CASE system is made up of stimulating transducers, an automatic traversing device for estimating VDT and touch-pressure detection threshold (TPDT), a microprocessor, an electronic controller, a visual display device (to present the numbers 1 and then 2 in forced-choice testing), a response key with which to enter the subject's responses, and a typewriter with which to enter instructions and print out results. The system has been described elsewhere in detail.[1] The testing arrangement is shown in Figure 15.1. CASE permits the evaluation of touch-pressure, vibratory, cooling, and warming detection thresholds on face, finger (hand), or toe (foot).

The algorithm in CASE employs (1) a range of quantitative stimuli large enough to test points with low thresholds in children and high thresholds in old people, (2) 21 levels of magnitude that increase exponentially, with steps based on a study of just-noticeable difference, and (3) preprogrammed rules for testing and finding threshold with use of a two-alternative forced-choice technique. CASE takes into account the

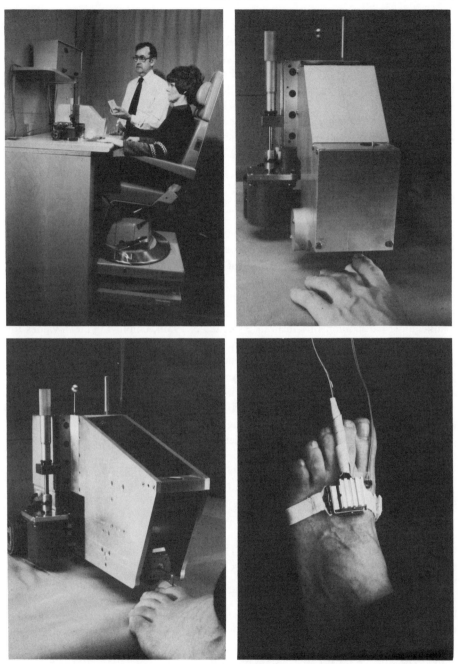

FIGURE 15.1 *Various components of CASE. Upper left: A subject being tested in the sensory laboratory. Upper right: Close-up view of the transducer used in assessing touch-pressure detection threshold. The stylus rests on the dorsal surface of the subject's index finger. Lower left: The transducer used to evaluate vibratory threshold. Lower right: The thermode used to evaluate warming or cooling detection threshold.*

number of supersensitive and insensitive points and the thresholds of sensitive points in expressing abnormality.

After initial positioning of the transducer and entry of biographic data and coded instructions, all aspects of testing and the printing out of results are automatic. The technician (or patient) enters the response for each stimulus pair presented. Since the same evaluation has been performed in more than 300 healthy subjects, percentiles for site, age, and sex have been estimated. The responses for a given patient can therefore be expressed as percentiles for these variables.

EFFECTS OF PATIENT VARIABLES AND DISEASE ON TEST RESULTS

Detection thresholds of touch pressure, vibratory sensations, and cooling sensations vary with site, age, and sex.[2] Site and age are major determinants of threshold. Some neurophysiologic measurements are thought to be influenced by height and weight. We have tested for the influence of height and weight on VDT by regressing the normal deviate of the combined percentile (number of insensitive points and threshold of sensitive points[4]) on a given height and on the ratio of the observed to ideal weight for that height (Metropolitan Life Insurance Co. table, 1959), employing mean values for medium frame in regression analysis. The study was based on VDT obtained on the great toe of 306 healthy subjects (i.e., without history of neurologic disease or diseases predisposing to neuropathy, and 8 to 81 years of age).

We found that threshold was greater with height ($P < 0.001$) but that the magnitude of this change was small ($< 1.8\%$ reduction in standard deviation). No significant association of threshold was found for weight. Of the variables site, age, sex, height, and weight, only site and age are major determinants of results. Sex and height contribute only minimally.

TPDT, VDT, and CDT are commonly abnormal in peripheral nerve or sensory tract disease. The distribution and pattern of abnormality may have diagnostic implications. Examples of such abnormality have been published.[2]

COMPARISON OF THRESHOLDS WITH USE OF OUR ALGORITHM AND AN AUTOMATED BÉKÉSY METHOD

In the development of CASE, various sequential methods for testing and scoring were simulated on the computer (as described in Chapter 16). According to the criteria of efficiency, repeatability, and adaptability to minicomputer, the chosen algorithm was found to be suitable for use in a system of finding threshold of TPDT, VDT, and CDT detection thresholds. In testing TPDT or VDT with forced choice at one site (e.g., toe or finger), it may be necessary to provide a series of 35 pairs of stimuli at each of nine points. The time required for all nine points averages between 20 and 25 minutes. Inherent problems are boredom and drowsiness, which adversely affect threshold. A more efficient algorithm would be highly desirable.

In our own testing, to reduce its time of administration, we used computer simulation and actual trials of normal subjects and patients with sensory loss. We found that decreasing the number of levels in testing or decreasing the number of turnarounds from six to four gave unacceptably divergent results as compared with those of the algorithm described above. With these alternative algorithms, the derived thresholds were sometimes spurious as compared with other types of nerve evaluation.

Two other approaches may be considered. The first is to test a single larger skin area rather than nine puntuate skin areas. We are currently testing this approach; results are not yet available. The second approach is to use the same nine points but to substitute a Békésy approach (also called "method of ups and downs" or "staircase method"). It employs the same stimulus, level at onset, and number of turnarounds, but it is not a two-alternative forced-choice approach.

Measurement of VDT by the algorithm employed in CASE was compared to that obtained by the Békésy method.[25] In healthy persons, the threshold was higher with the Békésy approach (Table 15.1). A more serious problem became obvious in the study of neuropathic patients. An occasional patient with severe sensory loss (as determined clinically and with the CASE algorithm) and severe neurophysiologic and morphometric abnormality of nerves had normal or supersensitive responses with the Békésy algorithm (Table 15.2). Such spurious results were not encountered with the CASE algorithm.

Table 15.1 Vibratory Detection Threshold (VDT) of Index Finger, Measured in 20 Healthy Subjects with the CASE Algorithm and with an Automated Békésy Approach

Determination	CASE	Békésy
Threshold of sensitive points (ln μm) (mean $\pm$ SD)	0.717 $\pm$1.000	1.588 $\pm$0.575
Number of supersensitive points in 9 subjects[a] (mean $\pm$ SD)	1.3 $\pm$1.8	0.2 $\pm$0.5

[a]Insensitive points were not found in these 20 subjects.

Table 15.2 Vibratory Detection Threshold (VDT) of Great Toe in Ten Patients with Peripheral Neuropathy,[a] Measured with the CASE Algorithm and with an Automated Békésy Approach

Determination	CASE	Békésy
Threshold of sensitive points (ln μm) (mean $\pm$ SD)	3.450 $\pm$1.018	2.792 $\pm$1.049[b]
Number of insensitive points in 9 subjects[a] (mean $\pm$ SD)	3.9 $\pm$3.2	5.9 $\pm$4.0

[a]The patients had inherited (5), chronic imflammatory-demyelinating (2), postgastrectomy (1), diabetic (1), and cause unknown (1) types of neuropathy.

[b]Four of ten patients had nine insensitive points. Two of the other six patients had one and two supersensitive points, respectively.

CONCLUSION

Clinical assessment of cutaneous sensation is not sufficiently standardized, quantitated, reproducible, or accurate to estimate detection threshold with anatomic site, development, age, sex, disease, or treatment. CASE can be used to estimate detection threshold with sensitivity and reliability. To decrease testing times and thus decrease spurious thresholds due to drowsiness, we have explored the sensitivity and reliability of testing one surface area rather than nine points. We have also compared thresholds measured with the CASE algorithm (with two-alternative forced choice) with those measured with a Békésy algorithm (without two-alternative forced choice). The threshold was higher and sometimes grossly in error with the Békésy approach.

REFERENCES

1. Dyck PJ, et al. Introduction of automated systems to evaluate touch-pressure, vibration, and thermal cutaneous sensation in man. Ann Neurol 1978; 4:502–10.
2. Dyck PJ, Karnes J, O'Brien PC, et al. Detection Thresholds of Cutaneous Sensation in Humans. In Dyck PJ, Thomas PK, Lambert EH, et al. eds. Peripheral neuropathy. Philadelphia: W.B. Saunders, 1984; 49:1103–38.
3. Selksular R, Nash D, Armstrong R. Sensitive, objective procedure for evaluating response to light touch. Neurology (Minneap) 1973; 23:1282–91.
4. Dyck PJ, Bushek W, Spring EM, et al. Sensitivity and specificity of vibratory cooling detection thresholds in the diagnosis of diabetic neuropathy. Diabetes Care 1987; 10:432–40.
5. Dyck PJ. Detection, characterization, and staging of diabetic polyneuropathy. Muscle Nerve 1987. (in press).
6. Dyck PJ, et al. Pathologic alterations of the peripheral nervous system of humans. In Dyck PJ, Thomas PK, Lambert EH, et al., eds. Peripheral neuropathy. Philadelphia: W.B. Saunders, 1984; 36:760–870.
7. Dyck PJ, Lambert EH, Nichols PC. Quantitative measurement of sensation related to compound action potential and number and sizes of myelinated and unmyelinated fibers of sural nerve in health, Friedreich's ataxia, hereditary sensory neuropathy, and tabes dorsalis. In Rémond A, ed. Handbook of electroencephalography and clinical neurophysiology. Amsterdam: Elsevier, 1971;9.
8. Guy RJC, Clark PN, Watkins PJ. Evaluation of thermal and vibration sensation in diabetic neuropathy. Diabetologia 1985; 38:131–7.
9. Dyck PJ, Daube J, O'Brien P, et al. Plasma exchange in chronic inflammatory demyelinating polyradiculopathy. N Engl J Med 1986; 314:461–5.
10. Service FJ, Rizza RA, Daube JR, et al. Near normoglycemia improved nerve conduction and vibration sensation in diabetic neuropathy. Diabetologia 1985; 28:722–7.
11. Barach JH. Test for quantitative vibratory sensation in diabetes, pernicious anemia and tabes dorsalis. Arch Intern Med 1947; 79:602–13.
12. Beutelsmann FW, Heimans JJ, Weber RJM, et al. Thermal discrimination thresholds in normal subjects and in patients with diabetic neuropathy. J Neurol Neurosurg Psychiatry 1985; 48:686–90.
13. Chochinow RH, Ullyot LE, Moorhouse JA. Sensory perception thresholds in patients with juvenile diabetes and their close relatives. N Engl J Med 1972; 286:1233–7.
14. Collins WS, Zilinsky JD, Boas LC. Impaired vibratory sense in diabetes. Am J Med 1946; 1:638–41.
15. Cornsweet T. The staircase method in psychophysics. Am J Physiol 1962; 75:485–91.

16. Mirsky IA, Futterman P, Broh-Kahn RH. The quantitative measurement of vibration perception in subjects with and without diabetes mellitus. J Lab Clin Med 1953; 41:221–35.
17. Nielsen VK, Lund FS. Diabetic polyneuropathy. Corneal sensitivity, vibratory perception and achilles tendon reflex in diabetics. Acta Neurol Scand 1979; 59:15–22.
18. Sosenko JA, Boulton AJM, Kubrualy DB, et al. The vibratory perception threshold in young diabetic patients: associations with glycemia and puberty. Diabetes Care 1985; 8:605–7.
19. Steiness IB. Vibratory perception in normal subjects. A biothesiometer study. Acta Med Scand 1957; 158:315–25.
20. Steiness IB. Vibratory perception in diabetics during arrested blood flow in the limb. Acta Med Scand 1959; 163:195–205.
21. Steiness IB. Influence of diabetic status on vibratory perception during ischaemia. Acta Med Scand 1961; 170:319–38.
22. Williamson RT. The vibrating sensation in affections of the nervous system and in diabetes. Lancet 1905; 1:855–6.
23. Williamson RT. The vibrating sensation in diseases of the nervous system. Am J Med Sci 1922; 164:715–27.
24. Wood EJ. A further study of the qualitative variations in the vibratory sensation. Am J Med Sci 1922; 163:19–30.
25. von Békésy G. A new audiometer. Acta Otolaryngol 1947; 35: 411–22.

Chapter 16

A Computer Evaluation of Quantitative Algorithms for Measuring Detection Thresholds of Cutaneous Sensation

Peter C. O'Brien, Peter James Dyck, and Jon L. Kosanke

Sensitive and accurate measurement of detection thresholds of sensation is needed to recognize differences among body parts and changes related to development, aging, and neurologic disease. It is also needed to assess risk factors in epidemiologic trials or treatments. Vibratory, cooling, or warming detection thresholds may be used as indicators of abnormality in large- and small-diameter afferent fibers of nerves.

Elsewhere in this book and in earlier reviews, we and others have provided evidence that detection thresholds vary, markedly with site and age and to a small degree with sex, height, and weight.[1-5] Detection thresholds also increase with disease of peripheral sensory neurons (axons).[1-5]

It is self-evident that for quantitative assessment of cutaneous sensation, the stimulus must be appropriate to the modality tested. Its waveform must be precisely described, invariant with magnitude, and available to be given at any magnitude over a wide range of amplitudes. It must also be the only sensory stimulus given during the test interval.[2] Bias of the subject or patient or observer can affect estimates of threshold.[2,6] To decrease response bias, forced-choice testing is employed.[2,6] One would expect a subject to guess correctly in 75% of forced-choice challenges (taken to be the criteria for threshold) when the stimulus is less than that for which the subject can confidently assert sensation. In accordance with this expectation, we have found that use of a forced-choice algorithm of testing provides lower thresholds than use of a staircase approach.

ALGORITHMS FOR A COMPUTER-BASED TESTING SYSTEM

On the basis of earlier trials, we recognize that results of a forced-choice algorithm may depend on the specific rules employed. In the investigation described in this chapter, we assess some of the rules we employ in the Computer-Assisted Sensory Examination (CASE) algorithm, using computer simulation to test the probability that a certain outcome will occur. For example, an algorithm for testing and finding threshold would be judged inappropriate if, by chance alone, estimated thresholds were often found to be very different than the true value.

In the CASE algorithm, what practical rules should be followed to ensure that estimates of threshold are sufficiently close to true values to be clinically useful? Ideally, it would be desirable to apply a variety of different approaches to a series of normal subjects and patients with a broad range of sensory impairment. However, the magnitude of the problem rendered such a patient-based evaluation infeasible, and we have therefore performed extensive computer-based simulations. The results of these simulations demonstrate dramatically the importance of carefully evaluating the rules of testing to find threshold in a variety of conditions when the true threshold is known.

This study was undertaken to optimize the algorithm for CASE. In the improved system to be developed (CASE IV), we plan to use 25 levels of stimulation by adding 4 levels to the 21 employed in CASE III.[2] The features of computer-assisted sensory examination have been described elsewhere.[2,7] The essential characteristics of the testing format are:

1.   The patient is presented with paired stimulus intervals indicated by the sequential visual display of the numbers 1 and 2. During a given pair of stimulus events, a cutaneous stimulus is given in one of the intervals and no stimulus (null-stimulus) is given in the other. The patient is required to indicate during which interval the stimulation occurred, regardless of whether or not he believes he felt anything.

2.   The up-down transformed-response rule proposed by Wetherill is used to move up and down among levels of stimulus magnitudes to identify the level at which awareness of the stimulus is correct 75% of the time, corrsponding to an actual awareness in 50% of forced-choice tests. The patient is presented with a series of forced-choice challenges at a given level. The pattern of observed responses (successes and failures) results in a decision that the patient has either succeeded or failed at that level of stimulation, and the next series of forced-choice testing is done at a harder or easier level, accordingly. If the next level to be tested is outside the levels available, we conceptually define additional levels as needed, with success or failure occurring with probability 1.

3.   The process in step 2 is repeated until K (a prespecified number) changes in direction occur, at which point the data are reviewed and an estimate of the true threshold is obtained.

This simulation study was designed to identify (1) suitable criteria for defining success or failure at a given level, (2) the most efficient manner for moving up and down among the 25 available levels, (3) the most suitable choice for K (the number of turnarounds to be used), and (4) the best method of estimating threshold once testing is completed.

The results of our investigation document the reliability and efficiency of CASE IV. More important, however, they suggest methods of developing and evaluating systems for the quantitative assessment of sensation that should be helpful to others.

TESTING SENSITIVITY

All our simulations required the specification of a model describing the true levels of sensation in a given patient. Three such models were used (Table 16.1), corresponding to sensitive patients with threshold at level 13 (model A), moderately insensitive patients with threshold at level 21 (model B), and grossly insensitive patients with threshold sufficiently beyond level 25 that the probability of success for any forced-choice pair, at any level, is 0.5—that is, the subject is guessing throughout (model C). The gradients used for how quickly the patient acquires sensation in models A and B reflect our experience in testing actual subjects. In evaluating each test procedure, we simulated the results for 1,000 hypothetical subjects for each of the models in Table 16.1 by generating a series of random numbers in the interval (0,1). For example, to simulate a forced-choice challenge at level 13 to a model A subject, we would consider the subject's response to be correct if the random number obtained was less than 0.75.

As we planned the simulation study, it was soon apparent that we could not evaluate all conceivable algorithms and then select the best, since the possibilities were virtually infinite. We therefore embarked on a series of evaluations in which each step was suggested by the preceding results.

Preliminary simulations indicated that a suitable starting point would be to fix K (the number of turnarounds) at 6, stepping in increments of 4, 4, 2, 2, 1, and 1 preceding turnarounds 1, 2, 3, 4, 5, and 6, respectively, and estimating threshold as the median of the levels tested at turnarounds 3, 4, 5, and 6. Our initial aim was to defer the evaluation of alternative schemes and to obtain criteria for defining whether the observed pattern of responses to forced-choice testing at a given level should be classified as success or failure. In considering possible candidates, we were constrained by the requirement that at threshold, the probability of success should be approximately 0.5. Four methods for defining success were considered. As indicated in Table 16.2, all produce success with probability approximately equal to 0.5 when testing at threshold. The probability of achieving success when the patient feels nothing (is guessing) varies from 0.188 to 0.033. In the simulations, it was assumed that forced-choice challenges occurred sequentially and that testing terminated as soon as the end result (success or failure) was apparent.

A comparison of the method's performances is provided in Table 16.3. The number of forced-choice challenges (trials) required to complete testing on a single subject did not include the challenges occurring below level 1 or beyond level 25. As expected, the time required for testing increases from one method to the next. In general, there is a corresponding gain in the accuracy of estimated thresholds, although the gain with method 4 appears unsatisfactory in view of the increased testing time required. Because the time required for method 4 was viewed as prohibitive, it was not evaluated further.

Table 16.1   Probability of Correct Response to a Single
Forced-Choice Challenge

	Model		
Level	*A*	*B*	*C*
1	0.50	0.50	0.50
2	0.50	0.50	0.50
3	0.50	0.50	0.50
4	0.50	0.50	0.50
5	0.50	0.50	0.50
6	0.50	0.50	0.50
7	0.50	0.50	0.50
8	0.50	0.50	0.50
9	0.50	0.50	0.50
10	0.50	0.50	0.50
11	0.55	0.50	0.50
12	0.65	0.50	0.50
13	0.75	0.50	0.50
14	0.85	0.50	0.50
15	0.95	0.50	0.50
16	0.98	0.50	0.50
17	0.98	0.50	0.50
18	1.00	0.50	0.50
19	1.00	0.55	0.50
20	1.00	0.65	0.50
21	1.00	0.75	0.50
22	1.00	0.85	0.50
23	1.00	0.95	0.50
24	1.00	0.98	0.50
25	1.00	0.98	0.50

Table 16.2   Methods of Defining Success at a Given Level of Testing[a]

	Probability of Success	
	At Threshold	*Guessing*
Method 1		
SSS, SSFS	0.527	0.188
Method 2		
SSSS, SSSFS, SSFSS	0.475	0.125
Method 3	0.495	0.074
i) 6 or 7 of 7 = S, or		
ii) 5 of 6 = *S*, 7 = *F*, 8 and 9 = *S*		
Method 4		
9 or more S in 11 trials	0.455	0.033

[a] S denotes success; F, failure.

Table 16.3 Simulation Results for Four Methods

| Method | Model | Actual Threshold Level[a] | Number of Trials | | Estimated Threshold | | | | % Within ±1 Level |
| | | | Mean | Max | Percentile | | | | |
					1	10	90	99	
1	A	13	26.1	55	7.5	11	14.5	15.5	64.6
	B	21	27.3	64	11	17	22	22.5	51.2
	C	Ins.	25.9	52	11.5	19.5	25.5	25.5	73.8
2	A	13	33.1	70	9.5	11.5	14.5	15.5	68.1
	B	21	33.7	73	14.5	18.5	22.0	23	64.3
	C	Ins.	19.7	60	14.5	23.0	25.5	25.5	85.4
3	A	13	56.2	101	9.5	11.5	14.0	14.5	77.5
	B	21	60.2	114	16.5	19.5	22.0	22.5	73.3
	C	Ins.	32.7	78	20.5	25.5	25.5	25.5	94.6
4	A	13	110.6	205	10.5	11.5	13.5	14.5	84.5
	B	21	120.6	214	17.5	19.5	21.5	22.5	78.3
	C	Ins.	62.1	154	23.5	25.5	25.5	25.5	98.2

[a]Ins. denotes insensitive.

REFINING THE ALGORITHM

The most important finding from these simulations is that an inordinate number of subjects have very low estimates of threshold for all methods. Additional simulations indicated that this problem could not be solved by increasing the number of turnarounds (K) to eight by changing the statistic used to estimate threshold (e.g., by using the mean of all six turnarounds or the mean of the last four). A review of data in the 1% of subjects with the lowest estimated threshold for each model indicated that modification of the stepping algorithm was the most promising approach to resolving this difficulty. Specifically, we adopted the convention that once a patient produced a pattern of responses resulting in failure, stepping would be by single-level increments whenever it was to a lower (more difficult) level. The rationale for this convention is apparent upon reviewing the models in Table 16.1 and recalling that correct response occurs with probability 1 beyond level 25. When a patient is tested at two or more levels above his true threshold, a correct response is virtually certain. Thus, when failure occurs at a given level, one can be reasonably sure that threshold is not far below, and one should proceed cautiously when moving to lower thresholds.

Evaluation of methods 1, 2, and 3 with the modified stepping algorithm (Table 16.4) indicates that estimation of threshold is markedly improved. This is particularly true for the lowest 1% of estimated thresholds, which is now much closer to the true threshold value. Comparison with the results obtained using eight turnarounds is provided in the lower half of the table. Clearly, the additional testing associated with eight turnarounds provides an additional gain in accuracy. However, the price of improved accuracy is a corresponding increase in the number of forced-choice challenges which, when translated into the patient time required to complete the test, may be prohibitive in some contexts. The data provided in Table 16.4 provide a basis for selecting a test algorithm appropriate to one's needs.

Since method 3 (with eight turnarounds) provided the most accurate estimates, we selected this algorithm for further evaluation. Specifically of interest was the best statistic for estimation, given the available data. Four statistics were evaluated: mean and median based on (1) all eight levels at which turnarounds occurred and (2) only the last six levels. It is apparent (Table 16.5) that using the mean of all eight turnaround points is inferior to the other three statistics, but no clear differences are apparent otherwise. Estimates based on means and medians of only the last four turn points (unpublished data) were quite similar to the three best statistics in Table 16.5.

RULES FOR THE ALGORITHM

The theoretical properties of the up-down transformed-response algorithm have been studied extensively by others.[8-15] However, these mathematical explorations have been related primarily to applications in bioassay. We are unaware of any evaluations relating to sensory testing other than those reported here. As our results show, it is essential that evaluations with specific applications be performed under circumstances appropriate to those applications. This is illustrated by the wide variations in the perfor-

Table 16.4 Simulation Results for Methods 1, 2, and 3 with Modified Stepping Procedure (K = 6 and 8)

| K | Method | Model | Actual Threshold Level[a] | Number of Trials | | Estimated Threshold | | | | % Within ±1 Level |
| | | | | Mean | Max | Percentiles | | | | |
						1	10	90	99	
6	1	A	13	32.3	70	10.0	12.5	14.5	16.5	63.4
		B	21	30.6	58	16.0	19.5	22.5	23.5	64.7
		C	Ins.	16.8	45	15.5	22.5	25.5	25.5	84.3
6	2	A	13	42.1	84	11.5	12.5	14.5	16.0	63.9
		B	21	39.4	75	18.0	20.0	22.5	23.5	66.3
		C	Ins.	17.3	47	17.5	25.0	25.5	25.5	93.8
6	3	A	13	69.5	138	11.5	12.5	14.5	15.5	78.0
		B	21	68.1	126	19.5	20.5	22.5	23.5	80.0
		C	Ins.	29.9	68	21.5	25.5	25.5	25.5	97.2
8	1	A	13	41.0	72	11.0	12.0	14.5	15.5	77.9
		B	21	38.9	73	16.5	19.5	22.5	23.0	75.6
		C	Ins.	20.0	52	16.5	24.0	25.5	25.5	89.4
8	2	A	13	51.9	90	11.5	12.5	14.5	15.5	74.6
		B	21	49.9	102	18.5	20.5	22.5	23.0	76.5
		C	Ins.	20.7	66	18.5	25.0	25.5	25.5	95.0
8	3	A	13	87.8	147	11.5	12.5	14.0	15.0	89.6
		B	21	86.6	159	19.5	20.5	22.0	22.5	89.5
		C	Ins.	34.4	88	23.5	25.5	25.5	25.5	98.9

K = 8 (4, 4, 2, 2, 1, 1, 1, 1)

[a] Ins. denotes insensitive.

Table 16.5 Comparison of Four Statistics for Estimating Threshold[a]

Statistic	Turnpoint Used	Model	Actual Threshold Level[b]	Percentiles					% Within ±1 Level
				1	10	90	99		
Mean	All	A	13	11.5	12.4	14.3	14.9		80.1
Mean	Last 6	A	13	12.0	12.5	14.2	14.8		88.4
Median	All	A	13	12.0	12.5	14.5	15.0		89.2
Median	Last 6	A	13	11.5	12.5	14.0	15.0		89.6
Mean	All	B	21	18.5	20.0	22.1	22.7		76.7
Mean	Last 6	B	21	19.7	20.5	22.0	22.7		89.2
Median	All	B	21	19.5	20.5	22.0	22.5		90.7
Median	Last 6	B	21	19.5	20.5	22.0	22.5		89.5
Mean	All	C	Ins.	20.3	23.9	26.0	26.0		86.4
Mean	Last 6	C	Ins.	22.8	25.5	25.7	25.7		97.2
Median	All	C	Ins.	21.5	25.5	25.5	25.5		97.4
Median	Last 6	C	Ins.	23.5	25.5	25.5	25.5		98.9

[a] Based on eight turnarounds, modified stepping, and method 3 for defining success.
[b] Ins. denotes insensitive.

mance of some of the algorithms we evaluated, according to which model of sensation (A, B, or C) was used. Moreover, any evaluation of a forced-choice approach to estimating thresholds of cutaneous sensation must reflect the fact that a correct response occurs with certainty when the stimulus is sufficiently strong but can never occur with a probability of less than 0.5 (unless, of course, a sensitive patient deliberately fails).

Our simulations indicated that the best way to deal with this feature of forced-choice testing was to adopt a somewhat unorthodox algorithm with a modified stepping procedure. The importance of this modification is reflected in Tables 16.3 and 16.4, which show that the lowest 1% of estimated threshold values among totally insensitive patients was 11.5 without modified stepping, as compared with 15.5 with that modification (using method 1 for defining success). By also incorporating an improved algorithm for defining success (method 3), the lower 1 percentile increased further to 21.5 and was further improved to 23.5 with use of eight turnarounds.

Which specific set of rules should be used? We believe that the answer to this question may vary with the circumstances. For example, in a clinical setting in which only a screen for gross abnormality is required and testing time must be minimized, a less precise algorithm may suffice. Conversely, in a research environment in which response to therapy must be accurately measured, method 3 with eight turnarounds would be the most appropriate—provided that testing does not take so long that because of boredom or fatigue, the subjects become unreliable in their responses.

CONCLUSION

The results of this investigation clearly demonstrate the importance of performing extensive computer simulations in the design and evaluation of quantitative methods for estimating thresholds of cutaneous sensation. Although a comprehensive evaluation must also include testing in both healthy human subjects and patients with sensory impairment, such testing should be preceded by simulations in which the true sensation of the "patient" is known. The importance of this finding is illustrated by supposing that an algorithm based on method 1 (using the original stepping procedure with six turnarounds) had been evaluated only in a patient population, without computer simulations. Among patients with no sensation within the ranges available for testing, 10% would have had thresholds estimated to be below level 20 (and 1% below level 12), and there would have been no way to identify the error, despite protestations of insensitivity by the patients.

REFERENCES

1. Steiness JB. Vibration perception in normal subjects and in diabetics. A biothesiometer study. Acta Med Scand 1957; 158:315.
2. Dyck PJ, Karnes J, O'Brien PC, et al. Detection thresholds of cutaneous sensation in humans. In Dyck PJ, et al., eds. Peripheral neuropathy, Philadelphia: W.B. Saunders, 1984: 1103–38.

3. Mirsby IA, Futterman D, Broh-Kahn RH. The quantitative measurement of vibration perception in subjects with and without diabetes mellitus. J Lab Clin Med 1953; 41:221.

4. Lindblom U. Quantitative testing of sensitivity including pain. In Stalberg E, Young RR, eds. Neurology: clinical neurophysiology. Butterworth International Medical Reviews. London: Butterworths, 1980; 1:168.

5. Pearson GHJ. Effect of age on vibratory sensitivity. Arch Neurol Psychiatry 1928; 20:482.

6. Sekular R, Nash D, Armstrong R. Sensitive objective procedure for evaluating response to light touch. Neurology (Minneap) 1973; 23:1282.

7. Dyck PJ, Karnes J, O'Brien PC. Detection thresholds of cutaneous sensation. In Dyck PJ, Thomas PK, Asbury AK, et al, eds. Diabetic neuropathy. Philadelphia: W.B. Saunders, 1987:107–21.

8. Choi SC. An investigation of Wetherill's method of estimation for the up-and-down experiment. Biometrics 1971; 27:961–70.

9. Davis M. Comparison of sequential bioassays in small samples. J R Stat Soc B 1971; 33:78–87.

10. Freeman PR. Optimal Bayesian sequential estimation of the median effective dose. Biometrika 1970; 57:79–89.

11. Hsi BP. The multiple sample up-and-down method of bioassay. 1969; 64:147–62.

12. Little RE. The up-and-down method for small samples with extreme value response distributions. J Am Stat Assoc 1974; 69:803–6.

13. Tsutakawa RK. Random walk design in bio-assay. J Am Stat Assoc 1967; 62:842–56.

14. Wetherill GB, Chen H, Vasudeva RB. Sequential estimation of quantal response curves: a new method of estimation. Biometrika 1966; 53:439–54.

15. Wetherill GB. Sequential estimation of quantal response curves. J R Stat Soc B 1963; 25:1–48.

Chapter 17

Quantitative Tests to Determine Peripheral Nerve Fiber Integrity

Pamela M. Le Quesne, Clare J. Fowler, and N. Parkhouse

In this chapter, the methods we use to assess the integrity of different types of peripheral nerve fibers will be described. To quantify independently the different aspects of peripheral nerve fiber function is important, as it permits the recognition of patterns of abnormality and the detection of changes that affect some but not all types of fibers. Differential assessment is also important in attempting to elucidate the etiology of the complications of some neuropathies (e.g., neuropathic ulcers and Charcot's arthropathy in diabetes). Furthermore, such methods of assessment must be established to allow longitudinal studies of neuropathy.

The protocol outlined here (and in Table 17.1) requires less than two hours and provides a quantitative assessment of all major subgroups of the peripheral nerves. Since peripheral neuropathy commonly affects the distal parts of the lower limbs most severely, we have concentrated on examination of the feet, and our tests have all been evaluated on feet. In many instances, other parts of the body can be satisfactorily examined with the same techniques, and normative data are available for some sites. In view of our current interest in diabetic neuropathy and the availability of many patients with this condition, most of the pathological data have been obtained through examination of diabetic patients.

For many years, the mainstay of quantitative evaluation of peripheral nerve function was electrophysiologic examination. However, routine clinical neurophysio-

We are grateful to Miss Marion Carroll for most of the control temperature threshold measurements, to Mrs. Fay Kaye for many biothesiometer measurements, and to Mr. Tarlok Gajree for assistance throughout the development of these tests. We also thank the Sir Jules Thorn Charitable Trust and ICI plc Pharmaceuticals Division for grants that enabled us to purchase and develop the apparatus used in these studies. N.P gratefully acknowledges the support of The William Scholl Foundation, administered through the London Foot Hospital. We are also indebted to Dr. A. Kurtz, The Middlesex Hospital, and Mr. K. Robertson, The London Foot Hospital, for allowing us to study patients under their care.

Table 17.1   Methods of Peripheral Nerve Assessment

Motor nerve fibers
  Evoked muscle action potential amplitude recorded from flexor hallucis
Sensory nerve fibers
  A-beta mechanoreceptors
    Vibration sensation assessed with biothesiometer
    Sural nerve action potential
  A-delta cold sensors
    Threshold for cooling
  A-delta fast pain sensors
    Pinch-pain threshold
  C warm sensors
    Threshold for warming
  C nociceptors
    Pinch-pain threshold
    Axon reflex flare induced by electrophoresed acetylcholine
Sympathetic nerve fibers
  Vasoconstrictors
    Cold pressor
    Deep inspiration
Sudomotor fibers
  Response to electrophoresed pilocarpine recorded by
    Humidity meter
    Dot count from bromphenol blue paper

---

logic methods involve stimulation of large-diameter nerve fibers and the recording of the evoked muscle action potential or the nerve potential in the same fibers. Many peripheral nerve fibers cannot be assessed by these techniques. Small myelinated and unmyelinated fibers predominate in peripheral nerves, and it is increasingly apparent that we must be able to quantify their function. It has been recognized for many years that during recovery from peripheral nerve damage, electrophysiologic recovery may lag behind clinical recovery. Thus, traditional methods are inappropriate for providing objective evidence of the course of a disease process. One of the main reasons is that both remyelinating and regenerating fibers are initially of small diameter and conduct slowly. They are therefore difficult to examine electrophysiologically. The ability to follow the progress of neuropathy has become particularly important since the recent and growing interest in possible therapies for various types of peripheral neuropathy. For a full assessment of fibers of different size and function, it is appropriate to combine electrophysiologic examination with quantitative functional testing.

MOTOR NERVE FIBERS

Quantitative measurement of muscle power provides valuable data about the functional state of motor nerves. However, the information obtained electrophysiologically by stimulation of motor nerves and recording of the amplitude of evoked muscle action potential is also valuable. In the lower limb, extensor digitorum brevis on the dorsum of the foot has frequently been used for recording the evoked muscle response. However, in moderate or severe neuropathy, it is common to find that no response can be elicited from this muscle. Motor units are also lost with aging. The amplitude of the action potential recorded from flexor hallucis, following stimulation of the posterior tibial nerve, has been found to provide a useful monitor of the state of the small muscles of the foot. Only in the most severe neuropathies is this potential unrecordable. In 17 control subjects, the mean ($\pm$ SD) amplitude was 7.8 $\pm$ 3.1 mV, as compared with a mean amplitude of 1.4 $\pm$ 1.4 mV in 12 diabetics with neurpathic foot ulcers and 0.2 $\pm$ 0.29 mV in 4 diabetics with Charcot's arthopathy.[1]

SENSORY NERVE FIBERS

Mechanosensitive Fibers

The main action potential recorded from a sensory nerve trunk is produced by a synchronous volley of nerve impulses in fibers subserving mechanosensation. The sural nerve is the nerve most easily accessible for examination in the lower limb. In patients with severe neuropathy and in some elderly subjects, no potential may be recordable, but the amplitude of the potential, when present, gives a valuable measure of the function of large-diameter nerve fibers. It is particularly useful in assessing a developing disorder but suffers from the disadvantages mentioned earlier in relation to the assessment of recovery.

Measurement of the vibration perception threshold (VPT) has proved valuable in assessing the functional state of A-beta mechanosensitive fibers. Sophisticated methods of measuring VPT have been evolved and described by Dyck and colleagues.[2] Precisely controlled graded stimuli are applied to nine points on the finger or toe and, with a forced-choice protocol, an accurate assessment of threshold is obtained. However, the method is time-consuming and requires an elaborate and expensive apparatus. It therefore has some limitations for routine clinical use, particularly in the field and in the survey of large numbers of subjects.

In assessing the suitability of a particular apparatus for this purpose, its sensitivity for detecting abnormality has to be weighed with the reproducibility of results and the speed of examination. We have found that the Bio-Thesiometer (Ohio) is a suitable apparatus as compared with two other commercially available machines.[3] It has been criticized for providing an uncontrolled stimulus, with threshold measurement dependent on the method of limits (i.e., the subject signals when the stimulus is felt or not felt during increasing or decreasing intensity) rather than a forced-choice procedure based on established psychophysical principles. However, we have shown an increase in threshold with age, thus demonstrating the sensitivity of the machine. We have also assessed the variability of repeated examinations in control and diabetic subjects.

The results for 155 control subjects are shown in relation to age in Figure 17.1, which also shows a linear relation of data after log transformation, and the calculated

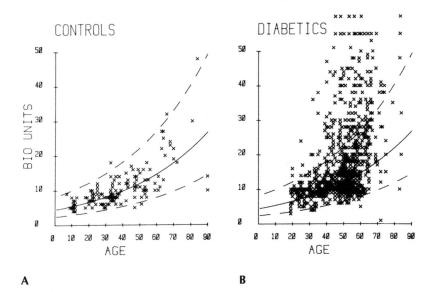

FIGURE 17.1 *Vibration perception threshold measured with a biothesiometer in control (A) and diabetic (B) subjects. Individual values are denoted by X. In each graph, the solid line is the calculated mean, and the dotted lines represent 95% confidence limits for the control subjects.*

mean and 95% confidence limits. The centile curves are almost identical to those obtained by Bloom et al.[4] from measurement of 519 control subjects, which further demonstrates the reliability of the apparatus. As a measure of reproducibility, an index (difference divided by the mean of two readings) was calculated for each subject in whom repeated measurements were made. The mean index was 0.17 ± 0.16 for 52 subjects. The calculated F value from log threshold measurements was 16.39, indicating a high signal-to-noise ratio for the method.

A further calculation was made concerning the ability of the machine to detect change in individual subjects. The observed change (from the mean of previous values to the current value) necessary to indicate a real change depends on the within-subject standard deviation (log scale), the number of previous observations, and the accepted risk of concluding that a change has occurred when in fact no change has occurred (type 1 error). In this calculation it is assumed that the within-subject standard deviation is constant, and the pooled value for the group is used. For a 5% type 1 error rate and two previous observations, the within-subject standard deviation is multiplied by a factor of 2.39. On this basis, a significant change would be +49% or −32%. This compares favorably with data obtained by others using other commercial machines.[5-7]

The Bio-Thesiometer has been used on 951 diabetic subjects routinely attending one of two diabetic clinics. Individual results are shown in Figure 17.1. In 215 diabetics (23%), VPT was more than 2 SD above the mean for age. The reproducibility of the results on successive examinations was comparable to that found in control subjects. The mean reproducibility index for 260 diabetics examined more than once was 0.21 ± 0.19, and the F value for log threshold was 12.16.

Thermal Sensory Fibers

Thermal sensation is often considered to be a continuum of a single sense, but this is not the case. Impulses induced by cooling stimuli are conducted in different fibers (A-delta) than those concerned with the sensation of warmth (C fibers). Moreover, the body regulatory functions are different, the response to cold being vasoconstriction, and that to heat being sweating.

Physiological studies in animals and humans have established that dynamic change in temperature is the effective stimulus to excite warm or cold sensors, and that rate of change is an important determinant of impulse discharge rate and recognition of temperature change.[8,9] Above the temperature range of 20 to 34 °C, the static impulse discharge rate from cold sensors is constant at a steady temperature. Warm afferents have a relatively low static firing frequency at 30 to 34 °C, below which they are silent.[10] Control of starting temperature is therefore unnecessary, provided that the subject is not vasoconstricted or in a condition of thermal discomfort. On this basis, Fowler et al.[11] have designed a thermal testing system (the Middlesex thermal tester) that delivers stimuli at a constant rate of change (1 °C/sec), the size of the stimuli depending on their duration. The thermode consists of a Peltier device sandwiched between cooling fins and a thin copper plate. The system is controlled by a small lap-held, battery-operated microcomputer (Epson HX20). This is connected to a thermode control unit via a standard RS232 port. The thermode control unit contains a serial input-output circuit, an A-D and a D-A converter, and a programmable power supply.

One advantage of this particular device is that it is portable. The computer is conveniently small, and the cooling fins attached to the thermode allow reequilibration over the range of temperatures used in testing. Most previous temperature testers have relied on water cooling or heating, which immediately makes them nonportable.

A 7.5-cm^2 thermode is used for testing the hand and face. However, when it was used to test the foot, many subjects were unable to appreciate an increase of 6 °C, the maximum change delivered. Fortunately, spatial summation of stimuli so greatly affects temperature appreciation[12] that by increasing the size of the thermode, the threshold for thermal appreciation was lowered to within the functioning range of the system. A thermode of 26 cm^2 is used for the foot. With this thermode, a threshold for warmth can be obtained in all control subjects. It is important that the whole surface of the thermode is in close contact with the skin for the stimulus to be effective, and a thermode of this size can make close contact when strapped over the medial surface of the sole of the foot. Contact is maintained by resting the thermode and the foot on a pillow. Thick skin and callosities could interfere with the passage of the stimulus to the sense organs, but it is rare to find any significant skin abnormality in the medial plantar region.

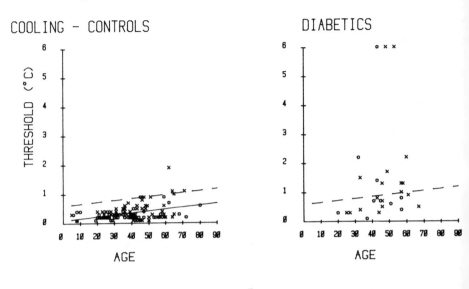

FIGURE 17.2 *Threshold for cooling stimulus in control (A) and diabetic (B) subjects. X denotes male, O denotes female. In (A), the solid line is the control mean and the dotted line is 2 SD above the mean. In (B), the dotted line is 2 SD above the control mean. (Redrawn from data of Fowler et al.[11])*

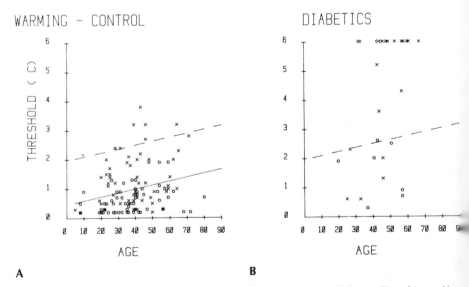

FIGURE 17.3 *Threshold for warming stimulus in control (A) and diabetic (B) subjects. X denotes male, O denotes female. In (A), the solid line is the control mean and the dotted line is 2 SD above mean. In (B), the dotted line is 2 SD above the control mean. (Redrawn from data of Fowler et al.[11])*

One other important advantage of the Middlesex thermal tester is that warm and cool thresholds can be estimated separately. In one popular device (the Marstock apparatus[13]), the difference between warm and cool appreciation is determined, but the two separate systems are tested together. The warm threshold is not tested in the system of Dyck et al.[2]

Data from 117 control subjects and 18 diabetics, obtained by Fowler et al.,[11] are shown in Figure 17.2 for cooling and Figure 17.3 for warming. The threshold for warming is higher than that for cooling in control subjects, and the threshold for both are higher in men than in women. In the diabetics, warmth appreciation was more often abnormal than was appreciation of cooling; 13 diabetics were unable to appreciate the maximum change of 6 °C for warmth, but only 3 were similarly insensitive to cooling.

Nociceptive Fibers

Pain

Many methods, using various types of stimulation, have been used to determine the threshold for pain appreciation. Although valuable information has been obtained about various aspects of pain appreciation in normal subjects with use of elaborate psychophysical testing procedures, these techniques have been difficult to apply to clinical problems.

Using a "pinchometer" designed and built by Dr. Bruce Lynn,[14] Le Quesne and Fowler[1] measured pinch-pain threshold on the dorsum of the foot in a series of diabetic subjects. A fold of skin was pinched between the metal plates of a pair of forceps. Force was transmitted by a stiff spring to a pair of strain gauges. The skin was pinched at a constant rate, and the patient signaled when the sensation changed from touch to pain. In control subjects, the first change in sensation was a sharp pain similar to the descriptions of "first pain" and presumably dependent on stimulation of A-delta fibers.

In diabetic subjects, the main abnormality was not an increase in threshold but an increased variability in threshold at the eight sites tested on the dorsum of the foot. In a proportion of the diabetic subjects, pain was not appreciated at one or more points when the maximum force (2.8 kg) was used. In other subjects, the quality of pain was altered. In some, a dull ache (presumably related to nociceptive C fiber activity) was felt instead of a sharp pain; in others, pain was referred to a site other than that stimulated, and in still others, pain was appreciated at an abnormally low level of stimulation. These abnormal findings were interpreted as being due to loss of A-delta fibers and to stimulation of collateral sprouts of surviving fibers or the abnormally sensitive tips of regenerating fibers or sprouts. Thus, this method gave better qualitative than quantitative information about disturbed appreciation of pain.

Flare

The dual sensory and secretory role of nociceptive C fiber afferents has become increasingly recognized in recent years. Their role in neurogenic inflammation has been widely explored since the recent interest in peptides, particularly in substance P, and the use of capsaicin as a tool to stimulate or destroy this system.[15] The currently favored concept is that substance P is released from nociceptive C fibers, and this in turn stimulates the release of histamine from mast cells and (possibly acting with other peptides) causes neurogenic vasodilatation. These events may contribute to the induction of local inflammation and repair as an adaptive response to injury.

We have devised an objective technique for quantifying the function of nociceptive C fibers on the basis of the cutaneous effector response (the axon reflex flare) rather than measurement of subjective pain in response to standard stimuli.

The characteristics and properties of the flare were well described by Lewis.[16] When the skin is injured by a scratch or prick, or when the subject receives the intradermal injection of histamine, a red flare develops, spreading for several centimeters beyond the limits of the injury. It is due to vasodilatation of the superficial vasculature and is abolished by the injection of local anesthetic prior to the injury and by nerve section followed by degeneration. It is not prevented by sympathectomy.

We stimulate the axon reflex flare by the electrophoresis of acetylcholine. Cutaneous blood flow is measured with a laser Doppler flowmeter, which produces a voltage signal directly proportional to microvascular blood flow in superficial skin vessels.[17] A 10% solution of acetylcholine is injected into the outer ring of a capsule 3 cm in diameter, which has three concentric compartments. This is attached to the skin over the instep on the sole of the foot. A current of 1 mA is passed for 5 minutes between the acetylcholine and an anode consisting of a metal plate covered with gauze and soaked in saline, which is attached to the opposite side of the foot. The flare spreads both outward and inward, and the laser Doppler probe, mounted in the middle of the inner capsule, continuously records the blood flow.

Electrophoresis for a predetermined length of time over a clearly circumscribed area ensures that the stimulus is constant and reproducible. This technique has the advantage of being noninvasive and therefore suitable for repeated measurements where the inflammatory pathways may already be disturbed. Topically applied, capsaicin is efficacious but takes up to 60 minutes to penetrate the skin, and on repeated application it damages the pathways being studied.[18] In searching for an atraumatic technique, we tried a variety of commercially available topical rubifacients, but with poor reproducibility, probably because of variable skin penetration. The use of the capsule ensures that the response is measured at a constant distance from the stimulus. The size of the response depends on the intensity of the reaction rather than the area of skin affected, an endpoint that is both difficult to quantify and variable but that has been used in many previous studies of the flare response. The method is sensitive, and a flare response can be recorded when none is visible to the naked eye. It can also be easily recorded from pigmented skin, which disguises the erythematous reaction.

There are several ways in which we have established that the response we are recording is an axon reflex flare. Acetylcholine is likely to be an effective stimulus; it has been established experimentally that this substance excites cutaneous C fibers.[19] The vasodilator response does not occur during electrophoresis of saline, nor does it occur after subcutaneous injection of local anesthetic (1% lignocaine) at a time when

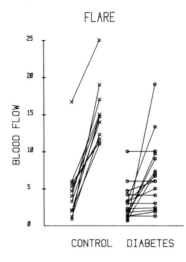

FIGURE 17.4   *Lines join values for resting blood flow and flow during axon reflex flare in individual control (X) and diabetic (O) subjects.*

direct vascular reactions still occur. The response is absent in skin that appears to be totally denervated in other ways.

The changes in blood flow during axon reflex vasodilatation are shown in Figure 17.4 for control and diabetic subjects. All the control subjects had a marked increase in blood flow. In a proportion of the diabetic subjects, flare was absent or markedly reduced.

Non-Neurogenic Vasodilation

In addition to neurogenic vasodilatation, Lewis[16] defined vascular reactions to stroking the skin that were non-neurogenically mediated. He called these the white reaction (vasoconstriction) and the red reaction (vasodilatation). We have used the latter to measure the capacity of vessels to dilate independently of any neurogenic influences. This is particularly important in the assessment of diabetic subjects in whom microvascular disease may be present. The reactions are produced by a single stroke with a dermograph, a purpose-designed blunt-pointed instrument with spring loading to assure standardization of force. The blood flow is then measured with the laser Doppler probe over the affected area.

In Figure 17.5, results for control subjects are shown, and it can be seen that the increase in blood flow is very similar to that occurring during the axon reflex flare. The increase in blood flow during the red reaction in diabetics with an abnormal flare response is also shown. Clearly, the vessels in the diabetic subjects were capable of dilating, so the abnormal flare response can be ascribed to degeneration of nociceptive C fibers; it is not due to intrinsic abnormality of the vessels.

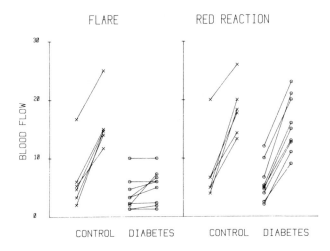

FIGURE 17.5   *Lines join values for resting blood flow and flow during axon reflex flare or red reaction in individual control (X) and diabetic (O) subjects. Flare and red reaction were measured in the same subjects.*

SYMPATHETIC NERVE FIBERS

Stimulation of sympathetic nerves to the limbs causes vasoconstriction and sweating. We measure functional responses of both these effects.

Vasoconstrictors

Microneurography in humans has confirmed that sympathetic neural discharges in skin nerves are associated with the maneuvers recognized to cause vasoconstriction (e.g., startle and inspiratory gasp tests, cold stimuli to a remote part of the body).[20] The presence or absence of these discharges in response to such stimuli gives some indication of the integrity of peripheral sympathetic nerve fibers.[21] However, although microneurographic studies have been valuable in demonstrating various aspects of the behavior of peripheral sympathetic nerves, they do not easily give a quantitative estimate of partial denervation.

In 1983, Low et al.[22] described the use of a laser Doppler flowmeter for measuring changes in skin blood flow after sympathetic activating stimuli and demonstrated diminished or absent responses in some neuropathic patients. We have used a similar technique to study the sympathetic vasomotor system.

We use two sympathetic stimuli: the inspiratory gasp and the cold pressor test, which consists of immersing one hand up to the wrist in ice-cold water for 10 seconds. Although it has long been recognized that sympathetic responses are variable, we have found that these two tests give more reproducible findings than do others, such as the

Table 17.2 Changes in Blood Flow Measured with Laser Doppler Probe after Sympathetic Stimulation in Control Subjects and Diabetic Patients.

	Cold Pressor Response			Gasp		
	n	% Fall	SD	n	% Fall	SD
Controls	11	59.8	22.8	9	56.4	27.8
Diabetics	13	36.4	29.0	13	38.0	27.0
P value		<0.02			>0.05	

startle response. The responses are obtained after acclimatization in an ambient temperature of 26 °C under comfortable and relaxed conditions. Measurements are made with the skin temperature at 34 to 35 °C. Recordings are made with the laser probe in the central well of the aforementioned capsule, which is attached to the sole of the foot. Sympathetic responses are measured before the axon reflex flare and pilocarpine reaction, which are subsequently studied without removing the capsule, so that all the measurements are made on the same part of the foot.

When recording resting blood flow, irregularity in the Doppler trace is a good indication of the intact sympathetic system. Conversely, smooth, regular oscillations of the trace are generally associated with diminished or absent responses to sympathetic arousal stimuli. We express our results in the same way as Low et al.,[22] i.e., with reduction in blood flow expressed as a percentage of the resting flow. As yet, our number of observations is small (Table 17.2). In control subjects, although resting blood flow varied considerably, a positive response to both tests was recorded in all. In 2 of 13 diabetic patients, there was no change following either stimulus, and in 2 there was only a small response—smaller than in any control subject. These patients all had other evidence of peripheral neuropathy. In both control and diabetic subjects, the results obtained with the two stimuli were always similar. The mean reduction in flow was less in the diabetics than in the control subjects, but this was only significant ($P < 0.02$) for the cold pressor test.

Sudomotor Fibers

In clinical practice, the presence or absence of sweating has often been determined by the topical application of a powder that changes color when moist (e.g., starch and iodine or quinizarine). More quantitative methods have depended on measuring changes in skin resistance (the psychogalvanic response). Quantitative evaporative techniques, dependent on measurement of the rate of moisture production, have been used for some years in physiological experiments but have only recently been applied clinically.[23]

The Quantitative Sudomotor Axon Reflex Test (Q-SART) technique described by Low et al.[23] depends on the stimulation of sweating by an axon reflex using acetylcholine, which is electrophoresed into the skin from the outer ring of the capsule previously described. The sweat produced in the inner capsule is evaporated into a stream

Table 17.3   Sweat Rate and Number of Active Sweat Glands after Electrophoresis of Pilocarpine

	Stimulated Sweat Rate			Activated Sweat Glands		
	n	$\mu l/cm^2$	*SD*	*n*	*no.*	*SD*
Controls	12	0.47	0.24	12	137	84.1
Diabetics	15	0.29	0.25	16	101	87.7
P value		<0.05			>0.05	

of dry nitrogen, the humidity of which is then measured. Using this technique, Ahmed and Le Quesne[24] found sweating to be absent on the dorsum of the foot in 27 of 52 diabetic feet, and reduced in 7. Sweating was absent in a higher proportion of feet with neuropathic ulceration (75%) than with Charcot's arthropathy (36%).

Axon reflex sweating produced by acetylcholine is short-lived, and volume is assessed from the integrated area of the humidity meter output. A steady state of sweating is not achieved. The volume of sweat produced is small. We have modified the Q-SART by taking advantage of the observation that denervated sweat glands do not respond to pilocarpine, this being a well-recognized exception to Cannon's law of denervation hypersensitivity. Kennedy et al.[25,26] have used this fact to study sweating in diabetics, measuring sweat production with an evaporimeter or by counting the number and measuring the volume of individual sweat drops by a Silastic imprint technique. Sweat output was reduced in many diabetic patients.

In order to stimulate sweat glands directly, we electrophorese 1% pilocarpine with a 1 mA current for 5 minutes. At the end of this period, the stimulated skin is dried, and a sudorometer capsule is placed directly over it. The moisture produced is evaporated into dry nitrogen, as previously described. The apparatus has been calibrated to measure the steady rate of sweat production, which continues for up to half an hour after stimulation. The number of active sweat glands is counted by an imprint technique, with use of paper soaked in bromphenol blue.[27] Active sweat glands appear as clearly defined blue dots on a yellow background and are easily counted under ×3 magnification. The paper is easy to prepare and store, and the method is sensitive and less messy than previously used contact methods of demonstrating sweating.

The rate of stimulated sweat secretion and the number of activated sweat glands in 12 control and 15 diabetic subjects are shown in Table 17.3. The means for both values were reduced in the diabetics, although the only significant reduction was in the sweat rate. Sweating was absent according to both methods of measurement in three diabetic subjects.

CONCLUSION

In the work described, our emphasis has been to design a battery of tests acceptable to large numbers of patients, many of whom have only mild neuropathy yet require repeated examination, and all of whom are short of time. The application of these relatively simple, noninvasive tests, carried out in less than 2 hours, gives a quantitative assessment of all the different subgroups of peripheral nerve fibers.

REFERENCES

1. Le Quesne PM, Fowler CJ. A study of pain threshold in diabetics with neuropathic foot lesions. J Neurol Neurosurg Psychiatry 1986; 49:1191–4.
2. Dyck PJ, Karnes J, O'Brien PC, et al. Detection threshold of cutaneous sensation in humans. In: Dyck PJ, Thomas PK, Lambert EH, et al., eds. Peripheral neuropathy, 2 ed. Philadelphia: WB Saunders, 1984: 1103–38.
3. Le Quesne PM, Fowler CJ. Quantitative evaluation of toxic neuropathies in man. In: Ellingson RJ, Murray N, Halliday M, eds. The London Symposium. EEG J Suppl, 1987; 39:347–54.
4. Bloom S, Till S, Sonksen P, et al. Use of a biothesiometer to measure individual vibration thresholds and their variation in 519 non-diabetic subjects. Br Med J 1984; 288:1793–5.
5. Fagius J, Warren LK. Variability of sensory threshold determination in clinical use. J Neurol Sci 1981; 51:11–27.
6. Salle HJA, Verberk MM. Comparison of five methods for measurement of vibratory perception. Int Arch Occu Environ Health 1984; 53:303–9.
7. Halonen P. Quantitative vibration perception thresholds in healthy subjects of working age. Eur J Appl Physiol 1986; 54:647–55.
8. Kenshalo DR. Correlations of temperature sensitivity in man and monkey, a first approximation. In: Zotterman Y, ed. Sensory functions of the skin in primates. New York: Pergamon, 1976: 305–30.
9. Davies SN, Goldsmith GE, Hellon RF, et al. Facial sensitivity to rates of temperature change: neurophysiological and psychophysical evidence from cats and humans. J Physiol (Lond) 1983; 344:161–75.
10. Hensel H, Kelshalo DR. Warm receptors in the nasal region of cats. J Physiol (Lond) 1969; 204:99–112.
11. Fowler CJ, Carroll MC, Burns D, et al. A portable system for measuring cutaneous thresholds for warmth and cold. J Neurol Neurosurg Psychiatry 1987; 50:1211–15.
12. Fruhstorfer H, Lindblom U, Schmidt WG. Method for quantitative estimation of thermal thresholds in patients. J Neurol Sci 1976; 39:1071–5.
13. Fruhstorfer H. Conduction in the afferent thermal pathways of man. In: Zotterman Y, ed. Sensory functions of the skin in primates. New York: Pergamon, 1976:305–30.
14. Lynn B, Perl ER. A comparison of four tests for assessing the pain sensitivity of different subjects and test areas. Pain 1977; 3:353–65.
15. Lembeck F. Sir Thomas Lewis's nocifensor system, histamine and substance P-containing primary afferent nerves. Trends Neurosci 1983; 6:106–8.
16. Lewis T. The blood vessels of the human skin and their responses. London: Shaw and Sons, 1927.
17. Nilsson GE, Tenland T, Obert PA. A new instrument for continuous measurement of tissue blood flow by light beating spectroscopy. IEEE Trans Biomed Eng 1980; 27:12–19.
18. Lynn B, Carpenter SE, Pini A. Capsaicin and cutaneous afferents. In: Chahl LA, Szolcsanyi J, Lembeck F, eds. 29th IUPS Satellite Symposium, Australia. 1984:83–92.
19. Douglas WW, Ritchie JM. The excitatory action of acetylcholine on cutaneous nonmyelinated fibres. J Physiol (Lond) 1960; 150:501–14.
20. Vallbo AB, Hagbarth K-E, Torebjork HE, et al. Somatosensory, proprioceptive, and sympathetic activity in human peripheral nerves. Physiol Rev 1976; 59:919–57.
21. Fagius J. Microneurographic findings in diabetic polyneuropathy with special reference to sympathetic nerve activity. Diabetologia 1982; 23:415–20.

22. Low PA, Neumann C, Dyck PJ, et al. Evaluation of skin vasomotor reflexes by using laser Doppler velocimetry. Mayo Clin Proc 1983; 58:583-92.
23. Low PA, Caskey PE, Tuck RR, et al. Quantitative sudomotor axon reflex test (Q-SART). Ann Neurol 1983; 14:573-80.
24. Ahmed ME, Le Quesne PM. Quantitative sweat test in diabetics with neuropathic foot lesions. J Neurol Neurosurg Psychiatry 1986; 49:1059-62.
25. Kennedy WR, Sakuta M, Sutherland D, et al. Quantitation of the sweating deficiency in diabetes mellitus. Ann Neurol 1984; 15:482-8.
26. Kennedy WR, Sakuta M, Sutherland D, et al. The sweating deficiency in diabetes mellitus: methods of quantitation and clinical correlation. Neurology 1984; 34:758-63.
27. Sakurai M. Use of bromphenol blue printing method for detecting sweat on the palm. J Hand Surg 1986; 11B:125-30.

Chapter 18

Evaluating the Motor Consequences of Cortical Injury

Deborah Claman and Thomas Zeffiro

In humans, lesions of the posterior parietal lobe (PPL) cause a number of complex disorders of behavior, including visuospatial disorientation, oculomotor dysfunction, constructional apraxia, hemispatial neglect, and an often dramatic disorder of reaching.[1-5] Various experimental approaches using animal models have been employed to discover the mechanisms underlying these disorders. Experimental parietal ablations in the subhuman primate have been found to cause a striking disturbance of goal-directed arm movements.[6-8] The results of recent anatomic,[9-12] electrophysiologic,[13-15] and behavioral[16,17] studies support the contention that the posterior parietal cortex plays a pivotal role in two related sensorimotor functions: the integration of sensory and motor coordinate systems and the control of visually guided movement.

In contrast, reports from the clinical literature have not emphasized the motor component of misreaching after PPL damage, concluding instead that in man, this disorder results from sensory disturbances, including loss of extrapersonal spatial relations.[18-20] Although it is possible that the observed species difference results from an elaboration or change in function of the posterior parietal region, it is also possible that this area subserves similar functions in both species and that the observed behavioral disorders would appear more similar if tested in analogous fashion.

In order to investigate the motor consequences of PPL injury in man, we studied trajectory properties of visually guided reaching movements in control subjects and in patients with unilateral parietal, frontal, or cerebellar lesions. Three questions were addressed: Does final position accuracy vary with hand or spatial hemifield in patients with PPL lesions? Do PPL lesions affect both the spatial and temporal properties of limb movements? Can a specific reaching disorder be identified by examining the trajectories of visually guided limb movements?

EFFECTS OF DAMAGE TO THE PARIETAL LOBE

The behavioral effects of PPL ablations in monkeys have been studied descriptively[6,7] and quantitatively.[8,16,21,22] These studies have shown that only the limb contralateral to a PPL lesion displays aberrant movements. The reaching disorder involves not only a decline in final position accuracy but also changes in the temporal properties of the movement.[17]

Several studies have examined the effects of visual guidance on reaching behavior after unilateral PPL ablations. In one study, the behavioral task involved reaching for peanut rewards in both light and dark.[8] With visual guidance, movements made with the contralateral limb were inaccurate; without visual feedback, misreaching occurred with both limbs. Two other studies of the spatial accuracy of monkeys' reaching movements after PPL lesions have indicated a directional bias of reaching errors toward the midline.[16,17] Without visual guidance, the monkeys showed a reaching bias to the left of targets presented to the right and to the right of targets presented to the left. Movements were inaccurate in both spatial hemifields, with slightly more errors made when reaching for targets in the contralateral spatial hemifield. With the contralateral limb, movements were inaccurate and uncoordinated. Kinematic analysis of visually guided forearm movements confined to the horizontal plane revealed that movements executed with the contralateral limb were of significantly shorter duration than those executed with the ipsilateral limb.[17] It was argued that these faster and less accurate movements resulted from loss of control over the contralateral limb. Similar findings were obtained in studies in which the PPL was reversibly inactivated by cooling, rather than ablated.[21]

Pure reaching deficits appear to result from lesions of the superior parietal lobule. After ablation of the inferior parietal lobule, visuospatial deficits have also been observed.[23-25] It has often proven difficult to determine whether an observed behavioral deficit results from a disorder of visuospatial analysis or from a disorder of motor planning and execution. Of two groups that studied the effects of inferior parietal lobe lesions and tested performance on variations of the same route-finding task, one interpreted the disorder as primarily an inability to navigate caused by visuospatial disorientation,[25] while the other interpreted the disorder as primarily an inability to execute fast and accurate movements, caused by motor retardation.[24] In the only study where ablations of discrete PPL subdivisions was attempted, misreaching resulted when both banks of the intraparietal sulcus were destroyed, whereas visuospatial and tactile discrimination deficits were observed after ablation of the inferior parietal lobule.[23]

In man, clinical studies have shown that (with some exceptions), the motor disorder resulting from unilateral PPL injury involves both hands and is most evident in movements terminating in the contralateral visual or spatial hemifield. The first accounts describing misreaching associated with parietal lobe damage came from Holmes et al. and Balint, who studied bilateral parietal lobe damage caused by penetrating head injuries.[2,3] These lesions resulted in spatial disorientation and what was termed optic ataxia, a disorder in which movements executed with either hand in either hemifield were slow and inaccurate.[1,2,26,27] Regarding the deficits observed after unilateral PPL damage in man, most studies have emphasized the inaccuracy of movements terminating in the contralateral field. Reports of unilateral PPL damage in man have emphasized that the misreaching is most severe for movements terminating in the contralateral spatial hemifield.[26,28-32] More recently, several cases have been reported in which misreaching was most prominent with the contralateral arm in either hemifield. Levine et al. described a patient with a right superior parietal lobe tumor whose reaching deficit was most severe when the contralateral hand was used and visual feedback was absent.[33] In another patient with a vascular lesion of the left posterior parietal lobe, the transient reaching deficit was less obvious with visual feedback, more severe with the contralateral hand, and most severe when reaching with the contralateral hand into the contralateral visual hemifield.[34]

Lesions of the parietal lobe in man also result in poor performance of tasks requiring appreciation of spatial relations. In an elegant study of patients who had undergone cortical excisions for the relief of intractable epilepsy, it was found that excision of the angular and supramarginal gyri (areas 39 and 40 of Brodmann) specifically caused such deficits.[18] Patients with unilateral damage of the PPL have also been shown to have deficits in various route-finding tasks.[19,35,36,38] These navigational disturbances, which have usually been explained with reference to disorders of visuospatial or memory functions, always result from lesions that include the inferior parietal lobule.

To summarize, the inaccurate reaching movements consequent to PPL lesions in monkeys are characterized by abnormal spatial and temporal trajectory properties. Specifically, the misreaching is most evident when movements are executed with the contralateral limb and visual guidance is allowed. In contrast, clinical reports have emphasized that motor performance is most impaired when movements terminate in the contralateral spatial hemifield. If the consequences of human PPL lesions were similar to those observed in the monkey, misreaching would be most prominent with use of the limb contralateral to the lesion site.[8] We hypothesized that the human reaching disorder would resemble that seen in subhuman primates if tested in similar fashion.

KINEMATIC ANALYSIS OF PLANAR ARM MOVEMENTS

In our study, multijoint limb trajectories were recorded for movements confined to a single plane; the subjects moved to various targets within that plane. The behavior of healthy control subjects was compared with that of patients with focal damage to the PPL, frontal lobe, or cerebellum. The effects of these lesions on spatial and temporal trajectory properties were studied.

The study included 10 healthy control subjects, 16 patients with unilateral PPL lesions, 6 patients with unilateral frontal lobe lesions, and 6 patients with cerebellar lesions.[39] All the patients were recruited from the Massachusetts General Hospital Neurology and Neurosurgery Services. Informed consent was obtained from each subject prior to participation. Lesion site was determined by computerized axial tomography and magnetic resonance imaging. Most of the patients had just had their first stroke. Patients who had had more than one stroke were excluded, as were any with marked weakness or neglect as detected by double simultaneous stimulation.

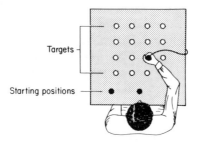

FIGURE 18.1   *The apparatus: a high-resolution digitizing tablet with light-emitting diodes mounted beneath.*

Patients were subclassified according to the presence (+VFD) or absence (−VFD) of visual field deficits. The data of those with somatosensory deficits were analyzed separately.

The testing apparatus consisted of a 20-inch-square (50.8 cm) horizontally mounted digitizing tablet and an attached stylus (Figure 18.1). This tablet and its controller determined the position of a search coil located within the pen with a spatial accuracy of 0.001 inch. The controller was connected to a MicroPDP 11/23 computer by means of a serial line that permitted a maximum data acquisition rate of 200 coordinate pairs per second. Beneath the translucent surface of the tablet was a board arrayed with 80 small light-emitting diodes (LEDs), which served as targets for visually guided reaching movements. Each LED could be lit individually under computer control but was otherwise invisible until activated. A data acquisition program was used to generate trials, to schedule all experimental events, and to sample and store the hand path for later analysis.

Behavioral Paradigm

The subjets performed a step-tracking task in darkness while comfortably restrained in front of the digitizing tablet. During a short practice session (usually 20 trials), the experimenter ascertained that the subject understood the procedure, which required his or her sliding the stylus along the surface of the tablet to specified target locations. The subject, holding a stylus in one hand or the other, was instructed to move to a starting position that appeared at various locations on the tablet's surface. Having attained this position, the subject initiated a trial by applying light downward pressure to the stylus tip. This resulted in the immediate appearance of a target LED.

Arm movements were recorded in blocks of 48 trials. Each block consisted of trials generated in pseudorandom order from each of three starting positions (left, center, and right) to each of 16 target positions arranged in a 4 × 4 array. Eight of the targets were to the left and eight were to the right of the tablet's midline, and were denoted as the left and right spatial hemifields, respectively. All movements were made from starting positions located near the subject (indicated by green LEDs) to target positions 2 to 22 inches (5 to 56 cm) from the subject (indicated by red LEDs). After each block of 48 trials, subjects were asked to transfer the stylus to the other hand, and the trial block was repeated. The subjects were instructed to move as quickly and accurately as possible and to avoid making corrective movements. They received no feedback as to the magnitude of the final position error.

The subjects were evaluated at least twice in this paradigm: once in a condition that permitted visual guidance, and once with no visual guidance. In the latter case (T_{off} condition), the task was performed in total darkness, and any movement of the subject from the starting position caused the target LED to be extinguished, so the subject was moving to a remembered location without being able to see his hand or the target. When visual guidance was permitted (T_{on} condition), each target LED remained lit throughout the trial.

Sensory cues available to the subjects under both conditions (with and without visual guidance) were maximized in a number of ways. Subjects were always allowed free and unrestricted eye and head movements; information about initial hand position was available in each trial, owing to the illumination of the starting-position LED; and response latency was measured but not controlled. Subjects could spend as much time as desired viewing the target before moving.

Data Analysis

An interactive computer program was used for data analysis. Each movement was displayed so that temporal events such as movement initiation and movement termination could be marked. Certain properties of the trajectories (e.g., peak velocity) could be extracted directly. Other properties (e.g., movement duration, length of the accelerative phase of the movement, length of the decelerative phase of the movement, and final position accuracy) were calculated for each trial. The position data were differentiated and double-differentiated with respect to time (using a 50-point digital filter, $-3dB$ point of 10 Hz, cutoff frequency of 7.5 Hz) to obtain tangential velocity and acceleration profiles for each movement; tangential velocity $= \sqrt{\dot{X}^2 + \dot{Y}^2}$; tangential acceleration $= \sqrt{\ddot{X}^2 + \ddot{Y}^2}$. Each hand-path, with its tangential velocity and acceleration profiles, was displayed on a graphics monitor (Figure 18.2). The data were examined trial by trial to mark and store points of movement initiation, termination, and peak velocity.

Movement initiation was defined as the point that corresponded to the first positive value along the tangential acceleration profile (ignoring tremor that sometimes caused small positive values prior to the beginning of the movement). Movement endpoints were measured at two positions. Because patients often did not terminate their movements at one unique point, a first endpoint (EP_1) was marked when tangential acceleration first crossed zero in the decelerative movement phase. A second endpoint (EP_2) was defined when velocity next crossed zero. In general, the control subjects terminated their movements at one unique point.

Movement time (MT) was obtained by subtracting the time of movement initiation from the time of the movement termination. Acceleration time (AT) was the time

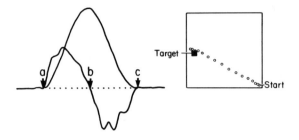

FIGURE 18.2   *Example of a single movement marked interactively during data analysis. The large square (right) is a scaled representation of the digitizing tablet surface, seen from above. The hand path (open circles) is displayed from a starting point to one of the 16 target positions (closed square). On the left are shown the tangential velocity and tangential acceleration profiles for that movement. The arrows mark initiation time (a), peak velocity (b), and the superimposed termination times, EP_1 and EP_2 (c).*

from movement initiation to the time at peak velocity, and deceleration time (DT) was the time from peak velocity to EP_1 or EP_2. Skew was calculated as $AT \div MT_1(SK1)$ and $AT \div MT_2(SK2)$. Peak velocity, peak acceleration, and peak deceleration were determined with maxima and minima detecting algorithms.

Movement endpoint was defined as the spatial location corresponding to the first zero crossing of the tangential acceleration profile during the decelerative phase of the movement (EP_1). The spatial coordinates of this position were compared with the actual target position for each movement. The difference between target position and final hand position was used as a measure of movement accuracy. Because movements to the same target were made repeatedly (though not in succession), it was possible to estimate the tendency to make errors in a particular direction as well as overall movement variability. To analyze the magnitude and direction of the reaching errors, a constant error vector (CEV)—the vector originating at each target position and terminating at the mean endpoint for that target (Figure 18.3)—was calculated for each of the 16 target positions. In order to analyze the magnitude of errors at various spatial locations, it was important to remove the effect of movement direction. This was accomplished by rotating the error vectors by the direction of movement, thereby transforming the vectors into a coordinate frame aligned with the direction of movement: $\theta_{\text{corrected}} = \theta_{\text{movement}} - \theta_{\text{error}}$. The vector components of the error were then displayed in the rotated coordinate system as normal and perpendicular to the direction of movement (Figure 18.3). Movements that terminated beyond a given target position were termed *hypermetric,* and those that terminated short of the target were termed *hypometric.* Therefore, positive values for the component of the CEV normal to the direction of the movement reflected hypermetric movements, and negative values reflected hypometric movements.

Using a similar procedure, the size and orientation of the cloud of corrected movement endpoints were determined with principal components analysis. The intersection of the principal component axes corresponds to the mean endpoint, and the distance from that point to the mean target position corresponds to mean constant error.

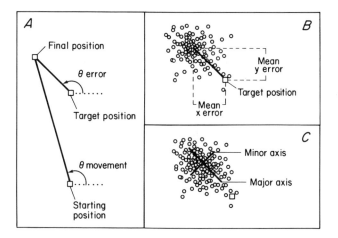

FIGURE 18.3 *Analysis of final position errors. (A) Vectors from the target position to each final hand position were rotated according to the direction of movement, thereby correcting the final position error vector for movement direction. (B) A constant error vector (CEV) has its origin at the target position and extends to the mean final hand position. (C) Principal components analysis was used to determine the eigenvectors for the population of final positions. The lengths of the major and minor axes equal 1 SD.*

Variable error was defined as the standard deviation of the endpoints for each target (Figure 18.3). Thus, the magnitude of the standard deviation of the data along either the major or minor axis represents the variable error in that direction. Multiplying the estimates of standard deviation along the major and minor axes results in a scalar quantity, referred to as *size,* that provides an estimate of the variable error in both spatial dimensions.

Inspection of the paths and tangential velocity profiles of individual movements revealed differences between patients with frontal or parietal lobe damage and control subjects. Representative movements from each of these groups are presented below, followed by the spatial and temporal characteristics of the movements. Then aggregate data for individual subjects are presented for one movement property, namely, errors of final position. Finally, measures of central tendency and variability for the spatial and temporal characteristics of the entire population of subjects are compared for the different groups and experimental conditions.

INDIVIDUAL MOVEMENT CHARACTERISTICS

The spatial and temporal characteristics of movements made by individual control subjects were remarkably similar in many respects (Figure 18.4). Goal-directed movements produced by the control subjects had the following general properties: (1) a strong nonlinear relationship between movement time and movement amplitude; (2) movement amplitudes ranging from 2 to 24 in (5 to 56 cm); (3) movement times

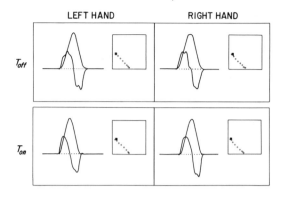

FIGURE 18.4   *Paths and tangential velocity profiles for individual movements performed by a control subject. The upper panels illustrate movements executed by the left and right hands without visual guidance (T_{off} condition). The lower panels illustrate similar movements executed with visual guidance (T_{on} condition).*

ranging from 300 to 900 msec; (4) average peak velocities of 40 in (101.5 cm) sec; 5 asymmetric velocity profiles with a trend toward greater symmetry when visual guidance was allowed; (6) slightly hypermetric endpoint errors (mean = 0.4 in [1 cm]) in the T_{off} condition, which corrected in the T_{on} condition; and (7) an absence of trajectory corrections near movement termination. In general, the control subjects exhibited movements of shorter duration, higher peak velocity, and smaller endpoint error when visual guidance was provided. For all movement properties analyzed, no significant differences were found between movements executed with either hand into either hemifield.

The trajectories of individual movements made by the patients with parietal lobe damage differed from those of control subjects (Figure 18.5). Similarly, the aggregate movement properties derived from the path and tangential velocity profiles of the patients had quite different characteristics when compared to those of control subjects, including (1) slightly shorter movement amplitudes; (2) prolonged movement times; (3) lower peak velocities; (4) symmetric velocity profiles, which became much more asymmetric when visual guidance was allowed; (5) hypometric endpoint errors; and (6) a tendency to make trajectory corrections during the decelerative phase of the movement. In the patients with parietal lobe damage, movements of similar sizes were of longer duration when visual guidance was provided, which was not the case in the control population. This reflects an increase in trajectory corrections, seen most clearly when vision of the target was allowed.

Figure 18.6 shows the path and tangential velocity profile of a typical movement made by a patient with a frontal lobe lesion. As in the patients with PPL injury, the analyzed movement properties also had characteristics different from those in control subjects, including (1) longer movement amplitudes, (2) prolonged movement times, (3) lower peak velocities, (4) asymmetric velocity profiles that did not alter when visual feedback was allowed, (5) hypermetric final position errors, and (6) smaller and

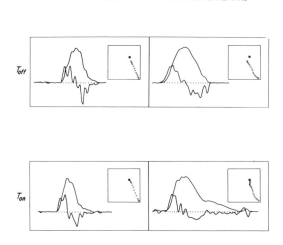

FIGURE 18.5   *Paths and tangential velocity profiles for individual movements performed by a patient with a posterior parietal lobe lesion. The upper panels illustrate movements executed by the hands ipsilateral and contralateral to the side of the lesion in the T_{off} condition. The lower panels illustrate similar movements executed in the T_{on} condition. The patient, a 62-year-old right-handed man, had a small infarct (presumed to be embolic) of the right middle cerebral artery. CT scan showed the lesion to be restricted mostly to the superior parietal lobule.*

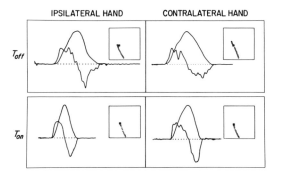

FIGURE 18.6   *Paths and tangential velocity profiles for individual movements performed by a patient with a frontal lobe lesion. The upper panels illustrate movements executed by the hands ipsilateral and contralateral to the side of the lesion in the T_{off} condition. The lower panels illustrate similar movements executed in the T_{on} condition. The patient, a 54-year-old right-handed man, had an infarct of the superior division of the right middle cerebral artery.*

fewer trajectory corrections during the decelerative phase of the movement. As in the control population, movements of shorter duration, higher peak velocity, and smaller final position error were seen when visual feedback was provided.

AGGREGATE DATA: FINAL POSITION ERRORS

The population characteristics of particular spatial movement properties, including constant and variable error, were analyzed in greater detail. Of particular interest was the degree to which an individual tended to overshoot or undershoot the target. Thus, a movement was referred to as hypermetric if the CEV had a positive component in the direction of movement, and hypometric if the CEV had a negative component in the direction of movement. Figure 18.7 displays the endpoint errors for a typical control subject. The errors have all been corrected for direction of movement, and movements to all targets have been pooled according to hand used or spatial hemifield. Although most control subjects made hypermetric movements in the T_{off} condition, T_{on} movements terminated in a cluster centering around the target position. The mean constant and variable errors did not vary between hands.

Examination of the final position errors made by patients with PPL lesions revealed strikingly different patterns (Figures 18.8 and 18.9). In contrast to control subjects, patients with PPL lesions made hypometric movements with and without visual guidance. This effect was most striking in movements made in the T_{off} condition by patients having both a PPL lesion and a visual field deficit. In both groups with PPL lesions, the hypometria tended to correct when vision of the target was allowed, suggesting that additional sensory cues were utilized to generate ongoing trajectory corrections. Consistent with this notion was the finding that the group of patients with both a PPL lesion and a visual field deficit tended to make the largest corrective

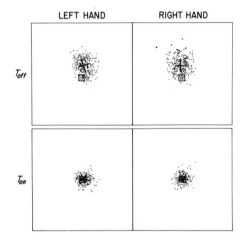

FIGURE 18.7 *Aggregate endpoint errors for a control subject. The data have been pooled to display endpoint errors made when movements were executed with either hand. The small central square in each panel represents the apparent target size. The upper panels show errors of the left and right hands in the T_{off} condition; the lower panels show errors of the left and right hands in the T_{on} condition.*

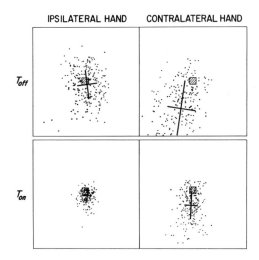

FIGURE 18.8 *Aggregate endpoint errors for a patient with a posterior parietal lobe lesion and a visual field defect. The data have been pooled to display final position errors made when movements were executed with either hand. The small central square in each panel represents the apparent target size. The upper panels show errors of the left and right hands in the T_{off} condition; the lower panels show errors of the left and right hands in the T_{on} condition. The patient, a 37-year-old right-handed man, had a small infarct (presumed to be embolic) of the posterior division of the middle cerebral artery. CT scan showed the lesion to be located in the right parietal-occipital cortex.*

movements of any group studied. There was no difference in the degree of hypometria when movements were sorted according to hand used or spatial hemifield.

POPULATION DATA: SPATIAL PROPERTIES

Differences between patient groups were apparent in the pooled final position error data (Figure 18.10). In contrast to the hypometria exhibited by the PPL patients in the absence of visual guidance, both cerebellar and frontal lobe patients were hypermetric. Although there was no difference between hands observed in the PPL lesion groups, both cerebellar and frontal lobe groups exhibited hypermetria that was more severe in the limb contralateral to the lesion. Patients with PPL lesions tended to make larger corrective movements than did patients with cerebellar or frontal lobe lesions.

Whereas the determination of constant error gave an estimate of the mean spatial error, the determination of the area covered by the population of final positions gave an estimate of the variability of the spatial error for the different groups (Figure 18.11). While patients with PPL lesions had increased variable error under both conditions of visual guidance as compared with control subjects, the patients with visual field deficits had larger variable error than did patients without visual field deficits under both

IPSILATERAL HAND   CONTRALATERAL HAND

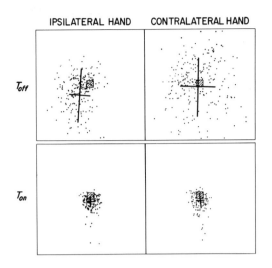

T_{off}

T_{on}

FIGURE 18.9   *Aggregate final position errors for a patient with a posterior parietal lobe lesion and no visual field defect. The data have been pooled to display final position errors made when movements were executed with either hand. The small central square in each panel represents the apparent target size. The upper panels show errors of the left and right hands in the T_{off} condition; the lower panels show errors of the left and right hands in the T_{on} condition. The patient, a 45-year-old right-handed woman, had a small infarct (presumed to be embolic) of the right middle cerebral artery. CT scan showed the lesion to be restricted mostly to the superior parietal lobule.*

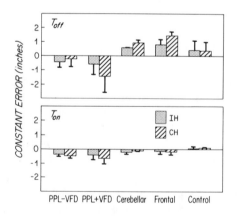

FIGURE 18.10   *Hypometria and hypermetria in the endpoint errors (EP_1). Ipsilateral and contralateral hands (IH and CH) are compared across groups. The top panel shows the results for the T_{off} condition, and the bottom panel shows the results for the T_{on} condition. The first endpoint (EP_1) was used.*

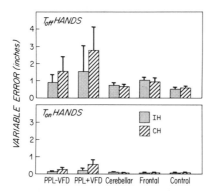

FIGURE 18.11 *Variable errors for all groups, comparing hands. Ipsilateral and contralateral hands (IH and CH) are compared. The top panel shows the results for the T_{off} condition, and the bottom panel shows the results for the T_{on} condition.*

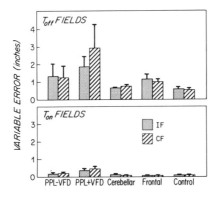

FIGURE 18.12 *Variable errors for all groups, comparing fields. Variable errors for ipsilateral and contralateral fields (IF and CF) are compared. The top panel shows the results for the T_{off} condition, and the bottom panel shows the results for the T_{on} condition.*

conditions. In contrast with the results of constant errors analysis, patients with PPL lesions had larger variable error in the hand contralateral to the lesion under both conditions. Variable error was larger in the spatial hemifield contralateral to the lesion in the PPL patients with visual field deficits when there was no visual guidance (Figure 18.12). This effect was not seen in patients without visual field deficits or when visual guidance was allowed. In comparison, cerebellar patients had variable error in the normal range under both conditions of visual guidance, and patients with frontal lobe lesions exhibited a small increase in variable error when visual guidance was absent. In cerebellar, frontal, and control groups, variable error was similar with either limb moving into either spatial hemifield.

POPULATION DATA: TEMPORAL PROPERTIES

The temporal movement properties analyzed were movement time and skew, a measure of the symmetry of the tangential velocity profile. Figure 18.13 shows pooled data for movement time. PPL patients exhibited increased movement time under both conditions of visual guidance. Without visual guidance, PPL patients with visual field deficits had longer movement times than those with no visual field deficits. All PPL patients had slightly longer movement times in the contralateral hand across all conditions. Corrective movements tended to be of longer duration in the PPL group with visual field deficits than in those without. The duration of the corrective movement was greater in the contralateral than the ipsilateral limb in PPL patients having no visual guidance (Figure 18.14). When visual guidance was provided, the interlimb difference

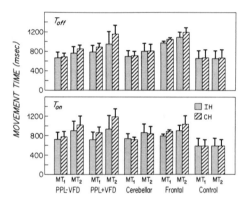

FIGURE 18.13   *Movement times (MT_1 and MT_2) for patient groups and control subjects. Ipsilateral and contralateral hands (IH and CH) are compared. The top panel shows the results for the T_{off} condition, and the bottom panel shows the results for the T_{on} condition.*

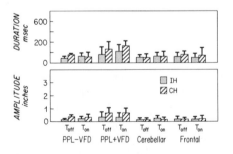

FIGURE 18.14   *Durations and amplitudes of corrective movements. The duration (upper panel) and amplitude (lower panel) of corrective movements, beginning at EP_1 and terminating at EP_2, are compared for the ipsilateral and contralateral hands (IH and CH).*

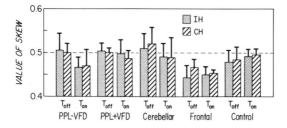

FIGURE 18.15   *Proportion of movement time spent in the accelerative phase (skew) under the two conditions of visual feedback. Skew is a measure of the symmetry of the tangential velocity profile. A value of 0.5 for skew would correspond to a symmetric velocity profile. Values less than 0.5 reflect prolongation of the deceralative phase of the movement. IH denotes ipsilateral hand, CH, contralateral hand.*

was apparent only in the group with visual field deficits. There was no difference between spatial hemifields in either group.

Whereas PPL patients with visual field deficits exhibited increased movement times with visual guidance, patients in the frontal group had decreased movement times with visual guidance. This decrease was similar to that seen in control subjects, although the movement times of the patients were greater. In contrast, patients with cerebellar lesions, and those with PPL lesions and no visual field deficits showed no difference in movement time with the addition of visual feedback. In patients with frontal but not cerebellar lesions the increased movement time was greater in the contralateral limb, which was also the case in PPL patients.

Figure 18.15 shows a measure of the symmetry of the tangential velocity profile under various conditions for different groups. The normal pattern was for the velocity profiles to become slightly more symmetric with the addition of visual guidance. In all PPL and cerebellar patients, visual guidance resulted in velocity profiles becoming more asymmetric and skewed toward the beginning of the movement. This effect was most prominent for the PPL group with no visual field deficits. In contrast, the velocity profiles of patients with frontal lobe lesions tended to be skewed toward the beginning of the movement under both conditions of visual guidance. No difference was observed between the ipsilateral and contralateral hands nor between the ipsilateral and contralateral spatial hemifields in any of the patients or controls.

CONCLUSION

What Characterizes the Reaching Disorder Seen after Posterior Parietal Lobe Injury in Man?

Unilateral PPL damage results in a global impairment of goal-directed limb movement, including bimanual abnormalities of spatial and temporal movement properties. Specifically, limb movements executed in the absence of visual guidance were hypometric, variable, and slowed. When visual guidance was provided, the hypometrial and variability in endpoint improved and there was an accompanying prolongation of the decelerative phase of the movement. This finding is consistent with the notion that these patients used the additional visual information to plan and execute a series of ongoing trajectory corrections during the decelerative phase of the movement. That is, the behavioral compensation that resulted in improved accuracy in final position was achieved at the cost of prolonged movement time.

Of note is the finding that the disorder was more severe in the limb contralateral to the lesion for most properties examined. Only those patients who had an obvious sensory impairment in the form of a visual field deficit exhibited an asymmetry in performance between spatial hemifields. This finding differs from previous reports,[40-42] in which movements of various kinds performed in the spatial hemifield contralateral to frontal or parietal lesions were more impaired.

How Specific Is the Syndrome of Parietal Misreaching?

The pattern of movement abnormalities seen in the patients with parietal lobe damage was different from that seen in the patients with either cerebellar or frontal lobe damage. Both of the latter groups tended to make movements that were hypermetric, although their performance also improved with the addition of visual guidance. The group with parietal lobe damage and no sensory deficit was the only group in which the addition of visual feedback resulted in prolongation of movement time. The movement disorder seen in the cerebellar and frontal groups was more lateralized, with larger errors and increased variability in th limb contralateral to the lesion.

Is there Truly a Species Difference?

If the effects of human PPL lesions were similar to those observed in the monkey, misreaching would be found mostly in the limb contralateral to the lesion site and would be influenced by the presence or absence of visual guidance.[8] Previous studies in the monkey had shown that the limb contralateral to a PPL lesion is more impaired than the ipsilateral limb.[6-8,16,21,22] It has recently been reported that the reaching disorder involves not only a loss of final position accuracy but also a loss of the proper coordination between various trajectory properties.[17] Hartje and Ettlinger[8] proposed that PPL ablations caused a primary reaching disorder specific to the contralateral limb, and a secondary, more generalized disorder affecting both limbs. In contrast, most previous clinical reports had not described any difference in the performance of either hand but instead had observed that patients with PPL lesions exhibited a bimanual reaching disorder that was most severe when moving into the contralateral spatial hemifield.[28,30,32.] More recently, cases were reported in which the movement disorder was greatest when moving the contralateral arm into both hemifields.[33,34]

The discrepancies among the clinical studies may reflect differences in patient populations and testing procedures. Most studies that reported misreaching only in the contralateral spatial hemifield after unilateral injury were based on single cases in which hemispatial neglect was a prominent feature. Because our aim was to determine the existence of a motor disorder that was dissociable from primary sensory or attentional deficits, we excluded patients with these additional impairments. It is notable that the two previously reported studies with features similar to ours[33,34] also involved patients with small, well localized lesions. Thus, it is possible that the more common finding of hemispatial neglect and misreaching is due to simultaneous damage to adjacent cortical areas, each of which subserves a different function in sensorimotor integration.

What Is the Mechanism of the Misreaching?

Before discussing possible mechanisms of misreaching, it is necessary to present an account of the process by which reaching movements may be normally planned and executed. First, the spatial and temporal properties of the trajectory are planned through the use of visual and proprioceptive information; the current location of the hand is determined, as well as its intended location relative to the body at the end of the movement in a body-centered frame of reference. The resulting spatial location information is used to generate a series of hand positions that specify the movement of the hand from the starting position to the final position, along a certain path and at a certain speed. This kinematic plan is translated into a series of neural commands, resulting in the use of the appropriate pattern of muscle forces to move the hand in the correct direction at the correct velocity.

A deficit in the analysis of visual space would therefore affect the earliest portion of the movement-planning process. Only the determination of the spatial location of the final position would be in error, and the other kinematic properties of the movement would be completely normal. It follows that final position errors without changes in other trajectory properties are consistent with a primary disorder involving the visual analysis of space. In contrast, a deficit involving either the trajectory planning process or its translation into a dynamic plan results in abnormalities in many of the kinematic properties of the movement, including movement time, peak velocity, and skew. Thus, findings of altered spatial and temporal movement properties in addition to final position error suggest a motor or combined sensory and motor disorder.

What Implications Do These Results Have Concerning Cortical Movement-Control Mechanisms?

The function or functions impaired after unilateral parietal lobe damage result in two behaviorally distinct reaching disorders of limb movement that are most pronounced in the limb contralateral to the lesion. The first, resulting from damage to the superior parietal lobule, is bimanual, with the most severe impairment in the contralateral limb. The second, resulting from damage to both the superior parietal lobule and adjacent visual areas, results in a more global impairment of movement, with poorer performance in both the contralateral limb and the contralateral spatial hemifield. The latter disorder cannot be caused by the primary sensory deficit alone, as patients with lesions involving only the occipital pole did not show the described pattern of results.[39] These findings are consistent with the notion that the process of spatial localization occurs very early in the movement-planning process and may be localized to the posterior parietal and anterior occipital cortex. The process is organized by spatial hemifield, with a particular area responsible mainly for the contralateral field; damage to this area alone may result in clinical neglect syndromes. The subsequent stages of trajectory planning and execution may involve functions localized to more anterior portions of the posterior parietal cortex, where the process is organized bilaterally, with a predominant influence on the contralateral limb. Damage to this area results in a bimanual reaching disorder consisting of abnormalities of movement in both the spatial and temporal spheres, consistent with a global impairment of movement planning and execution.

REFERENCES

1. Holmes G. Disturbances of visual orientation. Br J Ophthalmol 1918; 2:449-68.
2. Holmes G, Horrax G. Disturbances of spatial orientation and visual attention with loss of stereoscopic vision. Arch Neurol Psychiatry. 1919; 1:385-407.
3. Balint R. Seelenlahmung des Schauens, optische Ataxie, raumliche Störung der Aufmerksamkeit. Monatsschr Psychiatr Neurol 1909; 25:51-81.
4. Denny-Brown D, Chambers RA. The parietal lobe and behavior. Res Publ Assoc Res Nerv Ment Dis 1958; 36:35-117.
5. Critchley M. The parietal lobes. London: Edward Arnold, 1953.
6. Bates JAV, Ettlinger G. Posterior biparietal ablations in the monkey. Arch Neurol 1960; 3:177-92.
7. Ettlinger G, Kalsbeck JE. Changes in tactile discrimination and visual reaching after successive and simultaneous bilateral posterior parietal ablations in the monkey. J Neurol Neurosurg Psychiatry 1962; 25:256-68.
8. Hartje W, Ettlinger G. Reaching in the light and dark after unilateral posterior parietal ablations in the monkey. Cortex 1973; 9:346-54.
9. Jones EG, Coulter JD, Hendry SHC. Intracortical connectivity of architectonic fields in the somaticsensory, motor and parietal cortex of monkeys. J Comp Neurol 1978; 181:291-348.
10. Strick PL, Kim CC. Input to primate motor cortex from posterior parietal cortex (area 5). I. Demonstration by retrograde transport. Brain Res 1978; 157:325-30.
11. Petras JM. Connections of the parietal lobe. J Psychiatr Res 1971; 8:189-201.
12. Pandya DN, Selzer B. Intrinsic connections and architectonics of posterior parietal cortex in the rhesus monkey. J Comp Neurol 1982; 204:196-210.
13. Hyvarinen J, Poranen A. Function of the parietal association area 7 as revealed from cellular discharges in alert monkeys. Brain 1974; 97:673-92.
14. Mountcastle VB, Lynch JC, Georgopoulos A, et al. Posterior parietal association cortex of the monkey: command functions for operations within extrapersonal space. J Neurophysiol 1975; 38:871-908.
15. Sakata H, Shibutani H, Kawano K. Spatial properties of visual fixation neurons in posterior parietal association cortex of the monkey. J Neurophysiol 1980; 43:1654-72.
16. Lamotte RH, Acuna C. Defects in accuracy of reaching after removal of posterior parietal cortex in monkeys. Brain Res 1978; 139:309-26.

17. Faugier-Grimaud S, Frenois C, Peronnet F. Effects of posterior parietal lesions on visually guided movements in monkeys. Exp Brain Res 1985; 59:125–38.
18. Hecaen H, Penfield W, Bertrand C, et al. The syndrome of apractognosia due to lesions of the minor cerebral hemisphere. Arch Neurol Psychiatry 1956; 75:400–34.
19. Semmes J, Weinstein S, Ghent L, et al. Correlates of impaired orientation in personal and extrapersonal space. Brain 1963; 86:747–72.
20. DeRenzi E, Faglioni P, Scotti G. Hemispheric contribution to exploration of space through the visual and tactile modality. Cortex 1970; 6:191–203.
21. Stein JF. Effects of parietal lobe cooling on manipulative behavior in the conscious monkey. Oxford: Pergamon, 1978:79–90.
22. Faugier-Grimaud S, Frenois C, Stein DG. Effects of posterior parietal lesions on visually guided behavior in monkeys. Neuropsychologia 1978; 16:151–68.
23. Moffett A, Ettlinger G, Morton H, et al. Tactile discrimination performance in the monkey: the effect of ablation of various subdivisions of posterior parietal cortex. Cortex 1967; 3:59–96.
24. Milner AD, Ockleford EM, Dewar W. Visuo-spatial performance following posterior parietal and lateral frontal lesions in stumptail Macaque. Cortex 1977; 13:350–60.
25. Petrides M, Iversen SD. Restricted posterior parietal lesions in the rhesus monkey and performance on visuospatial tasks. Brain Res 1979; 161:63–77.
26. Ratcliff G. Disturbances of spatial orientation associated with cerebral lesions. New York: Academic Press, 1982.
27. Damasio AR, Benton AL. Impairment of hand movements under visual guidance. Neurology 1979; 29:170–8.
28. Riddoch G. Visual disorientation in homonymous hemifields. Brain 1935; 58:376–82.
29. Brain WR. Visual disorientation with special reference to the right hemisphere. Brain 1941; 64:244–72.
30. Cole M. Schutta HS, Warrington EK. Visual disorientation in homonymous hemifields. Neurology 1962; 12:257–62.
31. Costa LDL, Vaughan HG Jr., Horwitz M, et al. Patterns of behavioral deficit associated with visual spatial neglect. Cortex 1969; 5:242–63.
32. Ratcliff G, Davies-Jones GAB. Defective visual localization in focal brain wounds. Brain 1972; 95:49–60.
33. Levine DN, Kaufman KJ, Mohr JP. Inaccurate reaching associated with a superior parietal tumor. Neurology 1978; 28:556–61.
34. Ferro JM. Transient inaccuracy in reaching caused by a posterior parietal lesion. Neurol Neurosurg Psychiatry 1984; 47:1016–19.
35. Semmes J, Weinstein S, Ghent L, et al. Spatial orientation in man after cerebral injury. I. Analysis by locus of lesion. J Psychol 1955; 39:227–44.
36. Ettlinger G, Warrington E, Zangwill OL. A further study of visual-spatial agnosia. Brain 1957; 80:335–61.
37. Corkin S. Tactually guided maze learning in man: effects of unilateral cortical excisions and bilateral hippocampal lesions. Neuropsychologia 1965; 3:339–51.
38. Milner B. Visually-guided maze learning in man: effects of bilateral hippocamal, bilateral frontal, and unilateral cerebral lesions. Neuropsychologia 1965; 3:317–38.
39. Claman D. Motor consequences of posterior parietal lobe injury in man. Massachusetts Institute of Technology: Ph.D. dissertation, 1986.
40. Heilman K, Valenstein E. Mechanisms underlying hemispatial neglect. Neurol 1979; 5:166–70.
41. Heilman K, Bowers D, Watson R. Performance on hemispatial pointing task by patients with neglect syndrome. Neurology 1983; 33:661–4.
42. Meador KJ, Watson RT, Bowers D, et al. Hypometria with hemispatial and limb motor neglect. Brain 1986; 109:293–305.

Chapter 19

Assessment of the Primary Dystonias

Stanley Fahn

Dystonias are involuntary movements that are typically sustained, twisting, and repetitive, and can result in abnormal postures.[1] These movements and postures can affect all parts of the body. When dystonia affects only a single part of the body, it is referred to as *focal dystonia*. Many focal dystonias have been named according to the affected region: spasmodic torticollis, blepharospasm, oromandibular dystonia, lingual dystonia, spastic dysphonia, writer's cramp. When more than one focal region is affected, the disorder is described as segmental, multifocal, or generalized, or labeled a *hemidystonia*[1,2] if it involves one arm and one leg on the same side of the body. Hemidystonia is almost always due to an injury to the brain, such as encephalitis, head trauma, or stroke. The term *segmental dystonia* indicates that two or more contiguous parts of the body, such as an arm and the neck, are affected with dystonic movements. It is very common for focal dystonia to spread in a contiguous manner. For example, blepharospasm, when it spreads, involves other muscles of the head and neck region. *Generalized dystonia* involves at least one leg, the trunk, and some other body part. Almost all patients with generalized dystonia had onset of their symptoms in childhood.[1] *Multifocal dystonias* are those that do not fit into the above-described categories (e.g., dystonia) affecting just one leg and the neck.

When dystonia has such causes as birth injury, encephalitis, Wilson's disease, or head injury,[1] it is referred to as *symptomatic* or *secondary dystonia*. Many patients with symptomatic dystonia have neurologic signs, (e.g., corticospinal tract and cerebellar signs), which indicate that the dystonia is not pure but is accompanied by additional neurologic damage. In such a situation, rating scales for dystonia—particularly those assessing functional disability—cannot be used accurately as a quantitative measurement of dystonia alone. However, most cases of dystonia (about two thirds) are of unknown etiology, and are labeled *idiopathic* or *primary dystonia*. This category includes dystonias in individuals with a positive family history of the disorder. The genetics of dystonia are complex, examples of autosomal dominant, autosomal recessive, and X-linked recessive transmission having been reported.[1] Idiopathic dystonia is always a "pure" dystonia (i.e., no other neurologic signs are present).

Variants of classic or primary dystonia are also encountered. These include paroxysmal dystonia,[3] dystonic tics,[4] dystonia with parkinsonism,[5] and diurnal dystonia.[6] Although the severity of dystonic movements and postures in these variants could also be assessed by the scales described in this chapter, such application is often difficult.

RATING SCALE FOR GENERALIZED DYSTONIA

Fahn and Marsden developed a quantitative assessment for torsion dystonia that has proved to be statistically reliable and valid.[7] The scale (Appendix 19–A) has two sections: a movement scale based on examination of the patient, and a disability scale based on the patient's subjective impairment in activities of daily living.

The movement scale assesses nine body regions, including four cranial areas, the limbs, and the trunk. The score for each region is the product of two factors: the provoking factor, which quantifies the circumstance in which the dystonia appears (e.g., only with action or present at rest), and the severity factor, which quantifies the severity of dystonia regardless of the circumstances in which it appears. The severity factor is distinctly defined for each region, as severity differs according to the specific funtions served by the affected region.

Both the provoking factor and the severity factor are scored on a five-point scale of 0 (no dystonia present) to 4 (maximum severity, or present at rest). Since the product of the two factors provides the score for the region, the maximum score per region is 16 points. There are three exceptions: the products for the eyes, mouth, and neck regions are multiplied by 0.5 to downgrade the final scores for these regions relative to other regions, as their involvement appears relatively less important to the patient's overall disability.

The disability scale assesses the impairment of seven activities of daily living: speech, writing, feeding, eating, hygiene, dressing, and walking. Each is scored on a scale of 0 to 4 points with the exception of walking, which has a maximum score of 6.

The Fahn-Marsden scale has limitations. It cannot distinguish the disability of dystonia from that of spasticity, should the latter also be present. It is less sensitive for the various focal dystonias. I have therefore developed additional scales for the latter that allow "finer tuning" in their assessment. These scales, described below, eliminate the extraneous ratings of unaffected regions that would be included in the Fahn-Marsden scale for generalized dystonia. Assessment is not only more specific but more sensitive to slight changes.

RATING SCALE FOR BLEPHAROSPASM

Blepharospasm refers to contractions of the orbicularis oculi that result in closure of the eyelids. Marsden[8] was probably the first to suggest that blepharospasm is a form of focal dystonia. Idiopathic blepharospasm is referred to as essential blepharospasm if the disorder is limited to the facial muscles. If other regions of the cranial structures are involved, the usual designation is segmental cranial dystonia, or Meige syndrome.[9-12] Whereas essential blepharospasm is a focal idiopathic dystonia, reflex blepharospasm is due to either local eye irritation or neurologic disorders such as parkinsonism.

Like the Fahn-Marsden scale for generalized dystonia, the rating scale for blepharospasm is divided into two sections: a movement scale and a disability scale[13] (Appendix 19-B). The former has several parts. One measures the location of the abnormal contractions in individual muscles, with each involved muscle component receiving one point. Similarly, the scale provides one point for each influencing factor (e.g., sunlight, watching television, working). Any improvement with specific activities subtracts a point from the final score. Severity of eyelid closure is scored up to a maximum of 4 points. Spread of dystonia to other body parts is also evaluated. The disability scale evaluates the effect of the blepharospasm on activities of daily living, such as driving a vehicle, watching movies, going shopping, or walking in crowds. The validity and reliability of this rating scale has not yet been determined.

RATING SCALE FOR OROMANDIBULAR DYSTONIA

Oromandibular dystonia refers to contractions of the muscles of mastication and other muscles in or around the mouth. It can include lingual and pharyngeal dystonia. This oral region is a site to which blepharospasm commonly spreads,[14] but dystonia can also start in this region and remain isolated as a focal dystonia or spread to contiguous structures to become a segmental dystonia. Oromandibular dystonia is often mistaken for chorea because the movements of the jaw may be rapid and repetitive. In part, such movement develops because of discomfort in the jaw muscles caused by forceful, sustained contractions. Patients usually attempt to overcome these involuntary contractions by producing voluntary contractions of the antagonist muscles. Thus, if the involuntary contractions act to clench the jaw, the voluntary opposing contractions attempt to pull the jaw open. This results in a pattern of rapidly opening and closing the jaw. The examiner can usually distinguish between dystonia and other movements in this region by asking the patient to "let the muscle contractions occur without fighting them."[2]

The rating scale for oromandibular dystonia, like that for blepharospasm, comprises a severity scale and a disability scale (Appendix 19-C). The former evaluates the muscles involved, the influencing factors, and the severity of the contractions. The latter evaluates the impact of the dystonia on activities of daily living, such as the ability to speak, chew, swallow, and maintain body weight. The scales have not yet been validated.

RATING SCALE FOR TORTICOLLIS

Torticollis refers to contractions of the muscles of the neck that pull the head into abnormal postures. Torticollis is usually not a pure rotational movement. More often, one shoulder is elevated, and there is often some retrocollis and some tilting of the head toward a shoulder, as well as turning of the head. The term *spasmodic torticollis* is usually used for this disorder because many affected patients have jerky movements, and not just abnormal posturing, of the head. One of the fairly specific features of torticollis, as compared with dystonia elsewhere in the body, is the high frequency of nuchal pain that accompanies the abnormal movements and postures. Why pain should be so frequently associated with this type of focal dystonia but not with other types is unknown. Perhaps there are more pain fibers in the neck muscles than elsewhere. Or perhaps, as nuchal contractions occur commonly to produce tension headaches, such contraction (even if mild and not sufficient to produce headaches) may cause neck pain when combined with the involuntary contractions of torticollis.

The scale assessing torticollis evaluates the direction of muscle pulling, the influencing factors, the severity of the deformity, the presence of jerking movements, and severity of pain (Appendix 19-D). In addition to this movement scale, there is a disability scale that assesses the influence of torticollis on activities of daily living, such as the ability to drive, work, or fall asleep when lying down. These scales have not yet been validated. (A simple way to quantitate the severity of dystonia is to determine how long a patient can maintain the head in a straight position. This time measurement may reflect the degree of severity.)

RATING SCALES FOR ARM DYSTONIA, LEG DYSTONIA, AND TRUNK DYSTONIA

Arm dystonia usually begins as writer's cramp—the development of abnormal contractions of the hand, forearm, and arm muscles when the patient is using the arm for some voluntary motor activity, most commonly the act of writing. Other common acts that induce these abnormal contractions include playing a musical instrument and typing. As the dystonia progresses, other motor acts, such as buttoning and shaving, become involved. The abnormal movements often spread to the opposite arm.[15]

Involvement of the leg is predominantly a feature of childhood-onset dystonia.[2,16] Adult-onset dystonia ordinarily spares the legs. When the leg (or foot) is affected in adult-onset dystonia, the disorder is psychogenic in a high percentage of cases,[17] or may be a feature of parkinsonism. As with arm dystonia, childhood-onset dystonia involving the leg most often begins as an action dystonia. When the child walks, the leg twists in an abnormal manner. As the dystonia progresses, the leg shows the abnormal movements when the patient is at rest. Often, the disorder spreads to the trunk and the more rostral regions of the body.

Like leg dystonia, trunk involvement is more common with childhood-onset than adult-onset. Usually the abnormal posturing occurs when the child is walking and it commonly disappears when the child is lying down. With progression, the trunk can become deformed when the body is at rest, and kyphosis, scoliosis, and lordosis can be permanent.

Scales have been devised to assess the severity of arm, leg, and trunk dystonias (Appendixes 19-E through 19-G). These scales use a range of points from 0 to 4 to measure the severity specific to each region. For example, for arm dystonia, the ability to grasp is a major function and therefore is quantitated. For leg and trunk dystonia, the ability to walk is the major function, and this is similarly quantitated. Validation of these scales has not yet been attempted.

CONCLUSION

A simple clinical examination that does not require electronic or mechanical devices can be used to assess the severity of dystonia. The forerunner of our dystonia scales was designed to analyze generalized idiopathic dystonia.[7] Scales to quantitate the severity of many of the focal dystonias were subsequently developed, allowing more specificity and greater sensitivity of measurement. However, unlike the scale for generalized dystonia, those for the focal dystonias have not yet been validated.

REFERENCES

1. Fahn S, Marsden CD, Calne DB. Classification and investigation of dystonia. In Marsden CD, Fahn S, eds: Movement Disorders 2. London: Butterworths, 1987:332–58.
2. Fahn S. The varied clinical expressions of dystonia. Neurol Clin 1984; 2:541–54.
3. Bressman SB, Fahn S, Burke RE. Paroxysmal non-kinesigenic dystonia. Adv Neurol 1988; 50:403–13.
4. Fahn S. The clinical spectrum of motor tics. Adv Neurol 1982; 35:341–4.
5. Nygaard TG, Duvoisin RC: Hereditary dystonia-parkinsonism syndrome of juvenile onset. Neurology 1986; 36:1424–8.
6. Segawa M, Hosaka A, Miyagawa F, et al. Hereditary progressive dystonia with marked diurnal fluctuation. Adv Neurol 1976; 14:215–33.
7. Burke RE, Fahn S, Marsden CD, et al. Validity and reliability of a rating scale for the primary torsion dystonias. Neurology 1985; 35:73–7.
8. Marsden CD. The problem of adult-onset idiopathic torsion dystonia and other isolated dyskinesias in adult life (including blepharospasm, oromandibular dystonia, dystonic writer's cramp, and torticollis, or axial dystonia). Adv Neurol 1976; 14:259–76.
9. Paulson GW. Meige's syndrome. Geriatrics 1972; 27:69–73.
10. Tolosa ES, Lai C. Meige's diseases: striatal dopaminergic preponderance. Neurology 1979; 29:1126–30.
11. Meige H. Les convulsions de la face, une forme clinique de convulsion faciale bilatéral et médiane. Rev Neurol 1910; 21:437–43.
12. Tolosa ES, Klawans HL. Meige's disease: a clinical form of facial convulsion, bilateral and medial. Arch Neurol 1979; 36:635–7.
13. Fahn S. Rating scales for blepharospasm. Adv Ophthalmic Plast Reconstr Surg 1985; 4:97–101.
14. Fahn S. Blepharospasm: a focal dystonia. Adv Ophthalmic Plast Reconstr Surg 1985; 4:87–91.
15. Sheehy MP, Marsden CD. Writer's cramp—a focal dystonia. Brain 1982; 105:461–80.
16. Marsden CD, Harrison MJG, Bundey S. Natural history of idiopathic torsion dystonia. Adv Neurol 1976; 14:177–87.
17. Fahn S, William DT. Psychogenic dystonia. Adv Neurol 1988; 50:431–55.

The Fahn-Marsden Scale for Primary Torsion Dystonia

I. MOVEMENT SCALE

A. Provoking Factor Scores

1. All body parts except speech and swallowing:
   0 = No dystonia at rest or action
   1 = Dystonia on particular action
   2 = Dystonia on many actions
   3 = Dystonia on action of distant part of body or intermittently at rest
   4 = Dystonia commonly present at rest

2. Speech and swallowing:
   1 = Occasional either or both
   2 = Frequent either
   3 = Frequent one and occasional other
   4 = Frequent both

B. Severity Factors

1. Eyes:
   0 = No dystonia present
   1 = Slight; occasional blinking
   2 = Mild; frequent blinking, but without prolonged spasms of eye closure
   3 = Moderate; prolonged spasms of eyelid closure, but eyes open most of the time
   4 = Severe; prolonged spasms of eyelid closure, with eyes closed at least 30% of the time

2. Mouth:
   0 = No dystonia present
   1 = Slight; occasional grimacing or other mouth movements (e.g., jaw open or clenched; tongue movements)
   2 = Mild; movements present less than 50% of the time
   3 = Moderate dystonic movements or contractions present most of the time
   4 = Severe dystonic movements or contractions present most of the time

3. Speech and swallowing:
   0 = Normal
   1 = Slightly involved; speech easily understood, or occasional choking
   2 = Speech somewhat difficult to understand, or frequent choking
   3 = Speech markedly difficult to understand, or unable to swallow firm foods
   4 = Completely or almost completely dystonic speech, or anarthria, or marked difficulty in swallowing soft foods and liquids

4. Neck:
   0 = No dystonia present
   1 = Slight; occasional pulling of head
   2 = Torticollis obvious but mild
   3 = Moderate pulling of head
   4 = Extreme pulling of head

5. Arm:
   0 = No dystonia present
   1 = Slight dystonia, clinically insignificant
   2 = Mild; dystonia obvious but not disabling
   3 = Moderate; able to grasp; some manual function
   4 = Severe; no useful grasp

6. Trunk:
   0 = No dystonia present
   1 = Slight bending; clinically insignificant
   2 = Definite bending, but does not interfere with standing
   3 = Moderate bending; interferes with standing and walking
   4 = Extreme bending; prevents standing or walking

7. Leg:
   0 = No dystonia present
   1 = Slight dystonia, but does not cause impairment; clinically insignificant
   2 = Mild dystonia; walks briskly and unaided
   3 = Moderate dystonia; walking severely impaired, or requires assistance
   4 = Severe dystonia; unable to stand or walk on involved leg most of the time

II. DISABILITY SCALE

1. Speech:
   0 = Normal
   1 = Slightly involved; easily understood
   2 = Somewhat difficult to understand
   3 = Markedly difficult to understand
   4 = Completely or almost completely aphonic or anarthric

2. Handwriting (tremor or dystonia):
   0 = Normal
   1 = Slight difficulty; legible
   2 = Almost illegible

3 = Illegible
4 = Unable to grasp to maintain hold on pen

3. Feeding:
   0 = Normal
   1 = Uses "tricks"; independent
   2 = Can feed but cannot cut
   3 = Finger food only
   4 = Completely dependent

4. Eating:
   0 = Normal
   1 = Occasional choking
   2 = Chokes frequently; difficulty swallowing
   3 = Unable to swallow firm foods
   4 = Marked difficulty swallowing soft foods and liquids

5. Hygiene:
   0 = Normal
   1 = Clumsy but independent
   2 = Needs help with some activities
   3 = Needs help with most activities
   4 = Needs help with all activities

6. Dressing:
   0 = Normal
   1 = Clumsy but independent
   2 = Needs help with some
   3 = Needs help with most
   4 = Helpless

7. Walking:
   0 = Normal
   1 = Slightly abnormal; hardly noticeable
   2 = Moderately abnormal; obvious to naive observer
   3 = Considerably normal
   4 = Needs assistance to walk
   6 = Wheelchair-bound

Scales for Assessing Blepharospasm

BLEPHAROSPASM RATING SCALE

(Score 1 point for each positive answer unless directed otherwise.)

Location of Involuntary Movements

Upper face:
1. Frontalis or corrugator _____
2. Orbicularis oculi _____
3. Nasal muscles _____
4. Zygomatic muscles _____

Lower face:
5. Pursing of lips _____
6. Retraction of lips _____
7. Corner of mouth pulled sideways (risoris) _____
8. Buccinator (sucking in of cheeks) _____
9. Puffing out of cheeks _____
10. Mentalis _____
11. Platysma _____

When Present

12. At rest _____
13. Only with action (e.g., speaking) _____

Influencing Factors

(Compare with baseline [e.g., sitting in room light, not talking]: worse = +1, no change = 0, better = −1; if no information, write NA)

14. In sunlight _____
15. At movies _____
16. Watching Television _____

17. Walking ____
18. Talking ____
19. Writing ____
20. Reading ____
21. Sewing ____
22. Card playing ____
23. Working ____
24. Listening ____
25. Singing ____
26. Yawning ____
27. Wearing regular eyeglasses ____
28. Wearing sunglasses ____
29. Anger ____

Frequency of Involuntary Movements

30. (at baseline) ____

Movements constantly present at rest (>75% of the time)	(+5)
Movements present at rest 51–75% of waking time	(+4)
Movements present at rest 26–50% of waking time	(+3)
Movements present at rest 10–25% of waking time	(+2)
Movements present at rest <10% of waking time	(+1)

Severity of Involuntary Movements

(Select the maximum points from among the choices)

31. Upper face: ____

Increased blinking of eyelids	(+1)
Closure of eyelids	(+2)
Forceful closure of eyelids	(+3)
Severe, forceful closure of eyelids	(+4)

32. Mouth (excluding jaw): ____

Mild forcefulness	(+1)
Moderate forcefulness	(+2)
Severe forcefulness	(+3)

Dystonia Elsewhere in Body

(For information only, not for total score. Present with action only = +1, present at rest <75% of time = +2, present at rest >75% of time = +3)

33. Jaw ____
34. Tongue ____
35. Neck ____

36. Larynx ____
37. Pharynx ____
38. Right arm ____
39. Left arm ____

Thoracolumbar spine when sitting:
40. Tilt to right ____
41. Tilt to left ____
42. Kyphosis ____
43. Lordosis ____

44. Right leg ____
45. Left leg ____

BLEPHAROSPASM DISABILITY

Percent of Normal Activity

100% = Unaware of any difficulty

95% = Aware of some blepharospasm; some annoyance but no limitation of activities

90% = Completely independent; socially affected, but otherwise no limitation of activities because of blepharospasm; if there are any limitations of functional activities, the patient should check the ones listed below that apply

	Points (max = 2)
Sunglasses (check one or both of these if they apply:	
1. Need to wear sunglasses outdoors	1
2. Usually need sunglasses indoors	1

Driving (check those that apply):	(max = 5)
1. Uncomfortable but no limitation	1
2. Cannot drive at night because of blepharospasm	2
3. Can drive in daytime but need to prop eyelids open	2
4. Can drive only short distances	3
5. Cannot drive at all because of blepharospasm	4
6. Usually cannot ride in a car	5

Reading (check one if affected):	(max = 3)
1. Uncomfortable but no limitation	1
2. Mild to moderate limitation of reading	2
3. Marked limitation of reading	3

Television (check one if affected):	(max = 3)
1. Uncomfortable but no limitation	1
2. Mild to moderate limitation of viewing TV	2
3. Marked limitation of viewing TV	3

Movies (check one if affected):	(max = 3)
1. Uncomfortable but no limitation	1
2. Mild to moderate limitation of watching movies	2
3. Marked limitation of watching movies	3

Shopping (check one if affected):	(max = 3)
1. Uncomfortable but no limitation	1
2. Not able to shop alone in department store	2
3. Not able to shop, even when accompanied	3

Walking about (check one if affected):	(max = 4)
1. Uncomfortable but no limitation	1
2. Difficulty walking in crowds	2
3. Not able to walk alone outside	3
4. Not able to walk unassisted indoors	4

	Points
Housework or outside job (check one if affected):	(max = 3)
1. Uncomfortable but no limitation	1
2. Difficulty working because of blepharospasm	2
3. Not able to work because of blepharospasm	3
	(Total max = 26)

Calculations (total the points scored, divide by maximum possible for each patient, multiply the quotient by 90, and subtract from 90%):

$$90\% \ - \ 90(\text{score} \ \div \ \text{maximum possible}) \ = \ \text{Final score}$$

Scales for Assessing
Oromandibular Dystonia

OROMANDIBULAR DYSTONIA RATING SCALE

(Score 1 point for each answer unless directed otherwise.)

Location of Involuntary Movements

Lower face:
1. Pursing of lips ____
2. Retraction of lips ____
3. Corner of mouth pulled sideways
   (risoris) ____
4. Buccinator (sucking in of
   cheeks) ____
5. Puffing out of cheeks ____
6. Mentalis ____
7. Platysma ____

Jaw:
8. Mandible pulled down ____
9. Mandible pulled up ____
10. Mandible pulled sideways:
    right ____
11. Mandible pulled sideways:
    left ____
12. Mandible pulled in ____
13. Mandible pushed out ____

Tongue:
14. Present ____

Pharynx:
15. Present ____

When Present

16. At rest ____
17. Only with action (e.g., speak-
    ing) ____

Influencing Factors

(Compare with baseline, e.g., sitting, not talking; worse = +1, no change = 0, better = −1; if no information, write NA)

18. Walking _____
19. Talking _____
20. Writing _____
21. Reading _____
22. Singing _____
23. Humming _____
24. Eating _____
25. Yawning _____
26. Object in mouth _____

Frequency of Involuntary Movements

27. (at baseline) _____
     Movements constantly present at rest (>75% of the time)   (+5)
     Movements present at rest 51–75% of the time   (+4)
     Movements present at rest 26–50% of the time   (+3)
     Movements present at rest 10–25% of the time   (+2)
     Movements present at rest <10% of time   (+1)

Severity of Involuntary Movements

28. Mouth (excluding jaw): _____
     Mild forcefulness   (+1)
     Moderate forcefulness   (+2)
     Severe forcefulness   (+3)

29. Jaw: _____
     Mild forcefulness   (+1)
     Moderate forcefulness   (+2)
     Severe forcefulness   (+3)

30. Tongue: _____
     Mild forcefulness   (+1)
     Moderate forcefulness   (+2)
     Severe forcefulness   (+3)

31. Pharynx: _____
     Mild forcefulness   (+1)
     Moderate forcefulness   (+2)
     Severe forcefulness   (+3)

Dystonia Elsewhere in Body

(For information only, not for total score. Present with action only = +1, present at rest <75% of time = +2, present at rest >75% of time = +3)

32. Upper face ____
33. Neck ____
34. Larynx ____
35. Pharynx ____
36. Right arm ____
37. Left arm ____

Thoracolumbar spine when sitting:
38. Tilt to right ____
39. Tilt to left ____
40. Kyphosis ____
41. Lordosis ____

42. Right leg ____
43. Left leg ____

OROMANDIBULAR DYSTONIA DISABILITY

Percent of Normal Activity

100% = Unaware of any difficulty

95% = Aware of some oral dystonia; some annoyance, but no limitation of activities

90% = Completely independent; socially affected, but otherwise no limitation of activities because of oromandibular dystonia; if there are any limitations of functional activities, the patient should check the ones listed below that apply

	Points
Speaking (check one of these if affected):	(max = 3)
1. Mild impairment of speaking	1
2. Moderate impairment of speaking	2
3. Market impairment of speaking	3
Chewing (check one of these if affected):	(max = 3)
1. Mild impairment of chewing	1
2. Moderate impairment of chewing	2
3. Marked impairment of chewing	3
Swallowing (check one of these if affected):	(max = 3)
1. Mild impairment of swallowing	1
2. Moderate impairment of swallowing	2
3. Marked impairment of swallowing	3
Breathing (check one of these if affected):	(max = 3)
1. Mild difficulty breathing	1
2. Moderate difficulty breathing	2
3. Marked difficulty breathing	3
Weight loss (due to oromandibular dystonia):	(max = 6)
1. Currently 1–10% less than normal weight	2
2. Currently 11–20% less than normal weight	4
3. Currently >20% less than normal weight	6
Housework or outside job (check one of these):	(max = 3)
1. Uncomfortable but no limitation	1
2. Difficulty working because of oromandibular dystonia	2
3. Not able to work because of oromandibular dystonia	3
	(Total max = 21)

Calculations: Total the points scored, divide by maximum possible for each patient, multiply the quotient by 90, and subtract from 90%:

$$90\% - 90(\text{score} \div \text{maximum possible}) = \text{Final score}$$

Scales for Assessing Torticollis

TORTICOLLIS RATING SCALE

(Score 1 point for each positive answer unless directed otherwise.)

Direction of Movement

1. Retrocollis ____
2. Anterocollis ____
3. Torticollis: chin to right (R), chin to left (L) ____
4. Tilt of head: to right shoulder (R), to left shoulder (L) ____
5. Shift of head: to the right (R), to the left (L) ____
6. Shift of head: anteriorly (A), posteriorly (P) ____
7. Right shoulder: elevated (up), anteriorly displaced (ant) ____
8. Left shoulder: elevated (up), anteriorly displaced (ant) ____

When Present

9. Sitting, head unsupported ____
10. Sitting, head supported ____
11. Standing ____
12. Lying down ____

Influencing Factors

(Compare with baseline [e.g., sitting, head unsupported: worse = +1, no change = 0, less = −1)]

13. Standing ____
14. Walking ____
15. Talking ____
16. Writing ____
17. Lying down ____

Duration of Deviation When Sitting with Head Unsupported

18. Head constantly deviated (when patient is sitting): _____
     >75% of the time (yes = + 5; no = 0)
     Cannot voluntarily move head past midline (if not able = +2; if able = 0)
     Can voluntarily move head to the extreme opposite position (if able = −1;
     if not able = 0)
19. Head intermittently deviated (when patient is sitting): _____
     Head straight >75% of time (yes = +1)
     Head straight >50% of time but <75% of time (yes = +2)
     Head straight <50% of time (yes = +3)

Severity When Patient Is Sitting with Head Unsupported

20. Score _____
     Mild forcefulness: pulled <1/3 of maximum direction (+1)
     Moderate forcefulness: pulled 1/3 to 2/3 of maximum direction (+2)
     Severe forcefulness: pulled >2/3 of maximum direction (+3)

Pain When Patient Is Sitting with Head Unsupported

(unrelated to spasms; if pain occurs with spasms, see item 28)

21. Present: _____
         <10% of the time   (+1)
         10% to <25% of the time   (+2)
         25% to <50% of the time   (+3)
         50% to <75% of the time   (+4)
         >75% of the time   (+5)

22. Severity of pain: _____
     None   (0)
     Mild   (+1)
     Moderate   +3
     Severe   (+5)

Reduction of Severity with "Tricks"

(no relief = 0, partial relief = −1, total relief [>90%] = −2)

23. Hand on chin, jaw, or face _____
24. Hand on neck or back of head _____
25. Head resting against wall _____

Forceful Spasms

26. Average frequency: ____
Never	(0)
Rarely (< 1/day)	(+1)
Occasionally (1–3/day)	(+2)
Frequently (3–10/day)	(+3)
Very frequently (> 10/day)	(+4)

27. Average duration: ____
Not present	(0)
< 30 sec	(+1)
30–120 sec	(+2)
> 120 sec	(+3)

28. Average severity: ____
Not painful	(0)
Mild pain	(+1)
Moderate pain	(+2)
Severe pain	(+3)

Involuntary Movements of the Head

29. Tremor of the head (1 point for each): ____
    Horizontal
    Vertical
    (Note: both horizontal and vertical tremors = +2)

30. Gross jerky movements of the head:
Mild	(+1)
Moderate	(+3)
Severe	(+5)

Essential Tremor of the Hands

31. Score ____
Absent	(0)
Present	(+1)

Dystonia Elsewhere in Body

(For information only, not for total score. Present with action only or present at rest <75% of time = +1, present at rest >75% of time = +2)

32. Jaw (cranial nerve V) ____
33. Face (cranial nerve VII) ____
34. Tongue ____
35. Larynx ____
36. Pharynx ____
37. Right arm ____
38. Left arm ____

Thoracolumbar spine when sitting:
39. Tilt to right ____
40. Tilt to left ____
41. Kyphosis ____
42. Lordosis ____
43. Right leg ____
44. Left leg ____

TORTICOLLIS DISABILITY

Percent of Normal Activity

100% = Unaware of any difficulty

95% = Aware of some torticollis; some annoyance but no limitation of activities

90% = Completely independent; socially affected, but otherwise no limitation of activities because of torticollis; if there are any limitations of functional activities, the patients should check the ones listed below that apply

	Points
Driving (check those that apply):	(max = 5)
1. Uncomfortable but no special tricks needed	1
2. Can drive but need to use a sensory trick	2
3. Can drive only short distances because of torticollis	3
4. Usually cannot drive because of torticollis	4
5. Cannot ride in a car for long periods	5
Reading (check one of these if affected):	(max = 3)
1. Uncomfortable but no limitation	1
2. Mild to moderate limiation of reading	2
3. Marked limitation of reading	3
Television (check one of these if affected):	(max =3)
1. Uncomfortable but no limitation	1
2. Mild to moderate limitation of viewing TV	2
3. Marked limitation of viewing TV	3
Movies (check one of these if affected):	(max = 3)
1. Uncomfortable but no limitation	1
2. Mild to moderate limitation of watching movies	2
3. Marked limitation of watching movies	3
Shopping (check one of these if affected):	(max = 3)
1. Uncomfortable but no limitation	1
2. Not able to shop alone in department store	2
3. Not able to shop, even when accompanied	3
Walking about (check if affected):	(max = 2)
1. Uncomfortable but no limitation	1
2. Difficulty walking in crowds	2
Feeding (check one of these if affected):	(max =3)
1. Uncomfortable but no limitation	1
2. Mild to moderate impairment of feeding	2
3. Marked impairment of feeding	3
Falling asleep (check one of these if affected):	(max = 2)
1. Mild to moderate impairment of falling asleep	1
2. Marked impairment of falling asleep	2

	Points
Housework or outside job (check one of these if affected):	(max = 3)
1. Uncomfortable but no limitation	1
2. Difficulty working because of torticollis	2
3. Not able to work because of torticollis	3
	(Total max = 22)

Calculations: Total the points scored, divide by maximum possible for each patient, multiply the quotient by 90, and subtract from 90%:

$$90\% - 90(\text{score} \div \text{maximum possible}) = \text{Final score}$$

A Scale for Assessing Arm Dystonia

ARM DYSTONIA DISABILITY

Percent of Normal Activity

(Note: If an activity would not normally be performed by the patient, mark NA in left margin.)

100% = Unaware of any difficulty

95% = Aware of some finger, hand, or arm movements; some annoyance but no limitations of activities

90% = Completely independent; socially affected, but otherwise no limitation of activities because of arm dystonia; if there are any limitations of functional activities, the patients should check the ones listed below that apply

	Points
Writing (check one if affected):	(max = 3)
1. Mild difficulty writing	1
2. Moderate difficulty writing	2
3. Marked difficulty writing	3
Playing a musical instrument (check one if affected):	(max = 3)
1. Mild difficulty playing	1
2. Moderate difficulty playing	2
3. Marked difficulty playing	3
Buttoning (check one of these if affected):	(max = 3)
1. Mild difficulty buttoning	1
2. Moderate difficulty buttoning	2
3. Marked difficulty buttoning	3
Handling utensils and feeding (check one if affected):	(max = 3)
1. Mild difficulty with utensils or feeding	1
2. Moderate difficulty with utensils or feeding	2
3. Marked difficulty with utensils or feeding	3
Hygiene (check one if affected):	(max = 3)
1. Mild difficulty with shaving, brushing teeth, etc.	1

2. Moderate difficulty shaving, brushing teeth, etc.	2
3. Marked difficulty shaving, brushing teeth, etc.	3

Grasping objects (check one if affected):   (max = 3)
1. Mild difficulty grasping   1
2. Moderate difficulty grasping   2
3. Marked difficulty grasping   3

Housework or outside job (check one if affected):   (max = 3)
1. Uncomfortable but no limitation   1
2. Difficulty working because of arm dystonia   2
3. Not able to work because of arm dystonia   2

(max = 2)

Calculations: Total the points scored, divide by maximum possible for each patient, multiply the quotient by 90, and subtract from 90%:

90% − 90(score/maximum possible) = Final score

A Scale for Assessing Leg Dystonia

LEG DYSTONIA DISABILITY

Percent of Normal Activity

100% = Unaware of any difficulty

95% = Aware of some foot or leg movements; some annoyance but no limitations of activities

90% = Completely independent; socially affected, but otherwise no limitation of activities because of leg dystonia; if there are any limitations of functional activities, the patients should check the ones listed below that apply

	Points
Walking (check one if affected):	(max = 8)
1. Mild difficulty walking	1
2. Moderate difficulty walking; unable to keep up with peers	2
3. Marked difficulty walking but still independent	3
4. Uses some mechanical or personal aid to walk but can walk considerable distances	4
5. More limitation with walking; cannot walk more than one block without resting	5
6. Wheelchair used for traveling out of the house	6
7. Wheelchair used for getting around in the house most of the time	7
8. Not able to move about the house unassisted	8
Standing (check one if affected):	(max = 7)
1. Mild difficulty standing erect	1
2. Moderate difficulty standing erect	2
3. Marked difficulty standing erect	3
4. Unable to stand erect	4
5. Needs assistance to remain standing	5
6. Unable to stand alone	6
7. Unable to stand, even with assistance	7
Sitting (check one if affected):	(max = 4)
1. Mild difficulty sitting with legs down	1
2. Moderate difficulty sitting with legs down	2

3. Marked difficulty sitting with legs down   3
4. Unable to sit with legs down   4

Falling asleep (check one if affected):   (max = 2)
1. Mild to moderate impairment of falling asleep   1
2. Marked impairment of falling asleep   2

Housework or outside job (check one if affected):   (max = 3)
1. Uncomfortable but no limitation   1
2. Difficulty working because of leg dystonia   2
3. Not able to work because of leg dystonia   3
                                                                   (max = 3)

Calculations: Total the points scored, divide by maximum possible for each patient, multiply the dividend by 90, and subtract from 90%:

$$90\% - 90(\text{score} \div \text{maximum possible}) = \text{Final score}$$

A Scale for Assessing Trunk Dystonia

TRUNK DYSTONIA DISABILITY

Percent of Normal Activity

100% = Unaware of any difficulty

95% = Aware of some truncal movements; some annoyance but no limitations of activities

90% = Completely independent; socially affected, but otherwise no limitation of activities because of trunk dystonia; if there are any limitations of functional activities, the patients should check the ones listed below that apply

	Points
Walking (check one if affected):	(max = 8)
1. Mild difficulty walking	1
2. Moderate difficulty walking; unable to keep up with peers	2
3. Marked difficulty walking but still independent	3
4. Uses some mechanical or personal aid to walk but can walk considerable distances	4
5. More limitation with walking; cannot walk more than one block without resting	5
6. Wheelchair used for traveling out of the house	6
7. Wheelchair used for getting around in the house most of the time	7
8. Not able to move about the house unassisted	8
Standing (check one if affected):	(max = 7)
1. Mild difficulty standing erect	1
2. Moderate difficulty standing erect	2
3. Marked difficulty standing erect	3
4. Unable to stand erect	4
5. Needs assistance to remain standing in any posture	5
6. Unable to stand alone in any posture	6
7. Unable to stand in any posture, even with assistance	7
Sitting (check one if affected):	(max = 4)
1. Mild difficulty sitting erect	1
2. Moderate difficulty sitting erect	2
3. Marked difficulty sitting erect	3

4. Unable to sit erect   4
5. Needs assistance to remain sitting   5
6. Unable to sit even with assistance   6

Lying on back (check one if affected):   (max = 3)
1. Mild difficulty lying down without movements   1
2. Moderate difficulty lying down   2
3. Marked difficulty lying down   3

Falling asleep (check one if affected):   (max = 2)
1. Mild to moderate impairment of falling asleep   1
2. Marked impairment of falling asleep   2

Housework or outside job (check one if affected):   (max = 2)
1. Difficulty working because of truncal dystonia   1
2. Not able to work because of truncal dystonia   2
                                                              (max = 2)

(Calculations: Total the points scored, divide by maximum possible for each patient, multiply the quotient by 90, and subtract from 90%:

$$90\% \; - \; 90(\text{score} \div \text{maximum possible}) = \text{Final score}$$

Chapter 20

Assessment of Functional Capacity in Neurodegenerative Movement Disorders: Huntington's Disease as a Prototype

Ira Shoulson, Roger Kurlan, Allen J. Rubin, David Goldblatt, Jill Behr, Charlyne Miller, Judith Kennedy, Kathryn A. Bamford, Eric D. Caine, Daniel K. Kido, Sandra Plumb, and Charles Odoroff

The experimental therapeutics of neurodegenerative movement disorders is entering a new phase aimed at forestalling neuronal degeneration and clinical decline. This development is prompted by advances in understanding the pathogenesis of premature neuronal death and by improved prospects for attenuation of the neurodegenerative process with therapy. In this context, the mere assessment of short-term changes in disordered movement has proven inadequate for measuring long-term functional alterations that more closely reflect pathogenesis. Huntington's disease (HD) has served as a prototype for functional assessment by virtue of its completely penetrant autosomal dominant mode of inheritance, its relatively uniform clinical expression, and its predictable functional decline.[1]

The medium-sized spiny neurons in the striatum appear to be the most vulnerable and earliest sites of pathologic disruption in HD.[2,3] Neuronal degeneration is reflected partly by radiographic changes of striatal glucose hypometabolism, which are detected initially by positron emission tomography (PET)[4-6] and eventually by conventional computed tomography (CT).[7-10]

We thank the staff of the University of Rochester Clinical Research Center for their help in the evaluation of patients, and we thank Ruth Nobel, Donna LaDonna, and Carrie Irvine for their assistance in the preparation of this manuscript. This research was funded by grants (NS17978 and RR00044) to the University of Rochester Clinical Research Center from the United States Public Health Service, National Institutes of Health.

The time course and mechanisms responsible for triggering neuronal degeneration remain unclear, but various genetic and neurobiologic studies suggest that clinical expression may derive from excitotoxic processes, perhaps mediated by glutamate, that render the HD gene carrier susceptible to selective neuronal degeneration.[11] Continued advances in understanding the molecular genetic basis of HD, and the resulting ability to identify presymptomatic gene carriers,[12-14] should further enhance our knowledge of the disease's pathogenesis and provide a stronger basis for more sensible therapeutic strategies. Strategies to slow or halt neuronal degeneration and clinical decline now depend critically on the availability of quantitative measures to assess the functional correlates of HD longitudinally.

Ideally, a reliable in vivo measure of early striatal cell dysfunction would provide the most sensitive and valid therapeutic outcome variable for protective strategies. Although PET and possibly nuclear magnetic spectroscopy may one day provide such an index, these techniques require further validation and remain very expensive and cumbersome for application in large-scale clinical trials. Until reliable and feasible neurobiologic measures become available, longitudinal clinical assessment of functional capacity remains the most reasonable outcome variable for use in clinical trials.

HUNTINGTON'S DISEASE FUNCTIONAL
CAPACITY SCALE

During the 1976–1977 deliberations of the U.S. Commission for the Control of HD and Its Consequences,[15] investigators recognized the need for better characterization of the clinical course of HD resulting from both motor and mental deterioration. The focus of clinical assessment therefore shifted to an assessment of functional capacity, notwithstanding the motor and mental components thereof. Based on a cross-sectional analysis of the natural history of HD and heavily influenced by the experience of occupational and physical therapists, the HD Functional Capacity (HDFC) scale[16-18] was developed to assess the capacity of HD patients to function in five basic but related categories: occupational, financial, domestic, self-care, and level of care provided (Table 20.1).

The HDFC scale was designed so that a skilled health professional could evaluate the patient on the basis of a brief (15- to 20-minute) interview and functional examination. In practice, the clinician conducts separate interviews with the patient and a close family member or friend who is familiar with the patient's daily functioning. The examination is usually limited to what can be observed casually of the patient's functions during the course of the interview. On the basis of the interview and examination, the clinician rates the patient in each of the five categories according to what the patient is judged capable of doing. The patient often overestimates capacity, and the interview with family or friend helps to confirm actual function. A total functional capacity (TFC) score of 13 units on this ordinal scale indicates full capacity in all five categories, whereas a TFC score of 0 indicates total incapacity.

The HDFC scale focuses on assessment of the patient's capacity rather than actual performance. This places the emphasis on the clinician's judgment and does not require

Table 20.1 Criteria for Quantified Staging of Functional Capacities

A. Engagement in occupation
  3. *Usual level*—full-time salaried employment, actual or potential (e.g., job offer or qualified), with normal work expectations and satisfactory performance.
  2. *Lower level*—full- or part-time salaried employment, actual or potential, with a lower than usual work expectation (relative to patient's training and education) but with satisfactory performance.
  1. *Marginal level*—part-time voluntary or salaried employment, actual or potential, with lower expectation and less than satisfactory work performance.
  0. *Unable*—totally unable to engage in voluntary or salaried employment.

B. Capacity to handle financial affairs
  3. *Full*—normal capacity to handle personal and family finances (income tax, balancing checkbook, paying bills, budgeting, shopping).
  2. *Requires slight assistance*—mildly impaired ability to handle financial affairs, such that accustomed routine responsibilities require some organization and assistance from family member or financial advisor.
  1. *Requires major assistance*—moderately impaired ability to handle financial affairs, such that patient comprehends the nature and purpose of routine financial procedures and is competent to handle funds but requires major assistance in the performance of these tasks.
  0. *Unable*—patient is unable to comprehend the financial process and is totally unable to perform tasks related to routine financial procedures.

C. Capacity to manage domestic responsibilities
  2. *Full*—no impairment in performance of routine domestic tasks (cleaning, laundering, dishwashing, table setting, recipes, lawn care, answering mail, civic responsibilities).
  1. *Impaired*—moderate impairment in performance of routine domestic tasks, such that patient requires some assistance in carrying out these tasks.
  0. *Unable*—marked impairment in function and marginal performance; requires major assistance.

D. Capacity to perform activities of daily living
  3. *Full*—complete independence in eating, dressing, and bathing.
  2. *Mildly impaired*—somewhat labored performance:
  in eating (avoids certain foods that cause chewing and swallowing problems)
  in dressing (difficulty in fine tasks only, e.g., buttoning or tying shoes)
  in bathing (difficulty in fine performance only, e.g., brushing teeth); requires only slight assistance
  1. *Moderately impaired*—substantial difficulty
  in eating (swallows only liquid or soft foods and requires considerable assistance)
  in dressing (performs only gross dressing activities and requires assistance with everything else)
  in bathing (performs only gross bathing tasks, otherwise requires assistance)
  0. *Severely impaired*—requires total care in activities of daily living.

E. Care can be provided at:
  2. *Home*—patient living at home, and family readily able to meet care needs.
  1. *Home or extended care facility*—patient may be living at home, but care needs would be better provided at an extended care facility.
  0. *Total care facility only*—patient requires full-time, skilled nursing care.

Table 20.2   General Relationships of Stage of Illness to Total Functional Capacity (TFC) Scores and Estimated Duration of Illness

Stage	Corresponding TFC Score	Years from onset of illness: range (median)[a]
I	11–13	0–8 (3)
II	7–10	3–13 (7)
III	3–6	5–16 (12)
IV	1–2	9–21 (15)
V	0	11–26 (19)

[a] Estimated dates of illness onset were determined retrospectively on the basis of initial motor or mental symptoms; data were derived from 130 HD patients.[18]

rigorous documentation of performance. The examiner is required to arrive at a clinical rating of the patient's capabilities—a judgment that the clinician commonly makes in the day-to-day evaluation of disability. We have used a modified HDFC scale to assess functional performance as well as functional capacity, and our preliminary data reveal only minor discrepancies between capacity and performance ratings.

The TFC scores for this scale can be collapsed somewhat arbitrarily into five stages of illness (Table 20.2). The subdivision of illness into stages was formulated to detect changes in the earliest stages (I through III). This bias has proven helpful in therapeutic studies aimed at early intervention. However, the collapsing of TFC scores into stages of illness is useful only for descriptive purposes and not for statistical analysis in which the reduction of TFC scores into stages tends to waste data.

From the onset of illness to death, the average life expectancy of an HD patient is approximately 19 years. Since the onset of illness occurs at an average age of about 38 years, the prototypical gene carrier spends the first two thirds of life in a pre-symptomatic state and the last one third in a state of progressive disability.[19] The HDFC scale can therefore be considered a measure of disability spanning an average 19-year interval, although this concept is imprecise because of problems in reliably defining the onset of illness. In practice, onset is usually estimated retrospectively on the basis of the reported emergence of motor and/or mental features.

Several cross-sectional surveys have indicated that HD patients in the earliest stages (I through III) undergo an average functional decline of approximately one unit per year.[17,20] Since the HDFC scale is most sensitive to early changes in disability, the rate of functional decline appears to slow in the more advanced stages (IV and V). A precise determination of variance for the average rate of functional decline awaits the outcome of ongoing prospective studies on nonmedicated HD patients in the early stages of disease.[21]

VALIDITY TESTING

The neurobiologic relevance of the HDFC scale has been examined in several independent studies that compared the extent of functional capacity (or incapacity) to the severity of radiographic indexes of HD. The degree of caudate or striatal atrophy can be estimated with conventional CT by comparing the smallest distance between the heads of the caudate nuclei (caudate-caudate distance, or CC) to a reference dimension such as the outer table of the skull distance (OT) or the frontal horn distance (FH). By convention, these comparisons are expressed as the ratios CC/OT and FH/CC. In HD, the caudate-caudate distance increases disproportionately to the reference dimensions. Therefore, CC/OT increases and FH/CC decreases as a function of progressive caudate atrophy.[7-10] These radiographic indexes are subject to considerable variation if care is not taken to obtain objective measures that are standardized for level, thickness, and angle of the image. In our studies, linear measurements are calculated directly by the CT computer for axial images obtained at the level of the interventricular foramen, in slices 5 mm thick and at an angle parallel to the orbital roof.

Employing these standardized measures, we performed unenhanced head CT scans in 60 nonmedicated HD patients who were entering a clinical trial and who were considered to be in the earliest stages of illness. This cohort of HD subjects will also serve as a reference group for other studies to be discussed. The functional capacity of each patient was rated independently by six clinicians, and mean TFC was derived from the average of the six ratings.[22]

Mean TFC scores correlated to a greater extent with CC/OT ($r = 0.48$, $P < 0.0001$) and FH/CC ($r = -0.45$, $P < 0.003$) than with traditional retrospectively derived measures of HD, such as estimated duration of illness from initial symptoms ($r = 0.32$, $P < 0.02$ for CC/OT; $r = -0.39$, $P < 0.003$ for FH/CC). When the data were analyzed according to stages I (TFC = 11 to 13, n = 34) and II (TFC = 7 to 10, n = 26) and illness durations of 5 years or less (n = 33) and 6 years or more (n = 27), TFC was found to be a more reliable discriminator of caudate atrophy ($t = 3.95$, $P < 0.0005$ for FH/CC; $t = 3.59$, $P < 0.001$ for CC/OT) than were estimated duration of illness ($t = 3.70$, $P < 0.001$ for FH/CC; $t = 2.31$, $P < 0.05$ for CC/OT), present age, age at onset of illness, or maternal versus paternal descent of the HD gene (all $P < 0.05$).[22]

These strong radiographic relationships are not surprising, since functional capacity is assessed on the basis of prospectively derived information pertaining to the patient's current level of functioning rather than anamnestically derived estimates of when symptoms might first have emerged. Moreover, functional ratings are designed to assess specific categories of capacity or performance, in contrast to the vagaries surrounding the insidious onset of motor or mental features of HD. Functional ratings also provide useful information relevant to the clinical assessment of HD patients and their ongoing care.

To the extent that indexes of caudate atrophy reflect underlying neuronal degeneration in HD, functional ratings currently represent the most accurate clinical indexes of underlying disease. The radiographic validity of the HDFC scale has also been confirmed independently by other investigators. Stober and coworkers[23] compared the TFC ratings of 12 HD patients with a variety of CT indexes of caudate atrophy and, as in our study, they found that the HDFC scale correlated significantly with FH/CC ($r = 0.63$, $P < 0.05$) and CC/OT ($r = 0.56$, $P < 0.05$). Young et al.[6] applied the HDFC scale to the study of 15 nonmedicated patients with early to midstage HD who underwent PET scanning with fluorodeoxyglucose as well as conventional CT imaging. This population of subjects is of great interest, since most of the early-stage HD patients showed striatal glucose hypometabolism in the setting of normal CT indexes of caudate dimensions. This observation confirms the findings previously reported by others that cerebral metabolic dysfunction in HD precedes morphologic evidence of caudate atrophy.[4,5] Of relevance to clinical assessment, Young et al.[6] found that TFC ratings from the HDFC scale correlated strongly ($r = -0.91$, P < 0.001) with the degree of caudate hypometabolism. These data lend further support to the biologic validity of functional capacity ratings in HD.

RELIABILITY TESTING

We have also assessed inter-rater agreement in use of the HDFC scale.[24] Seven clinicians (two neurologists and a geneticist, psychiatrist, psychologist, nurse, and speech pathologist) conducted independent interviews of our 60 HD patients and their close family members or friends upon entry into our long-term clinical trial. Functional capacity data was analyzed by comparing the TFC scores for all possible permutations of differences between raters (60 subjects × 7 raters).

Agreement for TFC scores among all seven raters was completely concordant for 27% of the ratings, within 1 unit for 65%, within 2 units for 85%, and within 3 units for 96% (Figure 20.1). Spearman correlation coefficients for identical TFC scores among the seven raters ranged from 0.44 to 0.82 (mean, 0.62). The more conservative Kendall tau-B analysis generated correlation coefficients ranging from 0.38 to 0.70 (mean, 0.52). In this cohort of patients in the early stages of HD, the frequency of complete agreement for each of the five evaluation categories was 48% for occupational capabilities (category A), 57% for financial capacities (B), 68% for domestic and self-care skills (C and D), and 100% for level of care provided (E).

Taken together, these data indicate a high level of agreement among various types of health professionals in the use of the HDFC scale. The extent of agreement can also be viewed in the context of a stage of illness that corresponds to approximately three functional units. As such, agreement among all raters was discordant for the equivalent of a stage of illness in only 4% of 420 (60 × 7) total scores. Therefore, a decline of 2 to 3 TFC units is expected with great confidence to represent a reliable change in the progression of illness.

Longitudinal studies are in progress to assess the radiographic correlates of a 2- or 3-unit change in TFC. Our preliminary observations suggest that changes in CT indexes of caudate atrophy can be detected reliably over a follow-up period of 2 to 4 years, paralleling a functional decline of approximately 2 or 3 units, or the equivalent of one stage of illness.[25] On the basis of cross-sectional analysis of the PET studies of Young et al,[6] changes in fluorodeoxyglucose hypometabolism could be detected between groups of HD patients whose functional capacities differeed by 2 or 3 TFC units.

The cross-cultural reliability of the TFC scale has not been rigorously examined, but clinical investigation of the large HD families in Venezuela supports the applica-

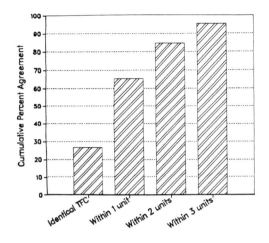

FIGURE 20.1   *Cumulative percent agreement for total functional capacity (TFC) ratings among 7 raters for 60 HD patients.*

bility of the HDFC scale to relatively diverse cultures. With only minor modifications to adapt for occupational capacity (A) and level of care provided (B) in the Venezuelan population, the HDFC scale has provided useful hallmarks of capacity, motor correlates, and progression of illness.[20] The nonmedicated cohort in Venezuela can be reasonably compared to nonmedicated HD patients examined in the United States. The motor and mental correlates of illness in the two populations are remarkably similar, suggesting that the general clinical expressivity of HD is relatively uniform.

MOTOR AND MENTAL CORRELATES

The HDFC scale was designed to avoid the pitfalls of short-term assessments that focus exclusively on the examination of motor and mental performance. An analysis of the motor and mental correlates of HD has been made more meaningful, now that the HDFC scale has undergone testing for validity and reliability.

In our 60 HD subjects, 13 motor signs (ocular motility, motor impersistence, cerebellar coordination, dysdiadochokinesia, finger-tapping, muscle-stretch reflexes, plantar responses, postural stability, walking, turning, parkinsonism, dystonia, and chorea) were rated by an independent examiner on an ordinal scale of 0 (normal) to 4 (severely abnormal).[26] According to calculations of Kendall tau-B coefficients, TFC correlated most strongly with severity of dystonia ($r = -0.40$, $P < 0.002$), postural instability ($r = -0.34$, $P < 0.003$), and chorea ($r = -0.27$, $P < 0.005$). FH/CC and CC/OT indexes of caudate atrophy correlated with the severity of dystonia ($r = 0.28$, $P < 0.005$) and hyperactivity of muscle-stretch reflexes ($r = 0.30$ for FH/CC and -0.24

for CC/OT; P < 0.004 and < 0.02, respectively). Therefore, severity of dystonic features was the motor sign that most consistently predicted the extent of functional impairment and caudate atrophy by CT. Although chorea is perhaps the most conspicuous motor sign of HD, the emergence and intensification of dystonic features appear to be important motor hallmarks of progressive neuronal degeneration in the earliest stages of illness.

In the PET studies of Young et al.,[6] bradykinesia and rigidity (parkinsonian features) correlated best with caudate hypometabolism (r = −0.69, P < 0.01), whereas chorea and oculomotor abnormalities were the most striking correlates of putamen hypometabolism (r = −0.84, P < 0.01, and r = −0.85, P < 0.01, respectively). The most robust motor correlates of TFC were oculomotor slowing (r = −0.91, P < 0.002), dysdiadochokinesia (r = −0.87, P < 0.002), and chorea and parkinsonism (r = −0.85, P < 0.002). That the motor correlates of TFC in our CT study and Young's PET study differed is most likely attributable to variability in the rating of motor parameters rather than to TFC, since the relationship between functional capacity and radiographic indexes was strikingly similar in both investigations. An interesting observation in the PET study was the significant correlation between dystonia and thalamic hypermetabolism of fluorodeoxyglucose (r = 0.62, P < 0.05), notwithstanding the lack of significant correlation between dystonia and caudate indexes by conventional CT.

We have also examined the neuropsychologic correlates of functional capacity and CT indexes in our cohort of HD subjects. A comprehensive battery of neuropsychologic tests was administered in standardized fashion at baseline evaluation.[27] Tests that assessed planning and sequencing operations (Stroop test, Trails B test) and visuospatial functions (visual copy test, WAIS-R block design test, visual recall test) showed the greatest discriminative power in distinguishing between patients with stage I and II HD. The Stroop and Trails B tests were also the most powerful correlates of the CC/OT (r = 0.46, P < 0.001) and FH/CC (r = 0.37, P < 0.01) indexes of caudate atrophy. Since cognitive impairment is thought to contribute greatly to the early functional decline in HD,[28,29] these preliminary findings provide clues for defining valid and reliable cognitive markers of early neuronal degeneration in HD.

Using a functional scale for assessing HD that was modeled after the scale for instrumental activities of daily living,[30] Brandt et al.[31] found that functional incapacity was most closely linked to cognitive impairment in HD, and that estimates of the duration of illness defined anamnestically were relatively poor predictors of dementia in HD. These observations lend further support to the applicability of functional scales in the assessment of neurodegenerative movement disorders.

APPLICATION TO CLINICAL TRIALS

As experimental therapeutics of movement disorders have become more focused on the process of underlying neuronal degeneration and on interventions to prevent or forestall neuronal death, the need has increased for meaningful and objective endpoints in the assessment of therapeutic efficacy. We have employed the HDFC scale in the design of a long-term clinical trial aimed at slowing clinical decline.[21]

Various animal and clinical studies have implicated glutamate-mediated excitotoxic neurodegeneration in the pathogenesis of HD.[11] A major assumption underlying the glutamate hypothesis of HD is that the responsible gene codes for one or more defects that predispose the gene carrier to the action of an actual or potential glutamate-mediated neurotoxin. Neural tissue, particularly striatal cells, are further presumed to possess a regional vulnerability to the toxin, and some yet unknown genetic influence(s) or extragenic factor(s), such as maturational events unique to the nervous system, are thought to account for the gradually evolving neurodegenerative process, the eventual onset of illness, and the inevitable clinical decline of HD. Accordingly, we have hypothesized that pharmacologic attenuation of glutamatergic neurotransmission, specifically in the corticostriatal pathway, will result in the slowing of neuronal degeneration and clinical decline.

In 1982–1983 we began a double-blind clinical trial in early-stage (I and II) nonmedicated HD subjects who were randomized to long-term baclofen (60 mg/day) or placebo.[21] In animal studies and at clinically relevant dosage, baclofen (beta [4-chlorophenyl]GABA) selectively inhibits the corticostriatal release of glutamate and aspartate.[32,33] Furthermore, short-term administration of baclofen to rodents exerts a weak protective effect against the potent neurotoxin kainic acid, as evidenced by the attenuation of kainate-induced reduction in striatal marker enzymes[34] and substantial moderation of kainate-induced stereotypy,[35] hypersalivation, and clonic seizures.[36] On the basis of these preclinical data and our encouraging pilot studies in a small group of HD patients, we embarked on a large-scale clinical trial.

Our preliminary studies suggested that we could reliably detect a change of 2 or 3 functional units in 30 months of observation. Therefore, in order to calculate sample size and statistical power for our trial, we selected the change in TFC at 30 months as our major endpoint variable. For our placebo-treated group, we estimated a decline of 1.25 functional units per year and defined a major protective effect of baclofen as a decline of 0.75 units per year (i.e., 40% less rapid than placebo-treated subjects) and a minor protective effect as a decline of 1.0 units per year (i.e., 20% less rapid than placebo-treated subjects). Since we do not yet have a reliable estimate of the variance in the rate of decline, we have calculated power based on the conservative assumptions of standard deviations of 1.0, 1.5, and 2.0 functional units. According to the curves generated in Figure 20.2, and assuming a two-sample normal distribution with a significance level set at 5% (alpha = 0.05), a total sample size of 60 subjects (30 on placebo, 30 on baclofen) will provide 99% power for detecting a major effect and 75% power for detecting a minor effect, using a standard deviation of 1.0 (Figure 20.2A). As the variance in the rate of functional decline increases, there is increasing loss of power for detecting major and minor therapeutic effects (Figure 20.2 B and C). Therefore, clarification of the variance for the rate of decline is of great importance in formulating sample size and power estimates for clinical trials employing this outcome variable.

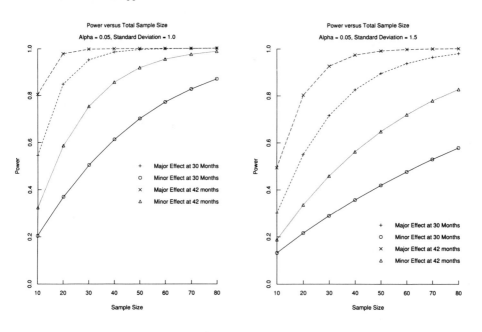

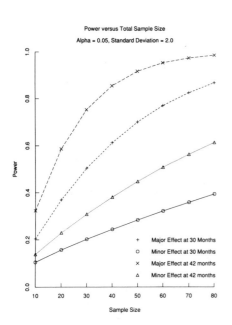

A

B

C

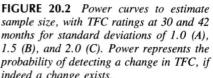

FIGURE 20.2 *Power curves to estimate sample size, with TFC ratings at 30 and 42 months for standard deviations of 1.0 (A), 1.5 (B), and 2.0 (C). Power represents the probability of detecting a change in TFC, if indeed a change exists.*

FUTURE APPLICATION OF THE HDFC SCALE

The HDFC scale will require reevaluation in light of the emerging techniques for reliable presymptomatic diagnosis of HD gene carriers through recombinant DNA linkage analysis.[13,14] Since presymptomatic individuals by definition have no disability, defining a neurobiologic correlate of early HD gene expression assumes greater significance. If we are eventually to expand therapeutic trials to presymptomatic individuals who carry the HD gene, then a sensitive neurobiologic correlate of HD gene expression is needed for assessment of the presymptomatic heterozygote. Radiographic techniques such as PET hold promise, but this method may not be as sensitive as was initially hoped.[5,6] As an interim measure, the emergence of clinical features might be used as an endpoint variable in clinical trials aimed at preventing or retarding the onset of symptoms and signs in presymptomatic individuals.

In the absence of well-defined biologic markers for neurodegenerative disorders, various scales have been formulated recently for application to Parkinson's disease,[37] dystonia,[38] and Alzheimer's disease,[39,40] as well as for assessing the normal process of aging.[41] We view the proliferation of clinical rating scales as a healthy sign of serious investigative interest. Testing of validity, reliability, and applicability to clinical trials is essential to the development of these scales. At present, it does not seem worthwhile to seek a unified functional scale for all neurodegenerative disorders, since diseases differ considerably in their clinical manifestations. Moreover, the development of reliable neurobiologic endpoints will in time replace the current reliance on functional scales. In the interim, the assessment of functional capacity fills a gap in the developing experimental therapeutics of neurodegenerative movement disorders.

CONCLUSION

The foregoing analysis underscores the importance of rigorously defining the validity, reliability, and variance of clinical endpoint variables for application to therapeutic trials. Because functional capacity is inevitably a subjective and operator-defined variable, the search for a more objective neurobiologic parameter is of high priority in clinical investigations of neurodegenerative movement disorders. A feasible method for reliably defining the extent of neuronal degeneration would substantially enhance the design of protective clinical trials. An alternative approach would be to define a time-dependent endpoint, such as the time required to reach a predetermined amount of neuronal degeneration. This criterion could then be employed in an analysis of time to neuron failure or survival.

REFERENCES

1. Shoulson I. Huntington's disease. In: Asbury AK, McKhann GM, McDonald W, eds. Diseases of the nervous system. Philadelphia: Ardmore Medical Books (WB Saunders), 1986: 1258–67.

2. Ferrante RJ, Kowall NW, Beal MF, et al. Selective sparing of a class of striatal neurons in Huntington's disease. Science 1985; 230:561-3.
3. Graveland GA, Williams RS, DiFiglia M. Evidence for degenerative and regenerative changes in neostriatal spiny neurons in Huntington's disease. Science 1985; 227:770-3.
4. Kuhl DE, Metter EJ, Riege WH, et al. Patterns of cerebral glucose utilization in Parkinson's disease and Huntington's disease. Ann Neurol 1984; 15:S119-25.
5. Hayden MR, Martin WRW, Stoessl AJ, et al. Positron emission tomography in the early diagnosis of Huntington's disease. Neurology 1986; 36:888-94.
6. Young AB, Penney JP, Starosta-Rubinstein S, et al. PET scan investigations of Huntington's disease: metabolic correlates of neurologic features and functional decline. Ann Neurol 1986; 296-303.
7. Sax DB, Menzer L. Computerized tomography in Huntington's disease. Neurology 1977; 27:388.
8. Terrence CF, DeLaney JF, Alberts MC. Computerized tomography for Hungtington's disease. Neuroradiology 1977; 13:173-5.
9. Barr AN, Heinze WJ, Dobben GD, et al. Bicaudate index in computed tomography of Huntington disease and cerebral atrophy. Neurology 1978; 28:1196-1200.
10. Neophytides AN, DiChiro G, Barron SA, et al. Computed axial tomography in Huntington's disease and persons at risk for Huntington's disease. Adv Neurol 1979; 23:185-91.
11. Schwarcz R, Shoulson I. Excitotoxins and Huntington's disease. In: Coyle JJ, ed. Experimental models of dementing disorders: a synaptic neurochemical approach. New York: Alan R. Liss, 1987:39-68.
12. Gusella JF, Wexler NS, Conneally PM, et al. A polymorphic DNA marker genetically linked to Huntington's disease. Nature 1983; 306:234-8.
13. Gusella JF, Tanzi RE, Anderson MA, et al. DNA markers for nervous system diseases. Science 1984; 225:1320-6.
14. Wexler NS, Conneally PM, Houseman D, et al. A DNA polymorphism for Huntington's disease marks the future. Arch Neurol 1985; 42:20-4.
15. Shoulson I, Commission for the Control of Huntington's Disease and Its Consequences. Clinical care of the patient and family with Huntington's disease. Washington, DC: National Institutes of Health 1977; 2:421-51.
16. Shoulson I, Fahn S. Huntington's disease: clinical care and evaluation. Neurology 1979; 29:1-3.
17. Shoulson I. Huntington's disease: functional capacities in patients treated with neuroleptic and antidepressant drugs. Neurology 1981; 31:1333-5.
18. Shoulson I. Care of patients and families with Huntington's disease. In: Marsden CD, Fahn S, eds. Neurology. Vol. II: Movement disorders (Butterworths International Medical Review). London: Butterworths, 1982:277-90.
19. Conneally PM. Huntington's disease: genetics and epidemiology. Am J Hum Genet 1984; 36:505-26.
20. Young AB, Shoulson I, Penney JB, et al. Huntington's disease in Venezuela: neurological features and functional decline. Neurology 1986; 36:244-9.
21. Shoulson I. Huntington's disease: anti-neurotoxic therapeutic strategies. In: Fuxe K, Roberts P, Schwarcz R, eds. Excitotoxins. London: Macmillan, 1983:343-53.
22. Shoulson I, Odoroff C, Kurlan R, et al. Huntington's disease: validity of clinical ratings and CT correlates of caudate atrophy. J Neurol 1985; 232 (Suppl.):134.
23. Stober T, Wussow W, Schimrigk K. Bicaudate diameter—the most specific and simple CT parameter in the diagnosis of HD. Neuroradiology 1984; 26:25-8.
24. Shoulson I, Bamford K, Caine E, et al. Inter-observer reliability of functional capacity ratings for Huntington's disease. Neurology 1985; 35 (Suppl. 1):176.
25. Shoulson I, Plassche W, Odoroff C. Hungtington's disease: caudate atrophy parallels functional impairment. Neurology 1982; 32:A143.
26. Shoulson I, Goldblatt D, Plumb S, et al. Motor correlates of early Huntington's disease. Neurology 1986; 36 (Suppl. 1):341.

27. Bamford K, Caine E, Kido D, et al. Neuropsychological impairment in early Huntington's disease: functional and CT correlates. Neurology 1986; 36:(Suppl. 1):102–3.

28. Fisher J, Kennedy J, Caine E, et al. Dementia in Huntington disease: a cross-sectional analysis. In: Mayeux R, Rosen W, eds. The dementias. New York: Raven, 1983:229–38.

29. Mayeux R, Stern Y, Hermann A, et al. The cause of disability in Huntington's disease. Ann Neurol 1984; 16:137.

30. Lawton MP. The functional assessment of elderly people. J Am Geriatr Soc 1971; 19: 465–75.

31. Brandt J, Strauss ME, Larus J, et al. Clinical correlates of dementia and disability in Huntington's disease. J Clin Neuropsychol 1984; 6:401–12.

32. Potashner SJ. Baclofen. Effects on amino acid release and metabolism in slices of guinea pig cerebral cortex. J Neurochem 1979; 32:103–9.

33. Cordingley GE, Weight FF. Non-cholinergic synaptic excitation in neostriatum: pharmacological evidence for mediation by a glutamate-like transmitter. Br J Pharmacol 1986; 88: 847–56.

34. McGeer EG, Jakubovic A, Singh EA. Ethanol, baclofen and kainic acid neurotoxicity. Exp Neurol 1980; 69:359–64.

35. Borison RL, Diamond BI. Kainic acid animal model predicts therapeutic agents in Huntington's chorea. Ann Neurol 1979; 6:149.

36. Bernard PS, Sobiski R, Dawson K. Comparative neurological and anticonvulsant effects of baclofen, muscimol, diazepam and gamma-butyrolactate (abstract). Brain Res Bull 1979; 4:695.

37. Montgomery GK, Reynolds NC, Warren RM. Qualitative assessment of Parkinson's disease: study of reliability and data reduction with an abbreviated Columbia scale. Clin Neuropharmacol 1985; 8:83–92.

38. Burke RE, Fahn S, Marsden CD, et al. Validity and reliability of a rating scale for primary torsion dystonia. Neurology 1985; 35:73–7.

39. Reisberg B, Ferris SH, Anand R, et al. Functional staging of dementia of the Alzheimer's type. Ann NY Acad Sci 1984; 435:491–3.

40. Rosen WG, Mohs RC, David KL. A new rating scale for Alzheimer's disease. Am J Psychiatry 1984; 141:1356–64.

41. Pfeffer RI, Kurosaki TT, Harrah CH, et al. Measurement of functional activities in older adults in the community. J Gerontol 1982; 37:323–9.

Chapter 21

Assessment of Parkinson's Disease

Anthony E.T. Lang and Stanley Fahn

It is possible that more attempts have been made to quantify the deficits of Parkinson's disease (PD), than those of any other neurologic disorder. Long before modern pharmacologic interventions became available, several methods of assessing the disability, symptoms, and signs of the disease had been developed. However, it was the introduction of levodopa (L-dopa) and the impact of this and subsequent drug therapies on the clinical features of the disease that created an urgent need for the development of accurate techniques for assessment of the diverse motor disturbances seen in parkinsonism.

The available methods of assessing PD can be subdivided as follows: (1) objective quantification techniques, which may be (a) complex physiologic assessments of different motor disturbances or (b) simple, timed tests of motor function that do not require complicated equipment; and (2) subjective assessments, including (a) patient functional disability scales and (b) subjective physician ratings of the severity of the signs of the disease. These methods have recently been reviewed in detail,[1-3] and it is not our intention to provide a comprehensive survey of this literature. Instead, we will briefly review the various techniques used in assessing PD and present a new rating scale—the Unified Parkinson's Disease Rating Scale (UPDRS)—that has been developed in an attempt to provide a standard format of assessment acceptable to a large number of investigators. Before proceeding, it is appropriate to emphasize certain aspects of the disease that interfere with the accuracy of any attempt to document its clinical deficits.

PROBLEMS ARISING IN THE ASSESSMENT OF PARKINSON'S DISEASE

As mentioned, the development of an effective means of treating PD precipitated the need to formulate scales that could accurately document clinical changes. In outlining some of the problems arising in our attempts to assess the features of the disease, it is important to consider how they will hamper the design and conduct of trials of newer pharmacologic agents. One must be extremely skeptical of reports that provide a series of numbers (independent of the method of assessment used) purporting to show "significant" reductions in the severity of the signs of the disease while failing to account for various factors that will now be discussed.

The natural variability in the features of parkinsonism were well known long before the introduction of levodopa. Stress and emotional upset increase the severity of the tremor and often make it impossible for the patient to relax completely to permit a consistent assessment of the severity of rigidity. The opposite phenomenon, "kinesia paradoxica," a short-lived improvement precipitated by sudden startle or fright, was also well recognized. The fluctuant nature of the signs and symptoms of the disease has been magnified greatly by "successful" L-dopa therapy. It is important to note that most of the clinical rating scales for PD were developed early in the levodopa era, before many of the late-stage problems—including fluctuations and dyskinesias—became evident.

Even when the physician is fully aware of the disease- and drug-related fluctuations and tries to overcome various contributing factors, it still may not be possible to obtain an accurate rating of clinical signs. In an inpatient environment, when plasma levels of L-dopa are maintained at a constant level with intravenous infusions, patients can "switch off" during even slight emotional upset.[4,5] Obviously, in outpatient drug trials, one cannot control for stress experienced during the trip to the clinic (which often includes driving through a busy downtown area), even with the most calming of ambulatory care settings. On the other hand, many patients perform better in the doctor's office than at home.

A medium- or short-duration response to L-dopa, followed by the so-called end-of-dose deterioration, or the wearing-off phenomenon, is a well-recognized pattern of response in most patients treated with L-dopa for two or more years. For ratings of the signs of parkinsonism to be meaningful in these patients, investigators often claim that scoring was done at the same time each day. However, in reality, it is often impossible to assess patients at the same fixed interval after ingestion of the medication (especially if a number of patients are being studied as a cohort in an experimental clinical trial). For one reason or another, either the appointment or medication timing will vary.

Even when the greatest care is taken to ensure consistency in stress level and drug timing, the efficacy of medication may still vary unpredictably. Later in the course of the disease, many patients find that the delay between taking medication and the onset of clinical response increases, and some doses may be followed by little or no clinical benefit.[6] In part, these problems may relate to the effects of food intake, which can interfere with local gastrointestinal drug absorption or cause competition for transport across the blood-brain barrier between L-dopa and ingested large neutral amino acids. This food-related variability is unpredictable, and differs from patient to patient,[5] and it is almost impossible to control for in an outpatient assessment of drug efficacy.

Multiple other factors also play a role in hampering the assessment of parkinsonism. For example, unbeknownst to the physician, patients with pronounced fluctuations may take an extra dose of L-dopa just before leaving home in an attempt to prevent severe, immobilizing "off" periods from occurring at the clinic. Subsequent assessments showing consistent improvement in mobility and increased dyskinesias may be attributed to other pharmacologic alterations, if the true drug history is not forthcoming.

It follows from the foregoing that a set of clinical rating scale numbers indicating reductions in such symptoms as tremor, rigidity, and bradykinesia may be entirely meaningless in pharmacologic studies of patients who have developed obvious fluctuations in their response to L-dopa. Although investigators must not be discouraged from attempting to rate the severity of the disorder, they must be mindful of the tremendous potential for variability in parkinsonian patients, particularly those who have been on dopaminergic therapy for some time. Knowledge of this variability emphasizes the need to incorporate some useful method of scoring the severity of fluctuations and assessing the disability experienced in both the "on" and "off" phases of drug response. This component is lacking in most commonly used subjective rating scales and is obviously impossible to obtain in any single objective quantitative assessment that is not carried out over a prolonged period.

Additional problems arise in assessing parkinsonism, even in patients whose symptoms show little variability. For example, an elderly individual with PD may demonstrate some disturbances of function due to the disease process and others that simply relate to nonpathologic aging. The latter, which can even include postural instability on tests for retropulsion,[7] do not respond to L-dopa[8] but may influence the scoring of parkinsonian severity and disability. It is also important to recognize that the uniformity of results provided by any method of assessment (either subjective or objective) will be influenced greatly by such factors as the thoroughness of instructions and degree of encouragement provided during testing. Even on a simple writing task, disturbances can vary considerably, depending on the instructions given to the patient.[3] Finally, it may be impossible to distinguish completely between motor disability and the altered psychological motivation so common in PD.

With these many factors in mind, we will now review briefly the techniques used to assess the signs and symptoms of the disease and introduce the UPDRS, which is provided in Appendix 21–A.

OBJECTIVE QUANTIFIED ASSESSMENT

Many methods have been used in attempts to quantify objectively the different motor deficits of PD. Most of these have involved the use of complicated or expensive physiologic equipment. As Marsden and Schacter[2] and Calne and coworkers[1,3,9] have recently reviewed these methodologies, only a brief discussion will be presented here, with emphasis on the techniques in common use today. Table 21.1 summarizes the various methods and includes references to a representative bibliography. Table 21.2 outlines some of the advantages and disadvantages common to most of the neurophysiologic assessment techniques listed.

Attempts to quantify the signs of parkinsonism date back to the early part of this century.[60,61] Since then, a number of methods have been applied to the quantification

Table 21.1 Objective Neurophysiologic Methods of Assessing Parkinson's Disease

Feature Assessed	Method[a]
Tremor	Optical recording[10]
	Electromyographic activity[11]
	Electromyography and computer analysis[12]
	Magnetic coils[13]
	Accelerometry (single-plane) (many examples)[14–16]
	Accelerometry plus telemetry (single-plane)[17]
	Computerized three-dimensional accelerometry[13,18,19]
Rigidity	Torque by which patient passively resists a constant velocity extension of the elbow[14]
	Torque measured with direct current motor for sinusoidal driving of flexion/extension of forearm[20]
	Servo-controlled electronic device flexing/extending elbow at constant angular velocities[21]
	Measurement of hysteresis loop of torque vs. displacement of forearm (representing workload):[21]
	"Activated Rigidity" measured in same fashion[22]
	Hysteresis loop for finger[23,24] and wrist[25] movement
	Long latency reflexes:
	Wrist[26,27]
	Forearm (biceps/triceps)[1,28]
	Thumb (long flexor)[29,30]
Bradykinesia[b]	Switch release to visual or auditory cue[16,31,32]
Reaction time (simple or complex choices)	Tracking task on oscilloscope[32–36]
	Pronation/supination to visual or kinesthetic cues[37]
Movement time	Touch or release switches (pads) to visual/auditory cues[16,31,32,40]
	Pronation/supination[38]
	Oscilloscope tracking[36,39]
Complex movements	Tapping tests[32,34,40]
	Pegboards[16,34,41]
	Functional tests (e.g., picking up small objects, putting on socks, other manipulative skills)[32,33,42]
	Fatigue[32,33]
	Handwriting—planimetric assessment[44]
Walking	Assessing number of steps and time to cover set distance[11,45]
	Sensor pads: assess number of steps, step length, and time[3,9]
	Optoelectronic camera system[46,47]
Miscellaneous	Blink rate[48]
	Blink reflex[49]
	Extraocular movements[50,51,52,53]
	Visual evoked potentials[54,55,56]
	Shortening reaction[57,58]

[a] Many investigators have reported the use of different objective methods of assessing PD. The references cited in this table provide examples of each technique and are not meant to represent a complete bibliography of the field.

[b] Several of these tests have been incorporated into the study of cognitive changes in PD, as well as the investigation of motor performance emphasized here.

Table 21.2 Objective Complex Quantitative Testing for Parkinsonism

Advantages	Disadvantages
Avoids inter-rater inconsistencies	Expensive and complicated
Avoids possibility of other signs influencing the scoring of feature in question	Time-consuming
	Not generally available
Provides a permanent record	Samples only a limited aspect of motor dysfunction
Provides information regarding the pathophysiologic basis of disordered motor control	Abnormal results in one motor behavior are not predictive of other motor deficits[34,59]
Not subject to the inaccuracies of other methods	May not be as accurate as subjective scoring for assessing parkinsonian disability[9]

of tremor, rigidity, several aspects of akinesia and bradykinesia, gait disturbances, and other less prominent components of the disease (Table 21.1). Although many of these techniques were designed to investigate the pathophysiology of one or more aspects of disordered movement, our focus is on their usefulness in assessing changes in the features of the disease over time in individual patients (e.g., in a trial of a new pharmacologic agent).

Accelerometer transduction with computer analysis is currently the most common method used for the quantification of tremor. Computerized triaxial accelerometry has provided a method of recording tremor in three dimensions, in contrast to the single-plane analysis originally available. Using triaxial accelerometry, Larsen and colleagues[3] have developed a program that analyzes power spectra in all three planes, gives a dominant peak frequency, and provides an index of the intensity of tremor as total distance (meters) traveled. Jankovic and Frost[19] used triaxial accelerometry to study movement vectors during the performance of voluntary arm abduction and adduction, as well as in the arm at rest. Under these dynamic conditions, they derived factors reflecting smoothness of movement and waveform of acceleration. Both factors were abnormal in almost all patients with PD, whereas only smoothness of movement was consistently altered in patients with essential tremor. They also found that intra-patient results remained consistent with repeated evaluation. For longer-term assessment, telemetry has been used in combination with single-plane accelerometry.[17] This technique has not yet been adapted to computerized triaxial recording.

Whereas many methods have been used to assess tremor and akinesia, attempts to quantify rigidity have been few. The leading investigator in this field has been Webster, who designed a servo-controlled electronic device (later computerized) that moves the elbow through flexion and extension at various constant angular velocities.[21,62,63] He found that the area of the hysteresis loop of torque required to displace the forearm versus the degrees of displacement (an area representing workload), averaged over a number of cycles of flexion and extension, was a much more sensitive measure of rigidity than torque alone. Mortimer and Webster[28] later showed that rigidity measured in this way decreased in response to L-dopa therapy. However, the increase in rigidity brought about by voluntary activation of the contralateral limb (activated rigidity) did not change. Recently, Teravainen and his colleagues in Calne's group applied a similar technique to the wrist,[25] finding that rigidity measured in this fashion correlates well with a subjective physician assessment. The technique is sensitive enough to detect an increase in rigidity with reinforcement and a decrease in response to L-dopa therapy. This group has found the optimal speed of rotation to be 140 to 190 degrees per second, with the range of movement ± 25 to 30 degrees. The type of movement (ramp waves versus sine waves) does not seem to make a difference, although the authors have primarily used sine waves in their studies (Tsui J, personal communication, 1986).

In recent years, long-latency electromyographic responses to muscle stretch have been studied extensively in PD. The amplitude of the second component of the long-latency responses is increased in parkinsonian patients with rigidity, and successful L-dopa therapy diminishes this response proportionally to the clinical benefit obtained.[64] However, this is probably not a useful method of evaluating patients on a routine or repetitive basis. In addition to the disadvantages listed in Table 21.2, there seems to be marked intra- and inter-patient variability, an inexact and unreliable correlation with the clinical features, and some overlap between parkinsonian patients and normal subjects (depending on the technique used).

Unlike tremor and rigidity, which are single, well-defined variables (relatively speaking), the motor disturbances described by the terms *akinesia, hypokinesia,* and *bradykinesia* are more complex and multifactorial. The **initiation** of movement may be slowed and occasionally arrested completely (e.g., "start hesitation"). The **speed** of repetitive or alternating movement is usually slower than normal. Ongoing movement **fatigues,** becomes **less precise,** and may be interrupted by frequent **arrests.** The performance of bimanual tasks may be particularly difficult. It is clearly impossible to assess all these disorders with use of a single technique or paradigm. Moreover, the disturbances observed during one motor task or in the study of one aspect of motor behavior are not predictive of the performance on other tasks. Therefore, any single measurement of a limited number of the aforementioned features probably will not reflect the overall disability caused by parkinsonian bradykinesia. To obtain a truly objective assessment of this complex disturbance, it is necessary to study several different aspects of motor behavior.

Reaction time (RT) and movement time (MT) have been the two most commonly assessed components of akinesia. Overall, RT is prolonged by about 30% in parkinsonian patients, as compared with controls, but individual patients show marked variation among themselves and considerable overlap with normals. Evarts and colleagues[37] found even less abnormality in complex or choice reaction times than on simple RT testing. Although RT tends to decrease with successful therapy, it does not seem to correlate well with the degree of clinical disability.

MT is more consistently abnormal in parkinsonism, particularly for large-amplitude movements involving proximal muscles. Studying this type of movement, Teravainen and Calne[1] found a correlation between MT and a subjective clinical score, as well as a larger improvement in MT than in RT with successful pharmacotherapy. These authors concluded that proximal MT provides one of the best indexes of parkinsonian bradykinesia. Various attempts have been made to assess rapid alternating movements (RAM) of the arms and fingers. Although RAM speed has been shown to increase with treatment, there is no consistent association between the degree of RAM disturbance and MT (as assessed in single movements)[1,36] and the correlation between changes in an observer's subjective assessment and RAM speed is poor.

Pressure-sensitive mats have been used to quantify disturbances in gait. They allow assessment of various factors, including the time taken to walk a specified distance, the number of steps taken, and the length and duration of each step. A map of an individual gait pattern can be reconstructed from this information, showing such features as start hesitation and freezing during the course of walking.[3] Despite its detail, this method of assessing gait may be no better than subjective rating, which integrates such additional information as arm swing, posture, and other upper body signs not evaluated with the pressure-sensitive mat.[9]

Formal quantification has been applied to a number of other disturbances seen in PD, (e.g., disturbances of oculomotor function, blink rate, blink reflexes, Westphal's phenomenon). Although clinical improvement (as documented by subjective testing) may be associated with changes in some of these parameters, there is little evidence that any of them provide an accurate measurement of parkinsonian disability.

Recently, Ward and colleagues[9] compared the sensitivity of objective measures of akinesia (RT, MT, and formal gait assessment) with a clinical subjective rating of the signs of parkinsonism, using a modified Columbia rating system (the scoring system from which the UPDRS was developed). They found MT alone to be the best objective assessment of akinesia and predictor of clinical disability. Overall, however, clinical observations were more sensitive than objective measurements in the detection of the motor disorder.

It must be concluded that objective quantification techniques are no substitute for good subjective clinical assessment of the disease. However, they provide complementary clinical information and important insights into the pathophysiology of disturbances in motor function. Data may be easily stored, retrieved, and analyzed. Finally, these methods of assessment avoid the inter-rater reliability problems inherent in subjective rating scales. Newer objective techniques are being actively developed. For example, a number of centers are beginning to use an opto-electric camera, or cell-spot system, to study parkinsonian motor dysfunction. This method permits the detailed assessment of simple movements and can also be applied to complex postural movements, as recently reported by Ingvarsson and colleagues from Sweden.[47] These investigators assessed the task of lifting a box from the floor, taking a few steps, and placing it on a high shelf. Three sequential phases were defined: postural, locomotor, and manual. They found variable alterations in each of these phases in late-stage parkinsonian patients with subsequent improvement occurring in response to a dose of L-dopa. It is probable that future developments in this field, such as the cell-spot technique, will provide better correlations with the clinical disturbances and further our understanding of the basic nature of the motor disorder of PD.

Among the simpler methods of quantification, timing of various activities may be used to assess motor disturbance in PD. These techniques commonly accompany the subjective rating scales to be discussed below. Little or no expensive or complicated equipment is required. For example, rapid repetitive and alternating movements may simply be counted over a fixed period of time. However, unless some method is used to document the completeness and accuracy of the movement, a simple record of the number of finger taps, pronation-supination movements, or foot taps performed in a specified number of seconds can be extremely misleading. Bradykinesia results in prominent fatigue, reduction in amplitude, and incompleteness of movement, all of which increase with persistent activity. Although these disturbances usually cause slowing of movement, the frequency of repetitive movements occasionally increases, as in the propulsive and hurrying (but shortened) stride of a festinating gait. Finally, it is possible to confuse voluntary, rapid, repetitive movement with underlying tremor, which, if pronounced, "takes over" the action (finger- or foot-tapping). In the UPDRS the assessments of finger-tapping, opening and closing the fist, pronation and supination of the forearm, and foot-tapping that rate the overall performance, taking into account the speed, amplitude, fatigability and completeness of movement, as well as interruptions in ongoing movement rather than simply counting the number of completed movements.

An assessment of functional activities (e.g., putting on a pair of socks, picking up small objects) has often been included in parkinsonian rating scales. However, because a single patient's performance is rarely uniform over a variety of tasks, several tests have to be carried out, each taking an average of two or more trials. An extreme example of this approach is the Simulated Activities of Daily Living Examination (SADLE) of Potvin and Tourtellotte,[2] which scores 19 different activities, including putting on a shirt, squeezing toothpaste from a tube, and dialing a telephone. This assessment is very time-consuming and is almost impossible to control for small-amplitude or incomplete but functional movements or for "tricks" that the patient has adopted to lessen the extent of disability. Another simple but more precise method of assessing the speed and accuracy of movement is the use of a pegboard test. The Purdue pegboard is perhaps the best known, and therefore is generally administered by a standardized method. Our group (AEL) has recently found that patients' performance on the Purdue pegboard (summing the number of pegs individually placed by each hand, and by both hands simultaneously, in 30-second intervals) correlates extremely well with their scores on a subjective rating scale (a modified Columbia scale) and an assessment of gait (Webster's step-seconds score).[65]

Gait may be assessed by recording the time and number of steps required to walk a set distance without the use of the automated pressure-sensitive mats discussed earlier. A simple and effective method was devised by Webster,[45] who measured the time required to rise from a chair, walk 4.5 m, turn around, and return to the chair. The time, in seconds, is multiplied by the number of steps taken with the right foot, providing a "step-seconds" product. Webster found that normal individuals score 50 to 100 step-seconds. Those with early PD often score over 100, whereas those with moderately advanced disease score between 200 and 400, and those with far-advanced disease score above 400. We (AEL) have found a significant correlation between this score and both the Purdue pegboard and the subjective rating of the severity of parkinsonism.[65] Because of its ease of application and good correlation with overall disability, our present assessment of parkinsonian patients combines simple quantification methods (i.e., the Purdue pegboard and the step-seconds assessment of gait) with the subjective assessment provided by the UPDRS.

SUBJECTIVE ASSESSMENT

The subjective assessment of PD has usually combined a scale that rates the disability experienced in the performance of various activities of daily living (ADL) with a physician's scoring of the signs of the disease observed on examination. There are almost as many subjective rating scales for PD as there are groups of investigators performing clinical trials in this disorder. Table 21.3 compares some of the more commonly used clinical rating scales. Some general comments regarding the problems and pitfalls specific to subjective rating are in order before we discuss the UPDRS and compare it to other scales.

Misunderstandings of the terminology used in the scoring of historical features are not infrequent. Despite careful descriptions and definitions of terms by the physician, patients may still confuse tremor with drug-induced involuntary movements, or freezing with "off" periods. Despite the very explicit criteria used in the grading of disability, it is common to obtain one score from the patient and another, more severe (and usually more accurate) score from the patient's spouse (or another friend or family member), who provides additional historical information. As mentioned earlier, most of the older ADL scales fail to take into account fluctuations in the level of disability. Even those (such as the UPDRS) that assess disability in the "on" and "off" states are hampered in assessing a function that the patient typically delays until the medication takes effect.

Many of the subjective rating scales for PD score the severity of various clinical features on a scale of 0 to 2, 3, or 4, using such terms as "minimal," "mild," "moderate," and "severe" with little or no further definition. In contrast to systems that utilize explicit descriptions of each scoring level, these scales encourage poor inter-rater reliability. In addition, scoring in one category of signs is more likely to influence the severity of other scores if there are no explicit behavior criteria for easy and regular reference. Some scales have used arbitrary weighting factors to indicate that certain features of the disease (e.g., gait) contribute more to the disability than others (e.g., facial expression). This type of weighting is often used with a nonexplicit scoring system—a combination that can enhance rather than reduce unreliability and the potential for poor inter-rater reliability. An alternative to the weighting approach has been to increase the emphasis on the more important clinical features by assessing certain aspects of the disease in several different ways (e.g., hand bradykinesia) and to lessen or remove the emphasis placed on others, as in the UPDRS.

Like many other subjective rating scales, the UPDRS includes the Hoehn and Yahr staging system[76] which was developed before the introduction of effective therapy for PD. A marked response to medication and variability in motor status is not represented by the staging unless a score is provided for both the "on" and "off" periods. A flaw in many recently published drug studies is the documentation of a single Hoehn and Yahr stage in patients with marked fluctuations (some from stage 2 to stage 5) without any mention of when in the course of fluctuations this value was obtained. Even when "on" and "off" stages are recorded, it is important to recognize that one cannot assume that the maximum Hoehn and Yahr stage reached (or any rating of "off"-

Table 21.3 Clinical Rating Scales

| | Subjective Rating | | | | Additional Objective Assessment | Functional Disability | | On-Off Assessment[b] | Side Effects Assessment[b] |
	Explicit Criteria	Undefined (Mild to Severe)	Weighted Scores	Equal Scores[a]		Explicit	Undefined		
Webster[45]	+	–	–	+	+	–	–	–	–
Columbia scale[66,67]	+	–	–	+	+	–	–	–	–
NYU scale[68]	–	+	+	–	+	–	+	–	–
UCLA scale[69]	–	+	+	–	–	–	+	–	–
NWU disability scale[70]	–	–	–	–	–	+	–	–	–
King's college scale[71,72]	–	+	–	–	–	–	+	–	–
UBC scale[c,73]	–	–	–	–	–	+	–	+	+
UPDRS	+	–	–	+	+	+	–	+	+

[a] Although some scores (e.g., facial characteristics, gait) are equal, there are usually more scores for disabling features of the disease in most of these systems.
[b] These assessments are part of the scale used. Workers using scales not assessing this aspect have developed other methods of actively assessing these features (e.g., on-off).[74,75]
[c] The UBC scale is used in combination with other subjective rating scales.

period disability, for that matter) is an indication of the maximum severity of disease. Most patients with fluctuations maintain a long-duration response in addition to their short- or medium-duration responses to L-dopa.[77] This is only evident after the drug has been withdrawn for a few days, at which time patients often experience a delayed increase in parkinsonism beyond that seen in their usual "off" periods.

THE UNIFIED PARKINSON DISEASE RATING SCALE

Diamond and Markham[78] recently compared the percent change relative to baseline score during a year's treatment with pergolide, using four different PD rating scales: the Hoehn and Yahr stage of disease scale, the Northwestern University disability scale, the New York University Parkinson Disease scale, and the UCLA disability scale. The changes recorded by these scales were frequently quite disparate. At times, some even showed improvement while others showed slight worsening. It was clear from this study that different scales measure different aspects of the disease. The authors concluded: "What is needed is a standard method of ranking parkinsonian disability that is sensitive to changes in clinical states in a logically consistent manner."

There are several advantages to developing a common method of rating PD, not the least of which is the facilitation of communication, both between investigators and in the final publication of results. Although a single PD rating scale may never satisfy all investigators, any attempt to formulate a universal scale must utilize very explicit behavioral criteria and remove as much ambiguity in scoring as possible. This would probably improve inter-rater reliability over that of currently available rating scales.

In October 1984, one of us (SF) organized a meeting of a group of experienced investigators in an attempt to formulate a unified clinical rating scale for PD. Since then, as clinicians have gained experience with the resulting UPDRS, a number of changes have been made; the most recent version is presented in Appendix 21-A, as is a list of the investigators involved.

The UPDRS includes six sections. The first deals briefly with psychological features associated with the disease or its treatment. The second offers a 13-point functional activities scale, to be completed for both the "on" and "off" states in patients experiencing motor fluctuations. To the usual ADL assessment of most similar scales, the UPDRS adds scores for freezing, disability caused by tremor (often providing a more accurate assessment of this feature than the severity seen on examination), and the presence of severity of sensory symptoms.

The third section deals with the rating of parkinsonian signs by examination. (It is important that the time since the last dose of medication be recorded with this score.) The basis for this section is the Columbia scale originally used by Yahr, Duvoisin, and their colleagues.[66,67] This scale and modifications of it[79-81] have probably been used more often than any other method for scoring parkinsonism. Montgomery[82] recently reviewed the history of the Columbia Scale; he and his colleagues have shown that several of its components have good inter-rater reliability.[83] These components have been maintained, and some have even been improved slightly, in the UPDRS. The UPDRS thus has an advantage over many other available scoring systems, most of which have not undergone such rigorous, formal observer-agreement testing. The UPDRS weights bradykinesia not by an arbitrary multiplication factor but through multiple assessments (i.e., three scores for hand bradykinesia, one for foot, one for global bradykinesia, one for facies, and one for gait). Certain nondisabling features have been de-emphasized; for instance, the score for seborrhea has been removed from the original Columbia scale. Other features not found in the original scale have been added; for example, a rating of action tremor.

Following the UPDRS clinical rating is a fourth section addressing complications of therapy, particularly dyskinesias and fluctuations. The UPDRS makes no attempt to rate the severity of dyskinesias as seen in the clinic. These often vary markedly from moment to moment. Even when scoring the same time period with videotape assessments, Montgomery et al.[83] found inter-rater reliability to be poor when simple criteria similar to those of the Columbia scale for tremor were used. Two observers may be less likely to bring a common subjective scale (i.e., based on personal experience) to the assessment of dyskinesias than to the assessment of tremor or rigidity.[83] In rating dyskinesias and fluctuations, the UPDRS only elicits general percentages; it does not attempt to assess the specific severity of dyskinesias in selected body parts or the number and duration of "off" periods. Although it would be ideal to have an accurate estimate of this latter information, it is surprisingly difficult to obtain. One approach, as seen in the University of British Columbia (UBC) scale,[73] involves direct questioning by the examiner regarding the distribution, duration, and severity of dyskinesias and the duration and frequency of "off" periods as they occur over a fixed period prior to assessment. However, when several members of one of our groups (AEL) consecutively assessed the same patients, using this approach, we found that the responses given by patients to the same questions often varied from one examiner to the next. Several attempts have been made to develop an hourly scoring system to be used by patients and their families at home.[68,74,75,84] The great variability of success that different patients have with this form of assessment argues against its inclusion in a unified scoring system.

The "complications" section of the UPDRS ends with questions on the presence or absence of sleep disturbances, gastrointestinal upset, and orthostatic lightheadedness, and with the recording of blood pressure and pulse in the sitting (or lying) and standing positions. Sections five and six include, respectively, a minor modification of the Hoehn and Yahr staging system and the Schwab and England ADL scale.

The Hoehn and Yahr system, well known to all PD investigators, provides a simple index of the distribution, severity, and progression of disease. Montgomery and colleagues[83] found excellent inter-observer agreement for the Hoehn and Yahr scale, with a strong correlation between the stages and the Columbia scores for bradykinesia, gait, and posture, but with no relation to resting or postural tremor scores.

The Schwab and England scale[85] provides an indication of the patient's capacity for ADLs as a percentage of normal. The patient and spouse are instructed to read the scale, from the top down, to just beyond the score that describes the patient's condition during the week prior to assessment. They then indicate the score, to the closest 5%, that best fits the level of disability. Patients with clinical fluctuations are asked to provide percentages for their best and worst states. There is good correlation between the rating determined by the physician upon reviewing the history and percentages provided by the patient and his or her family (unpublished observations of the Parkinson Study Group).

THE FUTURE

The investigators involved in the development of the UPDRS have reviewed videotaped patient assessments in order to assess the inter-rater reliability of the scale. Virtually all items in the UPDRS showed significant concordance, with most having a value of $P < 0.001$. Nonsignificant items in the ADL section were sensory symptoms and falling, and predictable "offs" and sleep disturbances in the section on complications of therapy.[88] There have been a number of changes in the scale since its inception, and it is likely that further modifications will be made in the future. One problem with a "unified" scale is that changes are difficult, as the agreement of many investigators is required.

Most investigators involved in PD research are experienced in the use of videotape for documenting movement disorders. There are clear advantages and disadvantages to the routine use of this technique.[2] The advantages are considerable: videotape provides a permanent record; reduces threats to reliability from boredom, distraction, and fatigue; allows blind assessments by several observers (sequences can be randomized); and is a convenient means of training new observers and validating rating scales.[2,83] Whether these advantages justify the inconvenience and expense involved remains to be seen.

Investigators will continue to use some type of subjective rating scale in combination with more objective measurements. With the increasing availability of personal computers and the decreasing expense of the necessary hardware, attempts will doubtless be made to develop unified objective assessment systems, particularly if more accurate techniques for measuring motor disturbances are developed.

More important than furthering our ability to score motor disability will be the development of reliable methods of assessing the severity of nigral cell loss. We are entering a new era in PD research , in which the mechanisms and prevention of nigral cell death will be emphasized over the mere treatment of its sequelae. If preventive or protective therapy is to become a reality, we require methods of assessing the function of nigral dopaminergic neurons, possibly even before dopamine loss reaches the critical 80% at which symptoms become manifest. Clearly, positron emission tomography with 6[18F]fluoro-L-dopa has the greatest potential in this area,[86,87] but future research may provide newer, more readily available techniques for obtaining the same information.

REFERENCES

1. Teravainen H, Calne D. Quantitative assessment of parkinsonian deficits. In: Rinne UK, Klinger M, Stamm G, eds. Parkinson's disease—current progress, problems and management. Amsterdam: Elsevier North-Holland, 1980:145-64.

2. Marsden CD, Schacter M. Assessment of extrapyramidal disorders. Br J Clin Pharmacol 1981; 11:129-51.
3. Larsen TA, LeWitt PA, Calne DB. Theoretical and practical issues in assessment of deficits and therapy in parkinsonism. In: Calne DB, Horoski R, McDonald RJ, et al., eds. Lisuride and other dopamine agonists. New York: Raven, 1983:363-73.
4. Shoulson I, Glaubiger GA, Chase TN. On-off response. Clinical and biochemical correlations during oral and intravenous levodopa administration in parkinsonian patients. Neurology 1980; 25:1144-8.
5. Nutt JG, Woodward WR, Hammerstad JP, et al. The "on-off" phenomenon in Parkinson's disease. Relation to levodopa absorption and transport. N Engl J Med 1984; 310:483-8.
6. Melamed E, Britton V, Zelig O. Episodic unresponsiveness to single doses of L-dopa in parkinsonian fluctuators. Neurology 1986; 36:100-3.
7. Weiner WJ, Nora LM, Glantz RH. Elderly inpatients: postural reflex impairment. Neurology 1984; 34:945-7.
8. Newman RP, LeWitt PA, Jaffe M, et al. Motor function in the normal aging population: treatment with levodopa. Neurology 1985; 35:571-3.
9. Ward CD, Sanes JN, Dambrosia JM, et al. Methods for evaluating treatment in Parkinson's disease. In: Fahn S, Calne DB, Shoulson I, eds. Advances in Neurology. New York: Raven, 1983; 37:1-7.
10. Beall CG. New method of recording muscular tremors. Arch Neurol Psychiatry 1925; 14: 751-5.
11. Schwab RS, Pritchard JS. Progression and progress in Parkinson's disease. J Nerv Ment Dis 1951; 65:489-501.
12. Calne DB, Lader MH. Electromyographic studies of tremor using an averaging computer. Electroencephalogr Clin Neurophysiol 1969; 26:86-92.
13. Nashold BS. Measurement of tremor. J Neurosurg 1966; 24(Suppl 1, Part II):320-3.
14. Agate FJ, Doshay LJ, Curtis FK. Quantitative measurement of therapy in paralysis agitans. JAMA 1956; 160:352-4.
15. Wachs H, Boshes B. Tremor studies in normals and in parkinsonians. Arch Neurol 1961; 4:66-82.
16. Velasco F, Velasco M. A quantitative evaluation of the effects of L-dopa on Parkinson's disease. Neuropharmacology 1973; 12:89-99.
17. Owen DAL, Marsden CD. Effect of adrenergic beta-blockers on parkinsonian tremor. Lancet 1965; 2:1259-62.
18. Dietrichson P, Langbretson OF, Houland J. Quantitation of tremor in man. In: Desmedt JE, ed. Progress in Clinical Neurophysiology. Basel: Karger, 1978; 5:90-4.
19. Jankovic J, Frost JD. Quantitative assessment of parkinsonian and essential tremor: clinical application of triaxial accelerometry. Neurology (Ny) 1981; 31:1235-40.
20. Boshes B, Wachs H, Brumlik J, et al. Studies of tone, tremor and speech in normal persons and parkinsonian patients. I. Methodology. Neurology 1960; 10:805-13.
21. Webster DD. A method of measuring the dynamic characteristics of muscle rigidity, strength and tremor in the upper extremity. IRE Trans Med Electr 1959; 6:159-64.
22. Webster DD, Mortimer JA. Failure of L-dopa to relieve activated rigidity in Parkinson's disease. In Messiha FS, Keeny Ad, eds. Parkinson's disease: neurophysiological, clinical and related aspects. New York: Plenum, 1977: 297-313.
23. Wright V, Johns RJ. Physical factors concerned with the stiffness of normal and diseased joints. Bull Johns Hopkins Hosp 1960; 215-31.
24. Long C, Thomas D, Crochetiere WJ. Objective measurement of muscle tone in the hand. Clin Pharmacol Ther 1964; 5:909-17.
25. Teravainen H, Tsui JK, Mak E, et al. Optimal indices for testing rigidity in Parkinson's disease. Neurology 1986; 36(Suppl. 1):244-5.
26. Tatton WG, Lee RG. Evidence for abnormal long-loop reflexes in rigid parkinsonian patients. Brain Res 1975; 100:671-6.
27. Tatton WG, Bedingham W, Verrier MC, et al. Characteristic alterations in responses to

imposed wrist displacements in parkinsonian rigidity and dystonia musculorum deformans. Can J Neurol Sci 1984; 11:281-7.

28. Mortimer JA, Webster DD. Evidence for a quantitative association between EMG stretch responses and parkinsonian rigidity. Brain Res. 1979; 162:169-73.

29. Marsden CD, Merton PA, Morton HB, et al. The effect of lesions of the central nervous system on long-latency stretch reflexes in the human thumb. In: Desmedt JE, ed. Progress in Clinical Neurophysiology. Basel: Karger, 1978; 4:342-60.

30. Rothwell JC, Obeso JA, Traub MM, et al. The behavior of the long-latency stretch reflex in patients with Parkinson's disease. J Neurol Neurosurg Psychiatry 1983; 46: 35-44.

31. Barbeau A. The problem of measurement of akinesia. J Neurosurg 1966; 24 (Suppl. 1, Part II):331-34.

32. Potvin AR, Tourtellotte WW. The neurological examination: advancements in its quantification. Arch Phys Med Rehabil 1975; 56:425-37.

33. Anden NE, Carlsson A, Kerstell J, et al. Oral L-dopa treatment of parkinsonism. Acta Med Scand 1970; 187:247-55.

34. Cassell K, Shaw K, Stern G. A computerized tracking technique for the assessment of parkinsonian motor disabilities. Brain 1973; 96:815-26.

35. Flowers KA. Ballistic and corrective movements in an aiming task: intention tremor and parkinsonian movement disorder compared. Neurology 1975; 25:413-21.

36. Flowers KA. Visual "closed loop" and "open loop" characteristics of voluntary movements in patients with parkinsonism and intention tremor. Brain 1976; 99:261-310.

37. Evarts EV, Teravainen H, Calne DB. Reaction time in Parkinson's disease. Brain 1981; 104:167-86.

38. Draper IT, Hohns RJ. The disordered movement in parkinsonism and the effect of drug treatment. Bull Johns Hopkins Hosp 1964; 5:465-80.

39. Angel RW, Alson W, Garland H. L-dopa and error correction time in Parkinson's disease. Neurology 1971; 21:1255-60.

40. Perret E, Eggensberger E, Siegfried J. Simple and complex finger movements of patients with parkinsonism before and after controlled stereotaxic thalamotomy. J. Neurol Nuerosurg Psychiatry 1970; 33:16-21.

41. Godwin-Austen RB, Tomlinson EG, Frears CC, et al. Effects of L-dopa in Parkinson's disease. Lancet 1969; 2:165-8.

42. Marsh DO, Schnieden H, Marshall J. A controlled trial of alpha methyl dopa in parkinsonian tremor. J Neurol Neurosurg Psychiatry 1963; 26:505-10.

43. Schwab RS, Chafetz ME, Walker S. Control of two simultaneous motor acts in normals and in parkinsonism. Arch Neurol Psychiatry 1954; 72:591-8.

44. Knopp W. Explorations in the assessment and meaning of the subclinical extrapyramidal effect of neuroleptic drugs. Pharmachopsychiatry 1968; 1:54-62.

45. Webster DD. Clinical analysis of the disability in Parkinson's disease. Mod Treat 1968; 5:257-82.

46. Knutsson E. An analysis of parkinsonian gait. Brain 1972; 95:475-86.

47. Ingvarsson P, Johnels B, Rydgren U, et al. Quantitative determination of posture and movement deficits in Parkinson's disease. Presented at the 1986 Congress of the International Medical Society of Motordisturbances, Lausanne, Switzerland, June 19-21, 1986.

48. Karson CN, LeWitt PA, Calne DB, et al. Blink rates in parkinsonism. Ann Neurol 1982; 12:580-3.

49. Kimura J. The blink reflex as a test for brain-stem and higher central nervous system function. In: Desmedt JE, ed. New developments in electromyelography and clinical neurophysiology. Basel: Karger, 1973; 3:682-91.

50. Lang AE, Marsden CD. Eye movements in basal ganglia diseases. In: Rose FC, ed. The eye in general medicine. London: Chapman and Hall, 1983:208-54.

51. White OB, Saint-Cyr JA, Sharpe JA. Ocular motor deficits in Parkinson's disease. I. The horizontal vestibulo-ocular reflex and its regulation. Brain 1983; 106:555-70.

52. White OB, Saint-Cyr JA, Tomlinson RD, et al. Ocular motor deficits in Parkinson's disease. II. Control of the saccadic and smooth pursuit systems. Brain 1983; 106:571–87.
53. Sharpe JA, Fletcher WA, Lang AE, et al. Smooth pursuit during dose-related on-off fluctuations in Parkinson's disease. Neurology 1986; 36(Suppl. 1):245.
54. Bodis-Wollner I, Yahr MD, Mylin L, et al. Dopaminergic deficiency and delayed visual evoked potentials in humans. Ann Neurol 1982; 11:478–83.
55. Gawel MJ, Das P, Vincent S, et al. Visual and auditory evoked responses in patients with Parkinson's disease. J Neurol Neurosurg Psychiatry 1981; 44:227–32.
56. Dinner DS, Luders H, Hanson M, et al. Pattern evoked potentials (PEPs) in Parkinson's disease. Neurology 1985; 35:610–13.
57. Angel RW. Shortening reaction in normal and parkinsonian subjects. Neurology 1982; 32:246–51.
58. Berardelli A, Hallett M. Shortening reaction of human tibialis anterior. Neurology 1984; 34:242–6.
59. Telland GA. Manual skill in Parkinson's disease. Geriatrics 1963; 18:613–20.
60. Lewy F. Die Lehre von Tonus und der Bewegung. Berlin: Springer, 1923.
61. Wilson SAK. The Croonian lectures on some disorders of motility and of muscle tone, with special reference to the corpus striatum: lecture II. Lancet 1925; 2:53–62.
62. Webster DD. The dynamic quantitation of spasticity with automated integrals of passive motor resistance. Clin Pharmacol Ther 1964; 5:900–8.
63. Webster DD. Rigidity in extrapyramidal disease. J Neursurg 1966; 24(Suppl. 1, Part III):257–82.
64. Lee RG, Tatton WG. Long-loop reflexes in man: clinical applications. In: Desmedt JE, ed. Progress in Clinical Neurophysiology. Basel: Karger, 1978; 4:342–60.
65. Taylor AE, Saint-Cyr JA, Lang AE. Frontal lobe dysfunction in Parkinson's disease: the cortical focus of neostriatal outflow. Brain 1986; 109:845–83.
66. Duvoisin RC. The evaluation of extrapyramidal disease. In: de Ajuriagerra J, ed. Monoamines, noyaux gris centraux et syndrome de Parkinson. Paris: Masson, 1970:313–25.
67. Yahr MD, Duvoisin RC, Schear MJ, et al. Treatment of Parkinsonism with levodopa. Arch Neurol 1969; 21:343–54.
68. Lieberman A, Dziatolowki M, Gopinathan G, et al. Evaluation of Parkinson's disease. In: Goldstein M, ed. Ergot compounds and brain function: neuroendocrine and neuropsychiatric aspects. New York: Raven, 1980:277–86.
69. Markham CH, Diamond SG. Evidence to support early levodopa therapy in Parkinson disease. Neurology 1981; 31:125–31.
70. Canter CJ, de la Torre R, Mier M. A method of evaluating disability in patients with Parkinson's disease. J Nerv Mental Dis 1961; 133:143–7.
71. Parkes JD, Ziklha KJ, Calver DM, et al. Controlled trial of amantadine hydrochloride in Parkinson's disease. Lancet 1970; 1:259–62.
72. Parkes JD, Zilkha KJ, Marsden P, et al. Amantadine dosage in the treatment of Parkinson's disease. Lancet 1970; 1:1130–3.
73. Larsen TA, Calne S, Calne DB. Assessment of Parkinson's disease. Clin Neuropharmacol 1984; 7:165–9.
74. Lees AJ, Shaw KM, Kohout LJ, et al. Deprenyl in Parkinson's disease. Lancet 1977; 2:791–5.
75. Schacter M, Marsden CD, Parkes JD, et al. Deprenyl in the management of response fluctuation in patients with Parkinson's disease on levodopa. J Neurol Neurosurg Psychiatry 1980; 43:1016–21.
76. Hoehn MM, Yahr MD. Parkinsonism: onset, progression and mortality. Neurology 1967; 17:427–42.
77. Muenter MD, Tyce GM. L-dopa therapy of Parkinson's disease: plasma L-dopa concentration, therapeutic response and side effects. Mayo Clin Proc 1971; 46:231–9.
78. Diamond SG, Markham CH. Evaluating the evaluations: or how to weigh the scales of parkinsonian disability. Neurology 1983; 33:1098–9.

79. Calne DB, Stern GM, Laurence DR, et al. L-dopa in postencephalitic parkinsonism. Lancet 1969; 1:744–6.
80. Teychenne PF, Bergsrud D, Rasy A, et al. Bromocriptine: low-dose therapy in Parkinson's disease. Neurology 1982; 32:577–83.
81. Weiner WJ, Koller WC, Perlik S, et al. Drug holiday and management of Parkinson's disease. Neurology 1980; 30:1257–61.
82. Montgomery GK. Parkinson's disease and the Columbia scale. Neurology 1984; 34:557–8.
83. Montgomery GK, Reynolds C, Warren RM. Qualitative assessment of Parkinson's disease: study of reliability and data reduction with an abbreviated Columbia scale. Clin Neuropharmacol 1985; 8:83–92.
84. Kartzome R, Calne DB. Studies with bromocriptine. Part I. "On-off" phenomena. Neurology 1976; 508–10.
85. Schwab RS, England AC. Projection technique for evaluating surgery in Parkinson's disease. In: Gillingham FJ, Donaldson IML, eds. Third symposium on Parkinson's disease. Edinburgh: Livingstone, 1969:152–7.
86. Nahmias C, Garnett ES, Firnau G, et al. Striatal dopamine distribution in parkinsonian patients during life. J Neurol Sci 1985; 69:223–30.
87. Calne DB, Langston JW, Martin WRW, et al. Positron emission tomography after MPTP: observations relating to the cause of Parkinson's disease. Nature 1985; 317:246–8.
88. Fahn S, Elton RL, and Members of the UPDRS Development Committee: Unified Parkinson's disease rating scale. In Fahn S, Marsden CD, Goldstein M, et al., eds. Recent developments in Parkinson's disease II. New York: Macmillan 1987:153–63.

Unified Parkinson's Disease Rating Scale[88]
(version 3.0, February 1987)
Definitions of 0–4 Scale

I. Mentation, Behavior, and Mood

1. Intellectual impairment:
   - 0 = None
   - 1 = Mild; consistent forgetfulness with partial recollection of events and no other difficulties
   - 2 = Moderate memory loss, with disorientation and moderate difficulty handling complex problems; mild but definite impairment of function at home, with need of occasional prompting
   - 3 = Severe memory loss with disorientation for time and often for place, severe impairment in handling problems
   - 4 = Severe memory loss, with orientation preserved to person only; unable to make judgments or solve problems; requires much help with personal care; cannot be left alone at all

2. Thought disorder (due to dementia or drug intoxication):
   - 0 = None
   - 1 = Vivid dreaming
   - 2 = "Benign" hallucinations with insight retained
   - 3 = Occasional to frequent hallucinations or delusions without insight; could interfere with daily activities
   - 4 = Persistent hallucinations, delusions, or florid psychosis; not able to care for self

3. Depression:
   - 0 = Not present
   - 1 = Periods of sadness or guilt greater than normal but never sustained for days or weeks
   - 2 = Sustained depression (1 week or more)
   - 3 = Sustained depression with vegetative symptoms (insomnia, anorexia, weight loss, loss of interest)
   - 4 = Sustained depression with vegetative symptoms and suicidal thoughts or intent

4. Motivation/initiative:
   - 0 = Normal
   - 1 = Less assertive than usual; more passive
   - 2 = Loss of initiative or interest in elective (nonroutine) activities
   - 3 = Loss of initiative or interest in day-to-day (routine) activities
   - 4 = Withdrawn; complete loss of motivation

II. ACTIVITIES OF DAILY LIVING (determine for "on"/"off")

5. Speech:
   - 0 = Normal
   - 1 = Mildly affected; no difficulty being understood
   - 2 = Moderately affected; sometimes asked to repeat statements
   - 3 = Severely affected; frequently asked to repeat statements
   - 4 = Unintelligible most of the time
6. Salivation:
   - 0 = Normal
   - 1 = Slight but definite excess of saliva in mouth; may have night-time drooling
   - 2 = Moderately excessive saliva; may have minimal drooling
   - 3 = Marked excess of saliva; some drooling
   - 4 = Marked drooling; requires constant use of tissue or handkerchief
7. Swallowing:
   - 0 = Normal
   - 1 = Rare choking
   - 2 = Occasional choking
   - 3 = Requires soft food
   - 4 = Requires nasogastric tube or gastrostomy feeding
8. Handwriting:
   - 0 = Normal
   - 1 = Slightly slow or small
   - 2 = Moderately slow or small; all words are legible
   - 3 = Severely affected; not all words are legible
   - 4 = The majority of words are not legible
9. Cutting food and handling utensils:
   - 0 = Normal
   - 1 = Somewhat slow and clumsy, but no help needed
   - 2 = Can cut most foods, although clumsy and slow; some help needed
   - 3 = Food must be cut by someone, but can still feed slowly
   - 4 = Needs to be fed
10. Dressing:
    - 0 = Normal
    - 1 = Somewhat slow, but no help needed
    - 2 = Occasional assistance needed with buttoning, getting arms into sleeves
    - 3 = Considerable help required, but can do some things alone
    - 4 = Helpless
11. Hygiene:
    - 0 = Normal
    - 1 = Somewhat slow, but no help needed
    - 2 = Needs help to shower or bathe; very slow in hygienic care
    - 3 = Requires assistance for washing, brushing teeth, combing hair, going to bathroom
    - 4 = Needs Foley catheter or other mechanical aids
12. Turning in bed and adjusting bedclothes:
    - 0 = Normal
    - 1 = Somewhat slow and clumsy, but no help needed

   2 = Can turn alone or adjust sheets, but with great difficulty
   3 = Can initiate attempt, but cannot turn or adjust sheets alone
   4 = Helpless

13. Falling (unrelated to freezing):
   0 = None
   1 = Rare falling
   2 = Occasionally falls, less than once daily
   3 = Falls an average of once daily
   4 = Falls more than once daily

14. Freezing when walking:
   0 = None
   1 = Rare freezing when walking; may have start hesitation
   2 = Occasional freezing when walking
   3 = Frequent freezing; occasionally falls because of freezing
   4 = Frequently falls because of freezing

15. Walking:
   0 = Normal
   1 = Mild difficulty; may not swing arms or may tend to drag leg
   2 = Moderate difficulty, but requires little or no assistance
   3 = Severe disturbance of walking; requires assistance
   4 = Cannot walk at all, even with assistance

16 Tremor:
   0 = Absent
   1 = Slight and infrequently present
   2 = Moderate; bothersome to patient
   3 = Severe; interferes with many activities
   4 = Marked; interferes with most activities

17. Sensory complaints related to parkinsonism:
   0 = None
   1 = Occasionally has numbness, tingling, or mild aching
   2 = Frequently has numbness, tingling, or aching; not distressing
   3 = Frequent painful sensations
   4 = Excruciating pain

III. MOTOR EXAMINATION

18. Speech:
   0 = Normal
   1 = Slight loss of expression, diction, and/or volume
   2 = Monotone, slurred but understandable; moderately impaired
   3 = Marked impairment, difficult to understand
   4 = Unintelligible

19. Facial expression:
   0 = Normal
   1 = Minimal hypomimia; could be normal "poker face"
   2 = Slight but definitely abnormal diminution of facial expression

3 = Moderate hypomimia; lips parted some of the time
4 = Masked or fixed facies, with severe or complete loss of facial expression; lips parted ¼ inch or more

20. Tremor at rest:
    0 = Absent
    1 = Slight and infrequently present
    2 = Mild in amplitude and persistent, or moderate in amplitude but only intermittently present
    3 = Moderate in amplitude and present most of the time
    4 = Marked in amplitude and present most of the time

21. Action or postural tremor of hands:
    0 = Absent
    1 = Slight; present with action
    2 = Moderate in amplitude; present with action
    3 = Moderate in amplitude; present with posture-holding as well as with action
    4 = Marked in amplitude; interferes with feeding

22. Rigidity (judged on passive movement of major joints with patient relaxed in sitting position; "cogwheeling" to be ignored):
    0 = Absent
    1 = Slight or detectable only when activated by mirror or other movements
    2 = Mild to moderate
    3 = Marked, but full range of motion easily achieved
    4 = Severe; range of motion achieved with difficulty

23. Finger taps (patient taps thumb with index finger in rapid succession with widest amplitude possible, each hand separately):
    0 = Normal
    1 = Mild slowing and/or reduction in amplitude
    2 = Moderately impaired; definite and early fatiguing; may have occasional arrests in movement
    3 = Severely impaired; frequent hesitation in initiating movements or arrests in ongoing movement
    4 = Can barely perform the task

24. Hand movements (patient opens and closes hands in rapid succession with widest amplitude possible, each hand separately):
    0 = Normal
    1 = Mild slowing and/or reduction in amplitude
    2 = Moderately impaired; definite and early fatiguing; may have occasional arrests in movement
    3 = Severely impaired; frequent hesitation in initiating movements or arrests in ongoing movement
    4 = Can barely perform the task

25. Rapid alternating movements of hand (pronation-supination movements of hands, vertically or horizontally, with as large an amplitude as possible, both hands simultaneously):
    0 = Normal
    1 = Mild slowing and/or reduction in amplitude
    2 = Moderately impaired; definite and early fatiguing; may have occasional arrests in movement

3 = Severely impaired; frequent hesitation in initiating movements or arrests in ongoing movement

4 = Can barely perform the task

26. Leg agility (patient taps heel on ground in rapid succession, picking up entire leg; amplitude should be about 3 inches):

0 = Normal

1 = Mild slowing and/or reduction in amplitude

2 = Moderately impaired; definite and early fatiguing; may have occasional arrests in movement

3 = Severely impaired; frequent hesitation in initiating movements or arrests in ongoing movement

4 = Can barely perform the task

27. Arising from chair (patient attempts to arise from a straight-backed wood or metal chair, with arms folded across chest):

0 = Normal

1 = Slow, or may need more than one attempt

2 = Pushes self up from arms of seat

3 = Tends to fall back and may have to try more than one time but can get up without help

4 = Unable to arise without help

28. Posture:

0 = Normal erect

1 = Not quite erect, slightly stooped posture; could be normal for older person

2 = Moderately stooped posture, definitely abnormal; can be slightly leaning to one side

3 = Severely stooped posture with kyphosis; can be moderately leaning to one side

4 = Marked flexion, with extreme abnormality of posture

29. Gait:

0 = Normal

1 = Walks slowly; may shuffle with short steps, but no festination or propulsion

2 = Walks with difficulty but requires little or no assistance; may have some festination, short steps, or propulsion

3 = Severe disturbance of gait; requires assistance

4 = Cannot walk at all, even with assistance

30. Postural stability (response to sudden posterior displacement produced by pull on shoulders while patient is erect, with eyes open and feet slightly apart; patient is prepared):

0 = Normal

1 = Retropulsion, but recovers unaided

2 = Absence of postural response; would fall if not caught by examiner

3 = Very unstable; tends to lose balance spontaneously

4 = Unable to stand without assistance

31. Body bradykinesia and hypokinesia (combining slowness, hesitancy, decreased arm swing, small amplitude, and poverty of movement in general):

0 = None

1 = Minimal slowness, giving movement a deliberate character; could be normal for some persons; possibly reduced amplitude

2 = Mild degree of slowness and poverty of movement that is definitely abnormal; alternatively, some reduced amplitude

3 = Moderate slowness; poverty or small amplitude of movement

4 = Marked slowness; poverty or small amplitude of movement

IV. COMPLICATIONS OF THERAPY (in the past week)

A. Dyskinesias

32. Duration: What proportion of the waking day are dyskinesias present? (historical information):
    0 = None
    1 = 1–25% of day
    2 = 26–50% of day
    3 = 51–75% of day
    4 = 76–100% of day
33. Disability: How disabling are the dyskinesias? (historical information; may be modified by office examination):
    0 = Not disabling
    1 = Mildly disabling
    2 = Moderately disabling
    3 = Severely disabling
    4 = Completely disabling
34. Painful dyskinesias: How painful are the dyskinesias?
    0 = No painful dyskinesias
    1 = Slightly
    2 = Moderately
    3 = Severely
    4 = Markedly
35. Presence of early morning dystonia (historical information):
    0 = No
    1 = Yes

B. Clinical Fluctuations

36. Are any "off" periods predictable as to timing after a dose of medication?
    0 = No
    1 = Yes
37. Are any "off" periods unpredictable as to timing after a dose of medication?
    0 = No
    1 = Yes
38. Do any "off" periods come on suddenly (e.g., within a few seconds)?
    0 = No
    1 = Yes
39. What proportion of the waking day is the patient "off," on average?
    0 = None
    1 = 1–25% of day
    2 = 26–50% of day
    3 = 51–75% of day
    4 = 76–100% of day

C. Other Complications

40. Does the patient have anorexia, nausea, or vomiting?
    0 = No
    1 = Yes
41. Does the patient have any sleep disturbances (e.g., insomnia or hypersomnolence)?
    0 = No
    1 = Yes
42. Does the patient have symptomatic orthostasis?
    0 = No
    1 = Yes

Record the patient's blood pressure, pulse, and weight on the scoring form

V. MODIFIED HOEHN AND YAHR STAGING

Stage 0   = No signs of disease
Stage 1   = Unilateral disease
Stage 1.5 = Unilateral plus axial involvement
Stage 2   = Bilateral disease without impairment of balance
Stage 2.5 = Mild bilateral disease with recovery on pull test
Stage 3   = Mild to moderate bilateral disease; some postural instability; physically independent
Stage 4   = Severe disability; still able to walk or stand unassisted
Stage 5   = Wheelchair-bound or bedridden unless aided

VI. SCHWAB AND ENGLAND ACTIVITIES OF DAILY LIVING SCALE

100% = Completely independent; able to do all chores without slowness, difficulty, or impairment; essentially normal; unaware of any difficulty

90% = Completely independent; able to do all chores with some degree of slowness, difficulty, and impairment; may take twice as long as normal; beginning to be aware of difficulty

80% = Completely independent in most chores; takes twice as long as normal; conscious of difficulty and slowness

70% = Not completely independent; more difficulty with some chores; takes three to four times as long as normal in some; must spend a large part of the day with chores

60% = Some dependency; can do most chores, but exceedingly slowly and with considerable effort and errors; some chores impossible

50% = More dependent; needs help with half the chores, slower, etc.; difficulty with everything

40% = Very dependent; can assist with all chores but does few alone

30% = With effort, now and then does a few chores alone or begins alone; much help needed

20% = Does nothing alone; can be a slight help with some chores; severe invalid
10% = Totally dependent and helpless; complete invalid
 0% = Vegetative functions such as swallowing, bladder and bowel functions are not functioning; bedridden

---

The following investigators contributed to the development of the Unified Parkinson's Disease Rating Scale: Yves Agid, Donald B. Calne, Roger C. Duvoisin, Stanley Fahn, Margaret M. Hoehn, Joseph Jankovic, Harold L. Klawans, Anthony E. Lang, Xavier LaTaste, Abraham Lieberman, Charles H. Markham, C. David Marsden, Richard Mayeux, Urpo K. Rinne, Gerald M. Stern, Paul Teychenne, and Melvin D. Yahr.

Chapter 22

Parkinson's Disease and Alzheimer's Disease: Differences Revealed by Neuropsychologic Testing

Suzanne Corkin, John H. Growdon, Gena Desclos, and
T. John Rosen

Parkinson's disease (PD) and Alzheimer's disease (AD) are chronic, progressive neurologic disorders of later life. Although PD was first described in 1817[1] and AD in 1907,[2] the possibility that they have a common etiology or share pathogenetic mechanisms was not entertained until recently. This chapter provides evidence from four disciplines regarding the similarities and differences between the two diseases. The questions raised here (which still await answers) are whether the similarities make a compelling case for the existence of a common etiology or pathophysiology underlying the diseases, and whether the cognitive manifestations of PD and AD overlap only slightly or to a considerable extent. Specifically, are the cognitive losses in PD qualitatively different from those in AD, or are the losses in PD similar in kind but milder than those in AD?

The conventional wisdom in neurology is that PD and AD are distinct nosologic entities, readily differentiable upon clinical examination. Except in rare cases, PD and AD are not confused, although they may coexist. It is therefore surprising that detailed data concerning the morphologic, chemical, neurologic, and cognitive correlates of these diseases reveal extensive overlap between them.[3] The communality of characteristics tempts brain scientists to speculate that PD and AD have a common etiology or pathophysiology, albeit with marked individual and group variations in the distribution of lesions. For example, Gajdusek[4] hypothesized that interference with axonal transport of the neurofilament is a common pathogenetic mechanism in AD, in a variant of PD, and in eight other neurologic diseases that bear little clinical resemblance to each other (Table 22.1). His speculation is supported by evidence that

Table 22.1 Gajdusek's Hypothesis (1985): Diseases in which Interference with Axonal Transport of the Neurofilament Is Postulated to Be the Pathogenetic Mechanism

Pugilistic encephalopathy
Pick's disease
Progressive supranuclear palsy
Down's syndrome
Werdnig-Hoffmann syndrome
Amyotrophic lateral sclerosis of Guam
Metal intoxication (dialysis dementia)
Motor neuron disease (Hirano)
Parkinsonism-dementia of Guam
Alzheimer's disease

unique antineurofilament autoantibodies appear in each of these degenerative diseases of gray matter. The links between the degenerative disorders of PD and AD are still poorly understood. This chapter reviews the evidence for similarities between PD and AD as adduced from studies in epidemiology, neuropathology, clinical neurology, and neuropsychology, and then shows how neuropsychologic methods can be used most effectively to determine whether the two clinical syndromes represent one disease process or two.

SIMILARITY OF EPIDEMIOLOGY AND GENETICS

PD and AD differ in their epidemiologic characteristics, suggesting that the diseases are etiologically dissimilar. The epidemiologic study of both diseases is complicated because accurate diagnosis is time-consuming and expensive and because incidence rates rise late in life, when mortality from other causes may preclude the onset of PD or AD. Caution is thus advisable in making comparisons.

AD is more common than PD. Rocca, Amaducci, and Schoenberg[5] estimated that there were approximately 1.4 million cases of AD in the United States in 1980, far above Kessler's[6] estimate of 150,000 to 400,000 cases of PD. Population-based studies suggest that age-specific indicence rates for PD peak around age 75.[7] Nearly two-thirds of PD patients first develop motor symptoms in the fifth or sixth decades of life; fewer than 20% of PD patients are first affected in the fourth or seventh decades.[8] The prevalence of AD increases sharply with age.[5] AD is more common in women than in men,[5] whereas PD shows the reverse pattern.[6] AD occurs in blacks at least as often as in whites,[9] but PD is reported to be relatively rare in blacks.[10] (Sampling bias may have influenced the results regarding PD.)

Besides age, the greatest risk factor for AD is a positive family history of dementia.[5] Although it is usually not possible to differentiate among causes of dementia in the deceased parents of current AD patients, it is clear that at least some families show a pattern of autosomal dominant inheritance of early-onset AD.[11] Mohs et al.[12] recently reported that regardless of patients' age at onset, relatives of AD patients showed a 46% cumulative incidence of probable AD by age 86, not far from the value of 50% to be expected from a fully penetrant dominant characteristic. Further, laboratories have assigned the putative "AD gene" for early-onset familial AD (FAD) to chromosome 21.[13] Whether all AD is inherited or whether there are sporadic forms remains uncertain; not all twins are concordant for AD,[14] and the region on chromosome 21 that is linked to FAD does not seem to be linked to AD with onset after age 65.[15,16] In contrast to the importance of heredity in AD, it is doubtful that PD is inherited. Duvoisin et al.[17] found zero concordance among 12 pairs of monozygotic twins, one of whom had been identified as having PD.

The preceding epidemiologic comparisons imply that AD and PD have different etiologies. It must be noted, however, that these studies have used diagnostic and neuropathologic criteria that do not differentiate between cases of PD with and without dementia. Almost no epidemiologic analyses of PD have focused on cases with dementia, although Gandy et al.[18] did report that the mean age at onset of dementia in PD is similar to the mean age at onset of AD. There is a need for epidemiologic studies that differentiate among PD patients according to whether they are demented.

SIMILARITIES OF NEURAL ALTERATIONS

The dominant trend during the last 10 years has been to assign PD and AD to dichotomous categories of dementia, called subcortical and cortical, respectively.[19,20] In the so-called cortical dementias (i.e., AD and Creutzfeldt-Jakob disease), language, perception, and praxis are said to be impaired, whereas in the subcortical dementias (i.e., PD, progressive supranuclear palsy, normal pressure hydrocephalus, Huntington's disease, Wilson's disease, multi-infarct dementia, and dementia associated with depression), mood disturbance and slowness of thought prevail but language, perception, and praxis are preserved. A compilation of the morphologic and chemical correlates of PD and AD, however, indicates that the subcortical-cortical distinction is simplistic and untenable.[21-23] The following paragraphs outline the evidence that cortical and subcortical regions are invaded substantially by both diseases.

In comparing the neuropathologic changes associated with PD and AD, it is vital to distinguish between PD patients that had been demented and those that had not. Most recent studies have made this distinction, and as a result, interest has focused on whether the dementia of PD is attributable to concurrent AD-type cortical neuropathology, or whether other patterns of neuropathology are associated with the dementia of PD. A previous review[24] identified three patterns of regional neuropathology in patients with idiopathic PD accompanied by dementia (Table 22.2). One pattern consisted of AD-type changes (i.e., neuristic plaques and neurofibrillary tangles in cortex.[25] A second pattern lacked cortical neuritic plaques and neurofibrillary tangles, but featured a loss of neurons in the nucleus basalis of Meynert and associated decreases in cortical choline-acetyltransferase activity.[26] A third pattern involved Lewy bodies within neurons distributed widely in the cortex and in subcortical nuclei.[27] Whether these three pathologic subtypes correspond to distinct patterns of clinical features and cognitive deficits has not been determined. The topic is worth investigating.

Table 22.2.   Regional Neuropathology in Parkinson's Disease with Dementia as Compared with Alzheimer's Disease[a]

Group	Cerebral Cortex	Substantia Nigra	Locus Ceruleus	Nucleus Basalis	Other Brainstem Structures
PD + D	Three Patterns 1. NP or NFT 2. No NP or NFT 3. Atypical with Lewy bodies	Always	Usually	Always	Usually
AD	Always NP and NFT	Never	Sometimes	Always	Rarely

[a]PD + D denotes Parkinson's disease with dementia; AD, Alzheimer's disease; NP, neuritic plaques; NFT, neurofibrillary tangles.

Like studies of the morphologic abnormalities in PD, most neurochemical studies now specify whether or not the patients were demented. The data are too sparse, however, to permit a comprehensive comparison of the neurochemical pathology in PD with and without dementia. Preliminary findings from Yves Agid's laboratory[28] indicate that the two PD groups do not differ with respect to striatal dopamine deficiency, but that only the demented patients show decreases of norepinephrine and serotonin in the cortex.

Table 22.3 compares the cortical neurochemical profile in PD with dementia to that in AD. The data summarized in the table are based on results from numerous investigators (for reviews, see references 29 and 30). The same four major ascending neurotransmitter systems (dopamine, acetylcholine, noradrenaline, serotonin) are affected in PD with dementia and in AD, even though the nature of the pathologic process may differ in the two disorders. Transmitter deficits are not necessarily found in all neurons in each system. For example, the cholinergic lesions in PD apparently involve only the innominatocortical system[31] and spare the striatum. The major difference between the two demented groups is the earlier and more extensive degeneration of the nigrostriatal dopamine system in PD than in AD. The currently available evidence suggests that neurons that synthesize neuropeptides seem to be affected similarly in PD with dementia and in AD, although neurotensin is apparently decreased in PD but normal in AD. A comparison of free amino acid levels in PD and AD awaits neurochemical analysis of brains from patients with PD. The leading neurotransmitter candidates for the regulation of behavioral capacities are acetylcholine, dopamine, norepinephrine, and serotonin.[24] Only acetylcholine has been linked to morphologic, chemical, and clinical features of dementia.[32]

In summary, the neuropathologic and neurochemical alterations in PD with dementia overlap considerably with those in AD, compromising cortical as well as subcortical brain tissue.

Table 22.3. Neurochemical Pathology in Cortex in Parkinson's Disease as Compared with Alzheimer's Disease[a]

Chemical System	PD	AD
Ascending systems		
Dopamine	↓	↓
Acetylcholine	↓	↓
Norepinephrine	↓	↓
Serotonin	↓	↓
Neuropeptide systems		
Somatostatin	↓	↓
Neuropeptide Y	→↓	↓
Vasopressin	?	↓
Corticotropin releasing factor	?	↓
Cholecystokinin	→	→
Vasoactive intestinal polypeptide	→	→
Met-enkephalin	→	→
Leu-enkephalin	→	?
Substance P	↓	↓
Bombesine	→↓	?
Neurotensin	↓	→
Free amino acids		
Glutamate	?	↓
Aspartate	?	→
Glycine	?	→
γ-Aminobutyric acid	?	↓

[a]PD denotes Parkinson's disease; AD, Alzheimer's disease; ↓, decreased; →, intact; ?, no data.

SIMILARITIES OF CLINICAL FEATURES

The extrapyramidal system is affected in both diseases, but motor signs and symptoms are the cardinal features of PD, even in early cases, whereas these findings are less prominent in early AD. Huff and Growdon[33] observed motor abnormalities (excluding those of balance and gait) in 15% of 165 patients with a clinical diagnosis of AD. The prevalence of balance and gait impairments was linked to dementia severity. One or both disorders occurred in only 13% of mild cases but in 41% of severely demented (though not institutionalized) cases, suggesting a progressive dysfunction of the striatal dopamine system. Other investigators have noted an even higher prevalence of extrapyramidal signs in AD.[34,35] One study stressed the similarity in the prevalence and severity of motor symptoms in AD and PD,[36] although qualitative differences in symptoms were evident. For example, PD patients showed cogwheel rigidity but not *gegenhalten,* whereas AD patients showed *gegenhalten* but not cogwheel rigidity.

The similarity of clinical features in PD and AD goes beyond the motor system. Specific cognitive deficits and dementia are now recognized characteristics of PD,[24] and they are the behavioral hallmark of AD. Even the patterns of cognitive test performance for the two groups are highly similar.[3,21,23,37]

SIMILARITIES OF COGNITIVE DEFICITS

The responsibility for measuring cognitive deficits in neurologic disease falls upon neuropsychologists. Neuropsychology contributes uniquely to the neurosciences in that it quantifies behavior. Ideally, each neuropsychologic measure should quantify a discrete and distinct aspect of behavioral function, thereby permitting the dissociation of specific behavioral capacities in neurologic disease as well as in experimentally produced brain abnormalities in animals. Analyses showing dissociations of function provide the basis of neuropsychology's impact in two arenas: clinical neurology and theoretical behavioral neuroscience. In the clinical arena, neuropsychologic testing extends the clinician's neurologic examination by quantifying the capacities that the neurologist assesses qualitatively in the office or at the bedside. In a laboratory setting, neuropsychologists can measure a plethora of abilities that fall under the broad headings of sensory function, motor function, attention, memory, language, visuospatial function, abstract reasoning, problem solving, affect, and so forth (Table 22.4). This rich sampling of a patient's behaviors, when compared with normative

Table 22.4   Functions that Can Be Evaluated by Neuropsychologic Tests

Test	Salient Function Tested
Raven Colored Progressive Matrices	Abstract reasoning
Geometric designs: Drawing	Praxis
	Nonverbal memory
	Recall and recognition
	Immediate and delayed
Benton Visual Retention	Nonverbal memory
	Recognition
Money Road Map	Spatial orientation
Luria Test of Mental Rotation	Mental rotation
Stroop test	Speed of reading
	Speed of color naming
	Ability to maintain set
Picture Arrangement	Sequencing, flexibility of set
Symbolic and Semantic Fluency	Verbal fluency
Boston Naming	Confrontation naming of objects
NYU Stories	Verbal memory
	Recall and recognition
	Immediate and delayed
Digit Span	Immediate memory
Recognition of Test Session	Incidental learning
	Recognition of content of tests
	Recognition of order of tests

standards, permits the quantitative definition of deficits and the distinction between spared and lost functions. Detailed information regarding many behavioral capacities permits the study of issues relating to the nature and extent of deficits, locus of lesion, course of disease, and response to treatment.

In the theoretical arena, demonstrations that two classes of behavior dissociate after an insult to the brain suggest that these behaviors have separate anatomical or chemical substrates. Ideally, we week double dissociations of function, such that lesion A impairs behavior X but not behavior Y, whereas lesion B impairs behavior Y but not behavior X.[38] Obtaining opposite patterns of spared and impaired functions with two different patient groups assures us that the differences between those groups do not reflect nonspecific factors, such as lower intelligence or greater disease severity in one group. The existence of a double dissociation implies that different behaviors depend on different brain regions. At the neural level, dissociations may be defined in terms of gross anatomy, cellular anatomy, or neurochemistry.

In summary, neuropsychology's contributions to neurology and neurosurgery yield a practical clinical payoff as well as an academic tonic. The remainder of this chapter illustrates the dual role of neuropsychology. The clinical problem addressed is the characterization of PD and AD; the theoretical issue is whether the two clinical syndromes represent one disease process or two.

NEUROPSYCHOLOGIC TESTS IN PD AND AD

Issues of Subject Selection

The results of any comparison of patients with PD and AD depend in part on how the two samples are selected. Subject selection, in turn, should depend on the questions to be addressed. In comparing PD patients with normal control subjects, the cleanest approach is to identify patients with PD who are neither demented nor depressed[39] and to separate them from patients with PD who are demented. The hope is that the performance of the nondemented group will predominantly reflect the effects of lesions of the dopamine systems, in contrast to the performance of the demented group, in which dopaminergic effects will be joined by, and will interact with, the effects of lesions involving other neurochemical systems. In comparing the dementia of PD with the dementia of AD, only PD patients with dementia should be selected. Although this point seems obvious, most published studies of cognition in PD include, but do not distinguish between, patients with and without dementia. As a result, the patterns of cognitive deficit probably reflect in part the proportion of demented and nondemented patients in each sample and may therefore be idiosyncratic to each study.

Three facts about the relation between PD and AD have strong implications for subject selection in studies comparing the two groups. First, all AD patients are demented by definition, whereas only about one third to one half of the PD population develops dementia. Current estimates of dementia prevalence in PD range from 2 to 93%, but the extreme figures (cited in reference 24) are certainly under- and overestimates, respectively. Second, most nondemented PD patients develop cognitive impairments, but these impairments are typically less severe than those seen in AD. Third, cognitive impairment progresses much slower among nondemented PD patients than among AD patients. This point was illustrated by a study[40] that compared the progression of memory impairments in PD and AD by administering the memory and information subscale of the Blessed dementia scale (BDS)[41] at least twice to 33 patients with PD and 70 with AD. These patients were consecutive cases examined in either the memory or movement disorders clinic of a general hospital and were retested at 6-month intervals. At the initial examination, the mean BDS score for the AD patients was 15.9 and increased at a mean rate of 0.365 points per month. The scores of the PD patients were essentially stationary, decreasing at a mean rate of −0.022 points per month from the initial mean of 2.1. The difference in rates was significant at $P < 0.001$. The greatest rate of change in any PD patient followed for 6 months or more was 0.210, about two thirds of the mean rate of change among AD patients. These differences persisted in a comparison of only the PD and AD patients who showed memory deficits of the same magnitude (initial BDS score between 3 and 22). The uniform failure to observe cognitive deterioration among PD patients suggests that PD patients who deteriorate at a rate typical of AD may have AD-type neuropathology or a related dementing disorder in addition to the characteristic nigrostriatal degeneration of PD.

The considerations cited above make it extremely difficult to equate groups of PD and AD patients with respect to severity of dementia. To do so would necessitate the choosing of samples that would misrepresent the overall populations. The best alternative to obtaining comparable population-based samples is to study a large number of consecutive cases from each disease group in the same medical setting. A further worry in this regard, however, is that patients with PD may come to research settings earlier in the course of disease than may AD patients. The tolerance of patients and their families for extrapyramidal motor disabilities may be lower than the tolerance of patients and their families for lapses of memory or word-finding difficulty, making the duration of disease before the first visit to a specialized clinic shorter in PD than in AD.

The choice of control subjects is complicated in its own right. For example, in a disease such as AD, which has a genetic component, should siblings who are at risk for the disease be included in a control group? We have answered this question in the affirmative, largely in order to be consistent with our definition of a control subject as someone who is free of clinically observable neurologic disease; preclinical disease states are, by definition, unobservable in either spouses or siblings, and thus their possible presence and likelihood should be ignored.

Issues of Test Selection and Administration

The following paragraphs highlight some characteristics of particular neuropsychologic tests that are in common use. Our purpose is to illustrate how test properties can influence performance differentially in patient groups (e.g., those with PD or AD) or in subgroups (e.g., men or women).

The motor symptoms of PD may handicap performance on timed cognitive tests, and examiners must be careful not to interpret poor performance due to bradykinesia as an indication of cognitive impairment.[42] For example, the Stroop test[43] has three parts, with 45 seconds allowed for each: reading color names aloud, naming the colors of the inks with which different-colored Xs are printed, and naming the colors of the inks with which discordant color names are printed. Our patients with PD without dementia were significantly slower than healthy control subjects at word reading and color reading ($P < 0.05$) (Figure 22.1). In contrast to the Stroop test, the Boston Naming Test[44] is untimed for practical purposes; the 20-second interval allowed to name each object was sufficiently liberal that PD patients were not handicapped. The same PD patients who were slower on the Stroop test did not differ significantly from the control subjects when asked to name pictures of objects or parts of objects; scores were based on accuracy rather than response time. In general, when using timed tests with PD patients, it is important (whenever the test format permits) to record two scores: the score achieved within the time limit and the score with the time limit disregarded.

Another task used with patients suspected of having dementia is category fluency. It is important to consider the choice of categories carefully because certain categories are more difficult for some subgroups than for others. For example, in our experience, men have greater difficulty than women in naming vegetables, whereas women are often thwarted in naming tools and vehicles. Similarly, subjects of lower socioeconomic status have a short supply of furniture names. The category of clothing is a poor choice because many items are within the subject's immediate view. Unfortunately, information about the appropriateness of different categories for testing fluency is rarely published and therefore must be acquired through testing experience.

A different sort of problem arises in administering the Money Road Map Test to patients with AD.[45] Subjects are shown a road map and are asked to pretend that they

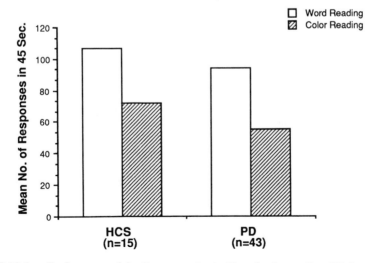

FIGURE 22.1   *Performance of the Stroop test is significantly slower (P < .05) in patients with Parkinson's disease without dementia (PD) in healthy control subjects (HCS).*

are taking a walk through a city, following a dotted line. At each corner they are asked to say whether they would turn left or right to stay on course. It is not uncommon for AD patients with aphasia to say ''left'' when they mean ''right,'' or vice versa. This problem can be circumvented by permitting subjects to raise the left or right hand to indicate the direction of each turn.

For AD patients with aphasia, the method of assessing learning may influence the results. Aphasic AD patients do disproportionately poorly at verbatim recall of stories as compared with recognition. Figure 22.2 compares the recall performance of control subjects, patients with PD without dementia, and patients with mild to moderate AD. The performance of the PD group did not differ from that of the healthy control group, but the performance of the AD group was significantly inferior to those of both the other groups. Immediately after the recall tests, a seven-item recognition memory test was given for the same material (Figure 22.3). In the recognition procedure, subjects were asked to point to the correct answer on a computer screen showing four response choices. The immediate recognition score of the AD group was still significantly lower than those of the other two groups (P < 0.05), but the gap between the PD and AD groups narrowed. On delayed recall, the AD group's score was no longer inferior to that of the PD group, suggesting that AD patients are especially helped by recognition testing. In general, it is usually preferable to use forced-choice recognition testing of memory with AD patients because on recall they often score poorly (i.e., show a floor effect), and they tend to respond ''yes'' with the method of continuous recognition.

Issues of Data Analysis

A number of statistical difficulties beset comparisons of the neuropsychologic and clinical characteristics of AD and PD patients. We focus here on two broad problems: (1) how to separate premorbid intellectual differences from the cognitive effects of the diseases, and (2) how to compare performance on different tests.

Premorbid Differences

In the sample of patients who attended our clinics, mean education and socioeconomic status were higher for PD patients than for AD patients. Our PD patients tended to be male by a two-to-one margin, and our AD patients showed the reverse pattern. Premorbid and demographic differences between diagnostic groups may lead to ambiguities in data interpretation. We have observed that PD patients have less severe deficits on all neuropsychologic measures. Does the explanation lie in the PD patients' greater premorbid faculties, or does PD impair cognition less than AD? Also, we believe that PD (but not AD) patients have a striking inability to switch cognitive sets.[39] Does the explanation lie in sex differences or in the particular effects of frontal lobe pathology in PD?

Our primary procedure for separating premorbid and demographic differences from disease-related effects has been to obtain separate control groups for the two diseases. Our AD control subjects (ADC) are the spouses and siblings of AD patients

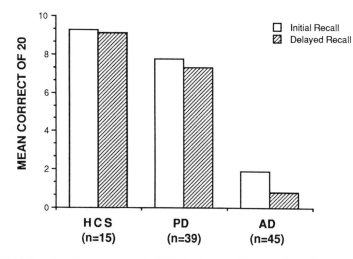

FIGURE 22.2 *Recall, as assessed by NYU Stories test, is poorer in patients with Alzheimer's disease (AD) than in nondemented parkinsonian patients (PD) and healthy control subjects (HCS). The performance of PD patients did not differ significantly from that of the controls.*

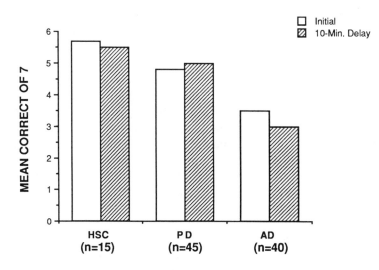

FIGURE 22.3 *Immediate recognition memory, as assessed by NYU Stories test, is poorer (P < 0.05) in patients with Alzheimer's disease (AD) than in healthy control subjects (HCS) or patients with Parkinson's disease without dementia (PD). When delayed recall was tested, the AD patients performed as well as the PD patients.*

seen in our clinic; similarly, PD control subjects (PDC) are the spouses and siblings of our PD patients. Data analyses follow a 2×2 factorial analysis of variance (ANOVA) design, in which disease (AD vs. PD) is crossed with status (patient vs. control). The interaction term represents the "difference of differences," the size of the quantity ([AD − ADC] − [PD − PDC]). The inner subtractions (AD − ADC) and (PD − PDC) scale patients with respect to their own controls, and the difference of these differences indicates whether the two diseases have similar effects relative to the proper control subjects.

Between-Test Comparisons

A recurring theme in data analysis is to compare patients' performance across tests. Do PD patients have greater deficits on timed tests than on untimed tests? Does AD affect naming ability before or after its affects sensitivity to grammatical relations? Is the pattern of AD patients' performance similar or dissimilar to that of PD patients? Necessarily, each such question requires the comparison of incommensurable variables—that is, variables measured on different response scales. On one test, the scores may correspond to the number of milliseconds required to respond; on another, to the total number of correct responses; and on a third, to a rater's judgment of the accuracy with which a picture was reproduced. Comparing such scores requires some prior transformation to a common scale. The statistical difficulties lie in how to perform the necessary transformations and how to then make the necessary comparisons.

Rosen and Corkin[46,47] have discussed both problems. In 1985 they recommended the use of a variance-components ANOVA to extract measurement error from estimates of the control subjects' between-subjects standard deviation (repeated measurements are necessary on each subject), and then the standardization of test scores with respect to the control subjects. Ordinary standard deviations alone are inadequate, because they represent a combination of between-subject variation in true scores and within-subject measurement error. In effect, standardizing by means of ordinary standard deviations causes the "scaling unit" to vary systematically as a function of each test's measurement error. In the present context, we recommend that for each test, pooled estimates of measurement error and the between-subjects sum of squares be derived with use of data from the two control groups (ACD and PDC). Subtracting the measurement error from the between-subjects sum of squares yields a variance that indicates "pure" error, and its square root equals the corrected between-subjects standard deviation (this process should be repeated for each test). Finally, each AD patient's score on each test should be normalized by subtracting the corresponding ADC mean from the raw score, and then dividing by the common (to both control groups) corrected standard deviation. Parallel calculations yield the corresponding scores for each PD patient. If adequate control data are unavailable, tests may be normalized by means of simpler (but less accurate) rank transformation procedures.[48]

The final difficulty consists of specifying and testing hypotheses about contrasting patterns of test performance shown by different patient groups. Rosen and Corkin[47] defined quantitative and qualitative hypotheses that describe between-group (AD vs. PD) and within-subject (e.g., test 1 vs. test 2) performance patterns. Rosen and Corkin discussed the analysis of these hypotheses within a repeated-measures ANOVA framework. Diagnostic group was treated as a between-subjects factor, and the several tests were treated as repeated measures. Because of the assumptions underlying ANOVA, their proposal was predicated on prior rescaling, such as that described in the preceding paragraph. Quantitative differences between the AD and PD groups corresponded to the main effect for diagnosis; AD and PD patients were said to differ quantitatively to the extent that, summing over tests, their overall means differ. Qualitative differences corresponded to the interaction of groups and tests and indicated the degree to which the groups had different test profiles. Multivariate profile analysis can be used to test similar hypotheses, but its requirements in terms of a high ratio of subjects to variables are usually excessive for neuropsychologic studies.

We have omitted a number of technical considerations. For example, the repeated-measures ANOVA must be corrected for the violation of certain covariance assumptions. For the present purposes, what is important is not so much the formal computational algorithms but rather the ability of the researcher to formulate hypotheses that pertain directly to comparisons between patient groups.

HOW MANY PATHOGENETIC MECHANISMS?

Pursuing the question of whether the mechanism of disease is single or dual seems advisable, because several investigators have called attention to common features of PD and AD. Our interim conclusion is that the pathogenetic mechanisms of the two diseases are difficult. Similarities in the neuropathology, neurochemistry, and clinical features of PD with dementia and AD do not constitute evidence of a common etiology; like appearances do not imply like mechanisms. Nor would a single disease process necessarily have uniform manifestations; embolic stroke illustrates that point well. Two other kinds of evidence, however, are relevant to the issue of multiple or single disease processes: the rate of progression of disease, and genetic predisposition. PD and AD differ markedly on both counts. The rate of cognitive decline in PD is a small fraction of that found in AD.[37,40] It is believed that many (perhaps most) cases of AD are familial, whereas a genetic component in PD is unlikely. These differences suggest that different etiologies underlie PD and AD. Whatever proves to be the case, the quest for answers will enhance our knowledge about both diseases.

REFERENCES

1. Parkinson J. Essay on the Shaking Palsy. London: Whittingham and Rowland, 1817.
2. Alzheimer A. Uber mine eigenartige Erkrankung der Hirnrinde [peculiar disease of the cerebral cortex]. Allg Zeitschr Psychiatr 1907; 64:146–8.
3. Corkin S, Growdon JH, Nissen MJ. Comparison of the dementias in Parkinson's disease and Alzheimer's disease. Vllth International Symposium on Parkinson's Disease, Frankfurt, Federal Republic of Germany, 1982.
4. Gajdusek C. Hypothesis: interference of axonal transport of neural filament as a common pathogenetic mechanism in certain diseases of the nervous system. N Engl J Med 1985; 312:714–19.
5. Rocca WA, Amaducci LA, Schoenberg BS. Epidemiology of clinically diagnosed Alzheimer's disease. Ann Neurol 1986; 19:415–24.
6. Kessler II. Parkinson's disease: an epidemiologic perspective. Adv Neurol 1978; 19:355–84.

7. Schoenberg, BS. Descriptive epidemiology of Parkinson's disease: disease distribution and hypothesis formulation. In: Yahr MD and Bergmann KJ. Advances in neurology, Vol. 45 New York: Raven Press, 1986.

8. Mawdsley C. Parkinson's disease. In: Matthews WB, ed. Recent advances in clinical neurology. London: Churchill Livingstone, 1975.

9. Schoenberg BS, Anderson DW, and Haerer AF. Severe dementia: prevalence and clinical features in a biracial U.S. population. Arch Neurol 1985; 42:740–3.

10. Reef HE. Prevalence of Parkinson's disease in a multi-racial community. In: Jager WA, Bruyn GW, Jeijstee APJ, eds. 11th World Congress of Neurology. Amsterdam: Excerpta Medica, 1977.

11. Nee L, Polinsky RJ, Eldridge R, et al. A family with histologically confirmed Alzheimer's disease. Arch Neurol 1983; 40:203–8.

12. Mohs RC, Breitner JCS, Silverman JM, et al. Alzheimer's disease: morbid risk among first-degree relatives approximates 50% by 90 years of age. Arch Gen Psychiatry 1987; 44:405–8.

13. St. George-Hyslop PH, Tanzi RE, Polinsky RJ, et al. The genetic defect causing familial Alzheimer's disease maps on chromosome 21. Science 1987; 235:885–90.

14. Nee LE, Eldredge R, Sunderland T. Dementia of the Alzheimer type: clinical and family study of 22 twin pairs. Neurology 1987; 37:359–63.

15. Roses A, et al. Linkage analysis in late onset familial Alzheimer's disease. Cytogenet Cell Genet (in press).

16. Perlcak-Vance M, et al. Late onset Alzheimer's disease excluded from locus of early onset familial Alzheimer's disease. Science (submitted).

17. Duvolsin RC, Eldridge R, Williams A, et al. Twin study of Parkinson's disease. Neurology 1981; 31:77–80.

18. Gandy SE, Barclay LL, Cedarbaum JM. Age of onset of dementia in Parkinson's and Alzheimer's disease and the role of levodopa. Ann Neuro 1986; 20:150.

19. Albert M. Subcortical dementia. In: Katzman R, ed., Alzheimer's Disease: Senile Dementia and Related Disorders New York: Raven, 1978:173–80.

20. Benson DF. Subcortical dementia: a clinical approach. In: Mayeux R, Rosen WG, eds. The dementias New York: Raven, 1983:185–94.

21. Mayeux R, Stern Y. Intellectual dysfunction and dementia in Parkinson's disease. In: Mayeux R, Rosen WG, eds. The dementias New York: Raven, 1983:211–27.

22. Whitehouse P. The concept of subcortical and cortical dementia: another look. Ann Neuro 1986; 19:1–6.

23. Pillon B, Dubois B, Lhermitte F, et al. Heterogeneity of cognitive impairment in progressive supranuclear palsy, Parkinson's disease and Alzheimer's disease. Neurology 1986; 36:1179–85.

24. Growdon JH, Corkin S. Cognitive impairments in Parkinson's disease. In: Yahr MD, Bergmann KJ, eds. Advances in neurology: Parkinson's disease. New York: Raven, 1986:383–92.

25. Hakim AM, Mathieson G. Dementia in Parkinson's disease: a neuropathological study. Neurology 1979; 29:1209–14.

26. Perry EK, Curtis M, Dick DJ, et al. Cholinergic correlates of cognitive impairment in Parkinson's disease: comparisons with Alzheimer's disease. J Neurol Neurosurg Psychiatry 1985; 48:413–21.

27. Woodward JS. Clinicopathologic significance of granulovacular degeneration in Alzheimer's disease. J Neuropathol Exp Neurol 1962; 21:85–91.

28. Agid Y, Javoy-Agid F, Ruberg M, et al. Progressive supranuclear palsy: anatomoclinical and biochemical considerations. In: Yahr MD, Bergmann KJ, eds. Advances in neurology: Parkinson's disease. New York: Raven, 1986; 191–206.

29. Price D. New perspectives on Alzheimer's disease. Rev Neurosci 1986; 9:489–512.

30. Beal MF, Martin JB. Neuropeptides in neurological disease. Ann Neurol 1986; 20:547–65.

31. Ruberg M, Rieger F, Villageois AMB, et al. Acetylcholinesterase and butyrylcholinester-

ase in frontal cortex and cerebrospinal fluid of demented and non-demented patients with Parkinson's disease. Brain Res 1986; 362:83–91.

32. Perry EK, Tomlinson BE, Blessed G, et al. Correlation of cholinergic abnormalities with senile plaques and mental test-scores in senile dementia. Br Med J 1978; 2:1457–9.

33. Huff FJ, Growdon JH. Neurological abnormalities associated with severity of dementia in Alzheimer's disease. Can J Neurol Sci 1986; 13:403–5.

34. Pearce J. The extapyramidal disorder of Alzheimer's disease. Eur Neurol 1974; 12:94–103.

35. Moisa PK, Marttila RJ, Rinne UK. Extrapyramidal signs in Alzheimer's disease. Neurology 1974; 34:1114–16.

36. Parkes JD, Marsden CD, Rees JE, et al. Parkinson's disease. Cerebral arteriosclerosis and senile dementia. Q J Med 43:49–61.

37. Mildworf G, Globus M, Melamed E. Alzheimer's disease and Parkinson's disease: strategies for research and development. In: Fisher A, Hanin I, Lachman C, eds. Advances in behavioral biology. New York: Plenum, 1986; 29:135–40.

38. Teuber HL. Physiological psychology. Ann Rev Psychol 1955; 6:267–96.

39. Ogden J, Growdon JH, Corkin S. Impaired ability of patients with Parkinson's disease to shift conceptual set in visuospatial tasks. (Manuscript in preparation.)

40. Rosen TJ, Growdon JH, Corkin S. Comparison of rates of progression in Alzheimer's disease and Parkinson's disease. J Neural Transm [Supp] 1987; 24:105–7.

41. Blessed G, Tomlinson BE, Roth M. The association between quantitative measures of dementia and of senile changes in the grey matter of elderly patients. Br J Psychiatry 1968; 114:797–811.

42. Boller F, Passafiume D, Keefe NC, et al. Visuospatial impairment in Parkinson's disease: role of perceptual and motor factors. Arch Neurol 1984; 41:485–90.

43. Stroop JR. Studies of interference in serial verbal reactions. J Exp Psychol 1935; 18:643–62.

44. Kaplan E, Goodglass H, Weintraub S. The Boston naming test, Experimental edition. Boston: Boston University, 1978.

45. Money J. A standard road-map test of direction sense. San Rafael: Academic Therapy Publications, 1976.

46. Rosen TJ, Corkin S. The definition and comparison of performance deficits: some statistical solutions. Pro Abstr Eastern Psychol Assoc 1985; 56:19.

47. Rosen TJ, Corkin S. On the analysis of disparate variables: assessing quantitative and qualitative group differences. Proc Abstr Eastern Psychol Assoc 1986; 43. (Abstr. no. 86-537.

48. Corkin S, Cohen NJ, Sullivan EV, et al. Analyses of global memory impairments of different etiologies. In: Olton DS, Gamzu E, Corkin S, eds. Memory dysfunctions; an integration of animal and human research from preclinical and clinical perspectives. Ann NY Acad Sci 1985; 444:10–40.

Chapter 23

Quantitative Aspects of Specific Developmental Disorders

Dorothy V.M. Bishop

Specific developmental disorders are defined as conditions in which, for no apparent reason, one specific aspect of development is impaired. Specific reading retardation (developmental dyslexia) and specific language impairment (developmental aphasia) are the commonest disorders of this kind. These conditions pose logical and methodologic problems in definition and assessment:

1. Is it valid to regard such disorders as cases of minimal brain damage?
2. Do these conditions constitute syndromes, or do they merely represent an extreme range of normal variation?
3. How can we quantify the behaviors on which our definitions are based? The focus of this chapter largely concerns the assessment of spoken language and the need to go beyond a simple dichotomy between expressive and receptive language.
4. How should we define impairment? Interpreting scores in terms of lag between test age and chronologic age can be misleading; a statistical approach using standardized scores is preferable.
5. How can we operationalize the exclusion criteria implicit in the definition of specific developmental disorders? Pitfalls are associated with a cutoff approach, which maintains that such variables as IQ and hearing level must be above a certain level to permit the diagnosis of specific developmental disorders. A regression-based approach, developed in studies of specific reading retardation, is more satisfactory.

THE CONCEPT OF SPECIFIC DEVELOPMENTAL DISORDER

Over the past three decades, there has been a gradual change in the population of children referred to pediatric neurologists. Thirty years ago, virtually all referrals were for conditions with a clear-cut physical basis (e.g., spina bifida, cerebral palsy, epilepsy). More recently, a new category of referrals has accounted for a small but significant proportion of cases. This category includes children who for no apparent reason fail to make normal progress in one specific area of mental development—typically, the mastery of spoken and/or written language. They do not fit the picture of intellectual retardation, because only isolated aspects of mental function are affected. In the third edition of *Diagnostic and Statistical Manual of Mental Disorders (DSM-III)*,[1] such disorders are labeled *specific developmental disorders* and defined as a subclass of "disorders of specific areas of development not due to another disorder" (p. 92).

Clinical and research studies with such children have been fraught with controversy and confusion. There is disagreement about terminology, about defining criteria, and about whether it makes sense to include such disorders in a medical diagnostic framework. Consider the following definition:

> Children with Specific Learning Disabilities exhibit a disorder in one or more of the basic psychological processes involved in understanding or in using spoken or written language. These may be manifested in disorders of listening, thinking, talking, reading, writing, spelling or arithmetic. They include conditions that have been referred to as perceptual handicaps, brain injury, minimal brain dysfunction, dyslexia, developmental aphasia, etc. They do not include learning problems that are due primarily to visual, hearing, or motor handicaps, to mental retardation, emotional disturbance, or to environmental disadvantage.[2]

This definition, which differs in many respects from the diagnostic criteria that can be applied to most medical conditions, has a number of problematic features:

1. The physical basis of the disorder is not understood.
2. The category is defined in terms of quantitative departures from normal functioning, not in terms of a constellation of symptoms.
3. The "basic psychological processes" are not easily quantifiable.
4. The definition of what level of performance constitutes a disorder depends on age.
5. The definition relies heavily on diagnosis by exclusion.

PHYSICAL BASIS OF SPECIFIC DEVELOPMENTAL DISORDERS

The apparent similarity between specific developmental disorders and the selective disturbances of higher mental functions that occur in association with localized cerebral lesions in adults led early workers to apply adult terminology to children, giving terms such as *developmental aphasia* and *developmental dyslexia*. However, the parallel with adult, acquired conditions is misleading in its implication of a clear-cut physical basis for the disorder. Research on this point is scant and controversial, but it seems that most learning-disabled children—except for those with profound comprehension problems or behavioral disorders—appear to be neurologically normal when studied with such techniques as electroencephalography or CT scan.[3] Given the lack of evidence for brain damage in these children, it is misleading to use the term *minimal brain damage* to describe their condition. *Minimal brain dysfunction* has been proposed as a more acceptable alternative, but this too implies that we have some understanding of the organic basis of the disorder. Although it is not implausible that a structural or biochemical abnormality in neurologic development underlies specific developmental disorders, it is impolitic to label a disorder in terms of a postulated cause for which there is no hard evidence.

SPECIFIC DEVELOPMENTAL DISORDER:
A SYNDROME OR A STATISTICAL ABNORMALITY?

Suppose we have two quantitative variables, such as reading ability and IQ, in a bivariate normal distribution. Inevitably, some children score 2 SD or more below the mean on the first measure. Furthermore, some of these children will score within the normal range on the second measure, the proportion depending on the correlation between the two tests. Is it valid to give this subset of children a medical diagnosis that distinguishes them from other children with poor reading scores, when they have no detectable physical abnormality and are defined as disordered purely on statistical grounds? In other words, is there a distinctive condition of "developmental dyslexia" that afflicts some children, or is this just a convenient label for children whose scores fall in a particular region of the bivariate normal distribution?

Yule and Rutter[4] used empirical data to address this issue, considering three basic questions. First: Does the number of children with a disproportionate impairment in reading skill exceed the number that would be expected on the basis of a normal distribution of reading scores and linear regression of IQ on reading? Using epidemiologic data, they demonstrated that this was indeed the case, lending justification to the notion that a specific condition accounted for selective reading impairment in some children. However, this particular result has been disputed.[5,6] Second: Do children with "specific reading retardation" (i.e., poor reading attainment discrepant with IQ) differ from other poor readers? The data gave a positive answer; differences in the pattern of associated deficits, in prognosis, and in sex ratio were found between these groups. Third: Does developmental dyslexia constitute a syndrome in the usual sense of the word (i.e., is there a particular constellation of symptoms that characterize this group)? Rutter[7] found no evidence for a unitary syndrome with the features traditionally regarded as characteristic of dyslexia. He concluded that although it is valid to distinguish between poor readers of low intelligence and children with disproportionately severe reading problems relative to IQ, the latter have a variable pattern of disorder and underlying causes. It therefore seems preferable to use a label such as *specific reading retardation,* which does not imply a unitary disease entity.

The epidemiologic approach adopted by Yule and Rutter has not yet been applied to other specific developmental disorders. However, the arguments against using medical terminology have been widely accepted and extended to developmental problems involving spoken lanuage, so that *specific language disorder* (or *impairment* or *disability*) is now frequently preferred over *developmental aphasia.*

There are subtle but important consequences of such a choice of terminology. A medical label can gain better educational provisions for a child (or even special dispensation when taking public examinations) and may elicit more sympathetic treatment from the general public by implying that the child is the unfortunate victim of a disease.

QUANTIFICATION OF LANGUAGE ABILITY

Most quantitative techniques in this field require training in psychology and linguistics, which few physicians are willing or able to undertake. My aim is not to provide an assessment protocol, but rather to demystify an area in which the terminology leaves many perplexed about the meanings of particular measures.

Spoken Language

The measurement of language skills is continually changing, reflecting developments in linguistic theory. A distinction has traditionally been made between expressive and receptive language, but many components of linguistic skill may be distinguished within each of these areas.

Expressive Language

The language spoken by a child can be evaluated under four main headings: phonology, grammar, semantics, and pragmatics.

Phonology: Mastery of the Speech Sound System

The term *phonological disorder* is now widely used for problems previously considered to be articulation disorders. This shift in terminology reflects a change of emphasis from the motor aspects of speech production to a linguistic conceptualization of these disorders.[8] Impairment of expressive phonology is extremely common in the child with a specific language disorder and may be the only noticeable linguistic deficit. Frequently, the child persists in using speech sounds in a very immature way. The following characteristics are particularly common:[9]

1. Some children make fewer distinctions between speech sounds than do adults. For example, many do not use the velar place of articulation, so that /k/ and /g/ are produced as /t/ and /d/ (e.g., *Goldilocks* is pronounced "doldilots").
2. Some children use only a consonant-vowel syllabic pattern ("open syllables"); e.g., *house* is pronounced "hou"; *cat* is pronounced "ca".
3. Some may reduce consonant clusters to a single consonant (e.g., *string* is pronounced "ting").

A child with more than one such immaturity may be highly unintelligble. Not all cases of phonological disorder can be classed as immaturities, but in most cases phonological analysis indicates that the child's use of speech sounds follows some consistent pattern (see Bishop and Rosenblom[10] for a discussion of the diagnostic significance of this). Because mastery of the adult sound system is nearly perfect in most children by the age of 4 years, it is seldom hard to decide whether or not a child has a phonological impairment unless the child is very young. Even an untrained ear can detect mispronunciations of words and recognize them as abnormal in a school-age child.

Expertise in phonetics is required for analysis of the nature and severity of a phonological problem. The simplest index of severity of disorder is some count of mispronounced sounds such as percentage of correctly pronounced consonants.[11] More complex qualitative analyses, which take into account the pattern as well as the number of phonological errors,[8] play an important role in the planning of therapy but are unnecessarily complex if the main concern is merely to determine whether or not a problem exists.

Grammar: Mastery of Language Form

Limited mastery of grammatical structure is another common feature of expressive language disorders in children. The child uses short, telegrammatic sentences as would a much younger child, and typically omits articles, prepositions, inflections, and auxiliary verbs in many contexts.

Techniques for assessing grammatical development range from simple counts of sentence length (suitable for giving a general estimate of severity of impairment) to complex grammatical analyses that give a much more detailed picture of the child's use of grammar.[12] Brown[13] popularized the use of mean length of utterance (MLU) as a simple summary index of level of grammatical development. MLU is a measure of average sentence length, in which the unit of measurement is the morpheme rather than the word. Morphemes, the most basic, indivisible elements of linguistic meaning, include grammatical inflections, prefixes, and suffixes, as well as uninflected words. A word may consist of a single morpheme (e.g., *dog, man*) or of several (e.g., *go-ing* consists of two morphemes; *un-man-ly,* three). In using the morpheme (rather than the word) as a unit, one can distinguish between a child who uses grammatical morphemes such as *-ing* and *-ed* and one who uses a similar number of words per utterance but does not produce inflections. MLU is widely used in research on language development and disorders, but its reliability and validity as a clinical tool have not yet been properly evaluated. Its value declines in older children because the increasing grammatical complexity of their speech is accomplished by devices that do not necessarily increase sentence length. Also, one's estimate of MLU may depend on the situation in which one chooses to record a child's language. Research on normal development usually aims to measure language in as natural a setting as possible, but this can be time-consuming and may yield very little data in a language-impaired child.

In a clinical setting, techniques for eliciting language from a child (e.g., a specific set of questions about pictures) are more convenient and may better indicate the child's capability, despite the artificial situation. A number of tests use this approach and provide criteria for scoring each response, depending on whether specific grammatical constructions are used. The final score can be related to normative data.[14-16]

The criterion for grammatical adequacy should be acceptability in the child's speech community, not some imposed standard of "correct grammar." For instance, "I ain't got nothing" is normal usage in many cultures, whereas an utterance such as "Me no got" is abnormal in any child over 4 years of age. Crystal et al.[12] point out that some tests penalize children if their response to a question omits elements of the sentence. For example, when asked "What's the girl doing?" the child obtains a higher score by responding, "The girl is sitting on the chair" than by giving the much more natural elliptical response, "Sitting on the chair." Clearly, such tests are undesirable.

There is debate in the literature regarding the extent to which phonological and grammatical problems are inter-related.[17] It seems that although the two types of disorder may be dissociated, they do tend to occur together with well-above-chance frequency.[18]

Semantics: Selecting Words and Combinations of Words to Convey Meaning

Grammatical analysis is concerned with the form of a child's language, whereas semantics is concerned with content. An expressive semantic problem exists when a child is poor at conveying meaning, even though his or her grammatical skills may be reasonable. For example, the child may have a limited vocabulary and use "filler" terms rather than precise words. Thus, whereas a 6-year-old with a grammatical deficit might say, "Goldilock sit chair. Eat porridge," a child with a selective semantic deficit might say, "The girl sat on something and ate some stuff." Note that although the first child's language is more likely to be identified as abnormal, the second child is far less effective at communicating information.

A number of tests assess a child's ability to convey information irrespective of his or her level of grammatical skill. The simplest approach is to assess the child's vocabulary by counting how many pictures or objects from a given set are named correctly. This approach can be extended to measuring how many "ideas" the child can convey when asked to describe a picture or tell a story. In Renfrew's Bus Story test,[19] for example, the child is told a story accompanied by cartoon pictures and is then asked to tell the story back to the tester, using the picture sequence to aid memory. The child is awarded points for each predefined "idea" that is produced. Bishop and Edmundson[18] found that expressive semantic ability, as measured by the Bus Story test, was the single best predictor of later outcome in a group of language-impaired 4-year-olds. Even in those with severe phonological and/or grammatical problems, outcome was good if they were able to convey the main content of the story adequately.

Pragmatics: Ability to Use Language Appropriately

The most recent linguistic development to influence the assessment of language disorder has been the rapid expansion of interest in pragmatics, the area of linguistics concerned with the skills needed to use language appropriately in a given situation. Some children have difficulties in this area, apparently because they are insensitive to the needs of the people listening to them. They may introduce a new topic without adequate explanation, failing to realize that the listener does not share their knowledge and needs some background information. A child telling a story may produce a sequence of sentences that is phonologically, grammatically, and semantically perfect, but the story will be hard to understand if the needs of the listener are not fulfilled. For example, the child may plunge into the middle of the story without introducing the characters properly. This child may digress so that the thread of the story is lost, or may use an inappropriately stilted style of speech, or may fail to respond to signs of incomprehension made by the listener. It is a moot point whether such difficulties should be conceptualized as deficits in social skills or language problems. Analysis of the complex range of pragmatic skills is still very much at the stage of qualitative description, but the considerable research interest in this area suggests that standardized quantitative assessment techniques are not far away.[20,21]

Receptive Language

In principle, receptive language can be subdivided in the same way as expressive language. Thus, a child's failure to understand what an adult says could represent difficulty in discriminating speech sounds (a phonological problem), difficulty in interpreting word order and inflections (a grammatical problem), difficulty in understanding the meanings of individual words (a semantic problem), or a failure to understand things that are implied but not directly stated (a pragmatic problem). Furthermore, the child may fail to understand a sentence because he or she did not pay attention to it or does not remember it. In practice, it often proves difficult to disentangle the sources of failure, since problems in one aspect of processing affect others. For example, a difficulty in discriminating speech sounds impairs the ability to understand word meaning. Less obviously, poor understanding of word meaning may affect speech discrimination (this will be discussed later). Rather than attempting to evaluate all aspects of receptive language in every case, it makes sense to adopt a hypothesis-testing approach by which different sources of comprehension failure are successively ruled out. If one can show, for example, that a child's understanding of word meanings is adequate, then it is safe to assume that the child has no serious problems in discriminating speech sounds.

Phonology

To understand language, it is not enough just to perceive that a sound has occurred; one must also be able to translate the acoustic waveform into linguistic units. Work in adult neurology has shown that certain brain lesions can interfere with this process, resulting in deficits ranging from inability to discriminate speech sounds to much more subtle impairments, such as inability to integrate information from the two ears or to understand distorted speech. Various elegant behavioral techniques have been developed for diagnosing lesions of the auditory pathway at the level of the brainstem and beyond.[22]

The notion that some kind of perceptual problem may be at the root of specific learning disabilities has long been popular, and at first glance may seem to be a fairly straightforward hypothesis to test clinically. However, there are difficulties.

The most obvious problem concerns the assessment of the ability to discriminate speech sounds. Two methods have been widely used. The first involves showing pairs of pictures with confusable names (e.g., *coat* and *goat*) and asking the child to point to the one named. However, a child may be able to discriminate the sounds of *coat* and *goat* yet not know what a goat is. In other words, failure on such a test may be a sign of a semantic rather than a phonological problem. An alternative is to present pairs of spoken words, to be judged by the child as "same" or "different." This technique is adopted in the Wepman discrimination test, which is widely used in the United States.[23] However, although this may be a useful way of assessing mild problems, young children and those with severe receptive problems may not understand the meaning of *same* and *different*.

Methodologic problems are not restricted to the assessment of children with severe comprehension difficulties. Suppose we are interested in looking for evidence of subtle auditory-perceptual problems in a language-impaired child who can understand a basic vocabulary and cope with simple task requirements. Unfortunately, there has been a tendency to assume that the diagnostic techniques developed for adults have a similar significance in children, and that poor performance implies dysfunction, if not an actual lesion of the central auditory pathways. The concept of central auditory dysfunction[24] has become a popular explanation for learning disabilities.

The extension of test methods from adults to children ignores the influence of language ability on the performance of central auditory tasks. Experimental psychologists have demonstrated that speech perception is not simply a "bottom-up" or "data-driven" process but is also subject to "top-down" influences (see Anderson[25] for a short, clear account). In other words, our knowledge of language affects our perception. As a simple example, consider how much easier it is to remember or discriminate a set of familiar words than words from a foreign language. Seymour et al.[26] note that a child's performance on a speech-sound discrimination task will be better with real words than with nonwords and will also depend on the familiarity of the words used. The clinical implication of this should be obvious: Any child who is weak in such areas as semantics and syntax will be less able to benefit by applying "top-down" processing in perceptual tasks and so will probably earn a low score on speech discrimination tests and measures of central auditory function. One cannot conclude with validity that a language disorder is the consequence of a perceptual disability or a central auditory dysfunction in such cases.

This logical problem is not insuperable. One possible solution is to compare the performance of a language-disordered child with the performances of younger, normal children of similar language level. If the language-disordered child performs more poorly than this group, a perceptual problem clearly exists that is not simply attributable to linguistic deficits.

Grammar

Several standardized tests are suitable for investigating the understanding of grammatical structure (e.g., part 5 of the Token Test,[27,28] the Test for Auditory Comprehension of Language,[29] and the Test for Reception of Grammar [TROG][30]). These tests demand little in the way of pragmatic or vocabulary skills. The child is presented with

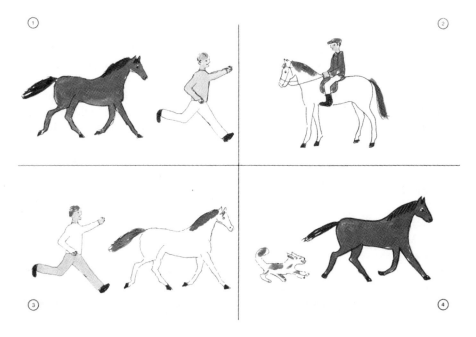

FIGURE 23.1   *Sample item from the Test for Reception of Grammar. The child must select the picture corresponding to the statement, "The horse is chased by the man." Selection of picture 1 is a grammatical error, whereas selection of pictures 2 or 4 indicates other reasons for poor comprehension, such as weak vocabulary, poor memory, or inattention.*

a circumscribed set of alternatives and given an instruction that uses simple vocabulary but increasingly complex grammar. Figure 23.1 shows a sample test item from TROG.[30]

One should beware of assuming that poor performance on such a test necessarily indicates a grammatical problem. Failure may occur because of inattention, poor memory, or failure to understand individual words used in the test. Although these causes of failure cannot be eliminated, it is possible to design a test so that errors due to these causes can be identified. In TROG, a vocabulary pretest is first given to see if the child knows the meanings of individual words used in the test. The pattern of errors reveals whether grammatical complexity is causing the most difficulty or whether the child tends to select a picture that shows a wrong noun or verb, indicating more general problems.

Semantics

Multiple-choice tests of understanding of individual word meanings (e.g., the Peabody Picture Vocabulary Test[31]) have been in existence for many years. Many children with specific language impairment who do not have obvious difficulties in understanding casual conversation can be shown to have comprehension problems when such tests are used (with understanding of grammatical structure being even more impaired).[32]

Pragmatics

Analysis of receptive pragmatic problems is still at a descriptive stage. A child with pragmatic problems may do well on any comprehension test where performance depends purely on a correct literal interpretation of complicated instructions, but may have difficulty in understanding what is not stated explicitly. If, for example, one says "John was at the beach. He stepped on some broken glass. He had to go to the hospital," a listener should be able to infer many things that have not been directly stated (e.g., John was not wearing shoes; the glass cut his foot). Some children appear to have difficulty in drawing these sorts of inferences and therefore have tremendous problems in understanding everyday conversation, even though they are apparently unimpaired when tested with more concrete, literal types of multiple-choice assessment.

Written Language

There are two basic approaches to evaluating reading ability: assessment of the child's oral reading of single words, and assessment of comprehension of sentences or longer passages that are read aloud or silently. The latter method is often preferred on the grounds that it provides a more meaningful estimate of the child's ability to make use of written information. However, single-word reading is more suitable if one is interested in analyzing the nature of a child's reading errors.[33]

CRITERIA FOR DEFINING IMPAIRMENT

Assessment of children is inevitably more complex than that of adults, since one cannot use any absolute standard as an index of impairment. Behavior that is abnormal in an 8-year-old may be normal in a 4-year-old. Thus, we need normative data on children of various ages before we can determine whether a score on a particular measure represents normal or impaired performance. All too often, these data are lacking. Test standardization is typically expensive, tedious, and time-consuming, and, for adequate standardization of a developmental test, the need for data on children of different ages means that the numbers involved are substantial. This problem is particularly acute in the field of language because new techniques of assessment are continually developing in the wake of theoretical advances in linguistics. McCauley and Swisher[34] have noted that many language assessments in current clinical use are poorly standardized and provide little or no information on reliability and validity.

Suppose, however, that there does exist a range of measures that have been adequately standardized on a nationally representative sample of children over a wide age range. How should we define impairment? One common method is to transform scores to age-equivalent scores and to rate impairment in terms of the discrepancy between such scores and chronologic age. This procedure is adopted by Stark and Tallal,[35] who propose a definition of "specific language impairment" in terms of the gap between chronologic age and "language age." There are, however, serious drawbacks to this approach.[36] The main difficulty is that it can give a misleading impression of severity of language impairment if (as is often the case) the variance of scores at any one age is high, relative to the variance associated with age.

Consider the hypothetical cases shown in Figures 23.2 and 23.3. Where variance within each age group is high relative to variance between age groups, it is not uncommon for children to obtain a score which would be average for a child one or two years younger. To say that an 8-year-old has a language age of 6 years sounds like a serious deficit, yet such a conclusion would be erroneous, as this type of score is common in normal 8-year-olds. However, when variance within an age group is small and variance between age groups is high (see Figure 23.3), a two-year lag in language attainment represents an unusual degree of impairment. For many language tests in common use, the situation is further complicated by the fact that the relationship between raw score and age is not a linear function but tends to level off at the upper age range (see Figure 23.4). Typically, ceiling effects become evident at the higher age levels, so within-age variance decreases with age. In such a situation, the clinical significance of a given lag in language age relative to chronologic age is not constant but depends on the age of

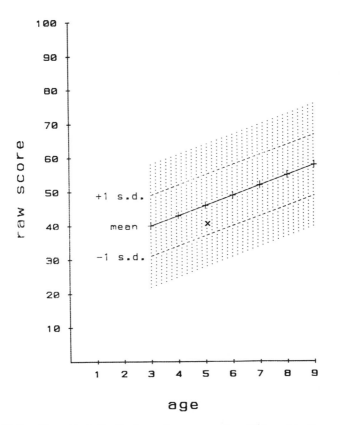

FIGURE 23.2 *Theoretical distributions of test scores for children 4 to 8 years of age. The variance within each age group is large relative to the variance between age groups, so it is not unusual for a child to obtain a score equivalent to the average score for children two years younger (point x).*

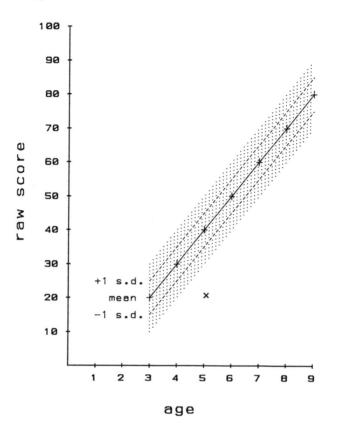

FIGURE 23.3   *Theoretical distributions of test scores for children 4 to 8 years of age, showing a situation in which the variance within each age group is small relative to the variance between age groups. It is very unusual for a child to obtain a score equivalent to the average score for children two years younger (point x).*

the child. As shown in Figure 23.4, a two-year lag at 9 years of age is a far less serious deficit than a two-year lag at 5 years of age. Nonlinear relationships between test score and age thus invalidate the use of chronologic age minus language age as a constant indicator of degree of deficit.

Similar arguments in the field of mental testing led designers of early intelligence tests to adopt a ratio measure, the IQ, in which "mental age" was expressed as a percentage of chronologic age. Analogous reading quotients or language quotients have sometimes been adopted in the assessment of specific developmental disorders, but there is little justification for this approach. Although it does mitigate some of the more obvious problems that arise when the function relating test score to age approaches a ceiling, it does not overcome the lack of comparability of language measures with different variances.

In intelligence testing, the solution has been to abandon the use of age-equivalent scores and instead to convert scores at each age to z-scores or some transformation

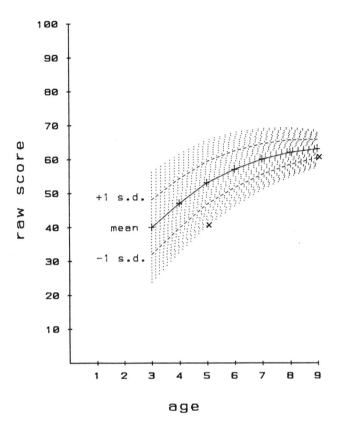

FIGURE 23.4 *Theoretical distributions of test scores for children 4 to 8 years of age, showing a situation in which mean scores start to level off and within-age variance decreases with increasing age. It is much more abnormal to obtain a score 2 years below age level at 5 years of age than at 9 years of age (see points marked x).*

of these—typically, standardized scores with means of 100 and standard deviations of 15. This approach gives a statistically defined index of severity of impairment that has the same meaning at different ages and across different tests. One can make a strong case for adopting a similar approach in language and reading assessment.

The particular cutoff point used to define impairment will vary. A fairly lenient cutoff (e.g., 10th percentile) may be appropriate when screening children for referral to a speech-language pathologist, whereas a much more stringent cutoff (e.g., 3rd percentile) may be used when deciding whether to recommend a child for special educational placement.

Deciding on criteria for impairment is straightforward enough if one is using a single test measure, but one often wants to make use of data from a whole battery of measures, particularly when assessing children with disorders of spoken language. This raises the question of how to combine information from different sources.

One solution is to average scores from different tests. Stark and Tallal[35] used scores from four expressive tests (mostly measuring grammatical ability) to arrive at an average "expressive language age." They used the Token test, the Test of Comprehension of Language, and two subtests from the Illinois Test of Psycholinguistic Abilities[37] to give an average "receptive language age." They then defined specific language impairment as a lag in expressive language age of at least 12 months and a lag in receptive language age of at least 6 months. There is, of course, no reason why a similar averaging approach should not be used with standard scores. However, average scores will give a misleading impression for children who have uneven patterns of language impairment, with some abilities in the normal range and others well below average. Stark and Tallal's study suggested that their definition may be over-restrictive. In a sample of children referred by specialists as cases of developmental language impairment, only half of those with normal nonverbal abilities fitted their criterion of specific language impairment. Many children were excluded because they had selective problems with isolated aspects of language function (e.g., those with severe expressive problems but normal comprehension were invariably excluded).

One may therefore prefer a less restrictive definition, whereby a child is regarded as language-impaired if his or her performance on any test falls well below normal limits. Bishop and Edmundson[18] evaluated a group of 4-year-olds on a range of expressive and receptive lanugage measures according to predefined quantitative criteria of impairment. There was variability from test to test in the number of children who scored in the impaired range. Expressive phonology and grammar were the most vulnerable language functions, whereas impairment was relatively uncommon on measures of expressive vocabulary and comprehension. Many children with problems severe enough to bring them to the attention of a specialist would not have been categorized as language-impaired if the average score on a language assessment were considered alone.

Clearly, a criterion based on an averaging procedure will result in a different sample of language-impaired children from one that looks for evidence of impairment in any one or more of several language functions. Which criterion, then, should one adopt? The answer will be determined partly by practical issues and partly by further empirical work. A restrictive criterion may be appropriate in a research setting, where one hopes—by selecting the most severe and unambiguous cases—to maximize any differences between experimental subjects and controls. However, where the aim is to identify children in need of therapy or special schooling, it seems more appropriate to use a method that picks out children who have severe difficulties in any area of functioning, irrespective of their average language attainment. In any case, we need more research on the practical implications of adopting one type of definition over another.

PROBLEMS OF DIAGNOSIS BY EXCLUSION

The definition of specific developmental disorder makes it clear that it is not enough to demonstrate that a child's performance on a language or reading test is poor for his or her age. One must also demonstrate that this impairment is not due to sensory or motor handicaps, mental retardation, emotional disturbance, or environmental disadvantage. These exclusions pose no problem when none of these factors apply, or when a condition such as profound hearing loss or severe subnormality is present and is clearly the main factor responsible for learning disability. Difficulties do arise, however, in less extreme cases. How severe a language or reading problem should we expect in a child with a 40-decibel hearing loss? Or in a child with a performance IQ of 70? In most cases, we do not know. The usual response to this problem is to choose an arbitrary cutoff point and exclude any child with a more severe handicap. Typically, a child is regarded as having a specific developmental disorder only if Wechsler Intelligence Scale for Children (WISC) performance IQ is at least 85, hearing threshold is no more than 20 decibels in the speech frequencies, and there is no evidence of any sensorimotor handicap or psychiatric disturbance. Such criteria provide a reasonable operational definition to use in a research study, as they yield a fairly homogeneous sample of children, but there are both logical and practical objections to their use in clinical diagnosis.

One problem is that one cannot assume that delayed language development or poor reading ability occurring in the context of a low IQ, hearing loss, or other handicap is necessarily caused by such conditions. It is logically possible for a child to have more than one disorder. We can only assume that a language/reading problem is totally explained in terms of another handicap if we know enough about the effects of that handicap on language development to specify whether the child's progress is within normal limits for children with that condition. Often, this is hard to judge. In practice, it is not uncommon to find children with moderate hearing loss or mild intellectual retardation whose severe reading or language problems seem disproportionate to the degree of handicap. However, when hearing or IQ falls below the cutoff level for defining a specific developmental disorder, these children are all too often placed in an educational limbo, denied access to suitable remedial help.

Yule and Rutter[4] pointed out that one can escape from the inconsistencies of using an IQ cutoff when defining specific reading retardation if one knows the correlation between reading score and IQ in the normal population. Epidemiologic data were used to compute the regression equation for predicting reading ability from IQ for children of different ages, so that children who were reading significantly below the level predicted on the basis of age and IQ could be identified. This approach defines a different subset of children from the cutoff approach, as can be seen in Figure 23.5. The figure shows that the regression-based approach selects all children falling below the line AB as cases of specific reading retardation; the more traditional cutoff approach would include only those backward readers (below line CD) with IQ scores above criterion (specified by line EF). Note that the regression criterion includes some children whose reading is only moderately below age level but who are nevertheless retarded, relative to the level expected on the basis of their high IQ (in area bounded by BHD). On the other hand, the criterion may exclude some children who would have been included in the original definition—those whose IQs are just above the cutoff point and whose low reading scores are not inconsistent with the level predicted by IQ (those falling in area EGH). Most important, the regression approach allows for the possibility of specific reading problems in children with low IQ (those falling in the area bounded by AGF, where reading is well below the level predicted, even given the low IQ).

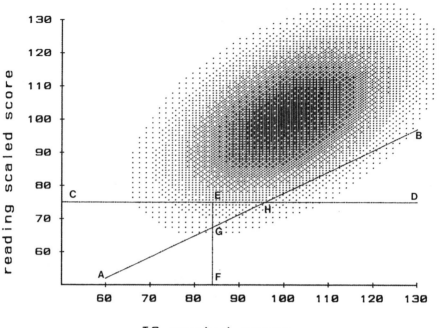

FIGURE 23.5   *Scatter plot of theoretical bivariate normal distribution of reading and IQ scaled scores. Cases falling below line AB have reading scores significantly below the level predicted on the basis of IQ ("specific reading retardation"). Cases below line CD obtain low reading scores irrespective of IQ ("backward readers"). Line EF divides the sample into cases of low IQ and the remainder. The area bounded by FED contains cases that would be defined as having specific learning disability by the conventional "cutoff" approach.*

FUTURE DIRECTIONS FOR RESEARCH

One message of this chapter is that language is not a unitary function but one that involves a range of different abilities, each of which may be selectively impaired. The reader may begin to wonder, however, where this process of subdivision and refinement of linguistic abilities will end. In the past, we were happy with one or two measures of expressive and receptive language skill. Now we are talking of subdividing each of these into component processes, with new concepts such as pragmatics threatening to spawn yet more new categories. Are we not in danger of becoming submerged under this welter of linguistic information?

What we need is research to evaluate the meaning and utility of various language measures in different settings. There is a tendency to assume that a complex, detailed measure must be superior to a short and simple one, but this is not necessarily so. The assessment method used should depend on the question being asked. Bishop and Edmundson[18] evaluated the efficacy of a battery of short tests assessing a range of language functions in predicting outcome in language-impaired 4-year-olds. It was found that outcome could be predicted with an impressively high degree of accuracy on the basis of performance on quick and simple tests that required little or no linguistic expertise. Furthermore, a large battery of tests was not necessary: there was only a small reduction in predictive accuracy when a single assessment was used. We need more research studies that look critically at the means we use to quantify language skills. A good measure is not necessarily one derived from a currently fashionable linguistic theory. Rather, it is one that tells us something about etiology or prognosis of the disorder or enables us to predict what type of treatment will be most effective.

REFERENCES

1. American Psychiatric Association. Diagnostic and statistical manual of mental disorders, 3 ed. (DSM-III) Washington, DC: American Psychiatric Association, 1980.
2. National Advisory Committee on Handicapped Children, cited in Gaddes WH. Prevalence estimates and the need for definition of learning disabilities. In: Knights RM, Bakker DJ, eds. The neuropsychology of learning disorders: theoretical approaches. Baltimore: University Park Press, 1976.
3. Bishop DVM. The causes of specific developmental language disorder ("developmental dysphasia"). J Child Psychiat 1987; 28:1–8.
4. Yule W, Rutter M. Epidemiology and social implications of specific reading retardation. In: Knights RM, Bakker DJ, eds. The neuropsychology of learning disorders: theoretical approaches. Baltimore: University Park Press, 1976.
5. Rodgers B. The identification and prevalence of specific reading retardation. Br J Educ Psychol 1983; 53:369–73.
6. Van der Wissel A, Zegers FE. Reading retardation revisited. Br J Dev Psychol 1985; 3:3–9.
7. Rutter M. The concept of "dyslexia." In: Wolff P, MacKeith RC, eds. Planning for better learning. Clinics in developmental medicine 33. London: Heinemann, 1969.
8. Grunwell P. Clinical phonology. London: Croom Helm, 1982.
9. Ingram D. Procedures for the Phonological Analysis of Children's Language. Baltimore: University Park Press, 1981.
10. Bishop DVM, Rosenbloom L. Classification of childhood language disorders. In: Yule W, Rutter M, eds. Language Development and Disorders. Clinics in Developmental Medicine (double issue). 101–102:16–41. London: MacKeith Press, 1987.
11. Shriberg L, Kwiatkowski J. Phonological disorders III: A procedure for assessing severity of involvement. J Speech Hear Disord 1982; 47:256–70.
12. Crystal D, Fletcher P, Garman M. The grammatical analysis of language disability. London: Edward Arnold, 1976.
13. Brown R. A first language: the early stages. London: Penguin Books, 1973.
14. Renfrew CE. Action picture test. 1966. Available from author at North Place, Old Headington, Oxford, England.
15. Lee LL. Northwestern Syntax Screening Test. Evanston, IL: Northwestern University Press, 1971.
16. Carrow E. Elicited Language Inventory. Boston: Ginn, 1979.
17. Panagos JM, Prelock PA. Phonological constraints on the sentence productions of language-disordered children. J Speech Hear Res 1982; 25:171–7.
18. Bishop DVM, Edmundson A. Language-impaired four-year-olds: distinguishing transient from persistent impairment. J Speech Hear Disord 1987; 52:156–73.
19. Renfrew CE. The bus story: a test of continuous speech. 1969. Available from author at North Place, Old Headington, Oxford, England.

20. Gallagher TM, Prutting CA. Pragmatic assessment and intervention issues in language. San Diego: College Hill, 1983.
21. Roth FP. Assessing the pragmatic abilities of children: Part 2. Guidelines, considerations, and specific evaluation procedures. J Speech Hear Disord 1984; 49:12–17.
22. Jerger J. Auditory tests for disorders of the central auditory mechanism. In: Fields WS, Alford BR, eds. Neurological aspects of auditory and vestibular disorders. Springfield, Ill: Charles Thomas, 1964.
23. Wepman JM. Auditory discrimination test. Chicago: Language Research Associates, 1973.
24. Keith RW. Central auditory dysfunction. New York: Grune & Stratton, 1977.
25. Anderson JR. Cognitive psychology and its implications. San Francisco: Freeman, 1980.
26. Seymour CM, Baran JA, Peaper RE. Auditory discrimination: evaluation and intervention. In: Lass NJ, ed. Speech and language: advances in basic research and practice. New York: Academic, 1981; 6.
27. De Renzi E, Vignolo LA. The Token Test: a sensitive test to detect receptive disturbances in aphasia. Brain 1962; 85:665–78.
28. Whitaker HA, Noll JD. Some linguistic parameters of the Token Test. Neuropsychologia 1972; 10:398–404.
29. Carrow E. Test for Auditory Comprehension of Language. Allen, TX: DLM Teaching Resources.
30. Bishop DVM. Test for Reception of Grammar, 1983. Available from author at Department of Psychology, University of Manchester, U.K.
31. Dunn LM. Expanded manual for the Peabody Picture Vocabulary Test. Minneapolis: American Guidance Service, 1965.
32. Bishop DVM. Comprehension in developmental language disorders. Dev Med Child Neurol 1979; 21:225–38.
33. Boder E. Developmental dyslexia: a diagnostic approach based on three reading-spelling patterns. Dev Med Child Neurol 1973; 15: 663–87.
34. McCauley RJ, Swisher L. Psychometric review of language and articulation tests for pre-school children. J Speech Hear Disord 1984; 49:34–42.
35. Stark RE, Tallal P. Selection of children with specific language deficits. J Speech Hear Disord 1981; 46:114–22.
36. McCauley RJ, Swisher L. Use and misuse of norm-referenced tests in clinical assessment: a hypothetical case. J Speech Hear Disord 1984; 49:338–48.
37. Kirk SJ, McCarthy J, Kirk WD. Illinois Test of Psycholinguistic Abilities. Urbana: University of Illinois Press, 1968.

Index

Abnormal findings report, 43
Acetylcholine
  electrophoresis of
    stimulation of axon reflex flare by,
      214–215
    stimulation of axon reflex sweating by,
      217–218
    Parkinson's with dementia vs. Alzheimer's
      and, 314, 315
Activities of daily living (ADL)
  Huntington's disease and capacity to
    perform, 273
  measures, 41–42
    data from simulated, 29
    decreases in normal functions with age
      for, 26
    Simulated Activities of Daily Living
      Examination (SADLE), 292
Adenosine diphosphate (ADP), 110, 114
Adenosine monophosphate (AMP),
  deamination of, 110
Adenosine triphosphate (ATP) support
  systems, 110
  NMR detection of, 114–116
Adrenocorticotrophic hormone (ACTH),
  multiple sclerosis and, 13–15, 164
Aerobic exercise, 103, 109
Age
  correction for, in standardization of
    scales, 82
  cutaneous detection thresholds and, 192
  effect on ambulation, 119–127
  mental, 338
  normal neurologic function and, 20–28
  variance in language ability and, 336–338,
    340
Age span, definition of normal neurologic
  function across, 24–28

Aging
  life-style risk factors in, 21, 22–23
  limits of, 22
  theoretical views on, 21–22
Akinesia in Parkinson's disease, quantifying,
  288, 290–292
Alpha, 57–58, 59
ALS. See Amyotrophic lateral sclerosis
  (ALS)
ALS score, 129, 130
Alternate-form reliability, 55–56
Alzheimer's disease (AD), Parkinson's
  disease and, 311–325
  clinical features, similarities of, 315–316
  cognitive deficits, similarities of, 316–318
  epidemiology and genetics, similarity of,
    312–313
  neural alterations, similarity of, 313–315
  neuropsychologic tests in, 317–323
Ambulation, effects of age and disease on,
  119–127
  adaptive capabilities, 120–126
  central vs. environmental factors in, 126
  data collection methods, 120–125
  experimental conditions, 125–126
AMP, deamination of, 110
Amyotrophic lateral sclerosis (ALS), 88,
  129–154
  natural history of, 133–137
  quantitative techniques to define, 94–98,
    129–142
    applications to clinical practice,
      137–141
    data reduction, 131–133
    data transposition, 130–131
    for motor performance, 93–94
    standardizing measurements in patients
      with, 82